RESCUE TECHNICIAN

Operational Readiness for Rescue Providers

The Maryland Fire and Rescue Institute of the University of Maryland is the state's comprehensive training and education system for emergency services. The Institute plans, researches, develops, and delivers quality programs to enhance the ability of emergency service providers to protect life, the environment, and property.

Training v. Tradition

Paradox or Partnership?

Is the tradition you're fighting to preserve,
worth more than the lives to be saved,
with the changes you're fighting to resist?

RESCUE TECHNICIAN

Operational Readiness for Rescue Providers

Maryland Fire and Rescue Institute
University of Maryland

STUDENT MANUAL

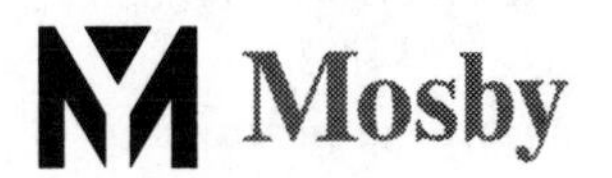

St. Louis Baltimore Boston Carlsbad Chicago Minneapolis New York Philadelphia Portland
London Milan Sydney Tokyo Toronto

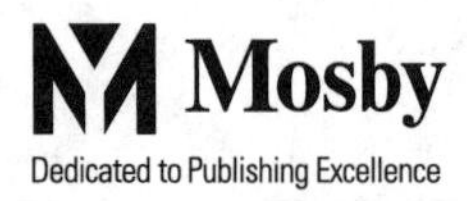

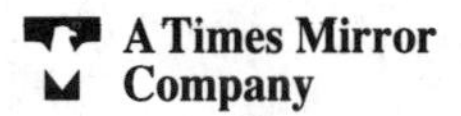

www.mosby.com

Editor-in-chief: Claire Merrick
Production Manager: Douglas Bruce
Senior Production Editor: Nadine Steffan

Mosby, Inc.
11830 Westline Industrial Drive
St. Louis, MO 63146

International Standard Book Number 0-8151-8390-9

Printing and Binding by Plus Communications
Composition by Maryland Composition, Inc.

98 99 00 01 02 / 9 8 7 6 5 4 3 2

Contents

Preface

The Maryland Fire and Rescue Institute developed this Rescue Technician Course offering all basic rescue providers the first of a tiered-level, didactic and practical training program. A quality team was assembled to chart the vision and substantive content of the program. This committee, comprised of the best rescue practitioners in their respective areas of expertise, addressed several key issues facing curriculum development: What do basic-level rescue providers actually respond to, and what level of operational/awareness training do they really need to carry out their tasks?

The Maryland fire service is a diverse entity because of the various types of apparatus that individual organizations use to respond to working incidents. There are rescue/squad companies that perform only rescue and extrication functions; suppression companies that house multitask vehicles and apparatus such as rescue-pumpers; truck companies that respond to both box and rescue assignments; and EMS companies that operate light- to medium-response vehicles that are equipped with rescue and extrication tools.

Historically, former rescue programs focused on the task-specific function of the rescue vehicle in a general perspective. *Rescue Technician* now addresses a broad-based approach to specialty training needs along with how these units will interface with each other during a rescue operation. It also provides an enhanced approach to classroom and practical laboratory sessions. *Rescue Technician* addresses the components of incident scene management, a new look at current and former materials, an overview on heavy-vehicle rescue, and an awareness of operational issues confronting basic-level rescue providers as they relate to confined space, trench, and excavation rescue scenarios and aquatic response emergencies.

Rescue Technician was structured to enable the student entering a rescue program to develop decision-making skills and the ability to properly assess a dangerous scenario and bring it to a safe and successful conclusion. The committee is confident that *you,* as a participant during this program, will benefit from a solid learning experience and up-to-date course content. The committee and the Institute Development Section extend a hearty welcome to those of you embarking on this 60-hour training endeavor, as it will be well worth your time and effort. We also wish you a successful course completion and encourage you to continue on to the next level.

Robert J. Schappert, III
Coordinator
Rescue Course Development

Acknowledgments

Managing rescue operations presents a myriad of challenges for the rescue providers and officers of any fire service organization. As the 21st century rapidly approaches, the dynamics associated with the mission of the fire service dictate a need for highly skilled rescue providers and a proactive vision to keep the grassroots memberships of these organizations in step with the times.

The Maryland Fire and Rescue Institute gratefully acknowledges the professionalism, commitment to excellence, and vision shown by the following quality team developers representing MFRI faculty and staff, and career, volunteer, and private sectors. The quality of this revised rescue program could not have been possible without them.

S. Rebecca Spicer, Manager
Institute Development Section
Maryland Fire and Rescue Institute

Robert J. Schappert, III
Rescue Revision Project Coordinator
Maryland Fire and Rescue Institute

A. J. Esposito
Rescue Instructor, MFRI
Coordinator, North East Regional Office
Maryland Fire and Rescue Institute

Ramon E. Hodgson
Rescue Instructor, MFRI
Special Programs Section
Maryland Fire and Rescue Institute

Stoyan (Llynn) Russell
Rescue Instructor, MFRI
Retired Safety Director
Genstar Corporation

Battalion Chief Ronald Horn
Rescue Instructor, MFRI
City of Hagerstown Fire Department

Sergeant Michael W. Collins
Rescue Instructor, MFRI
Montgomery County Department of Fire/Rescue Services

Lieutenant Thomas Carr
Heavy Vehicle and Specialty Rescue Instructor
Montgomery County Department of Fire/Rescue Services

Bob Howarth
Rescue Instructor, MFRI
Anne Arundel County Training Division

Lieutenant Robert Moody
Rescue Instructor, MFRI
Montgomery County Department of Fire/Rescue Services

Lieutenant William F. Luebberman
Rescue Instructor, MFRI
Manager, Carroll County Emergency Services Training Center

Michael A. McNeill
Rescue Instructor, MFRI
Safety Engineer, NASA/Goddard Space Flight Center

Gregory R. Valcourt
Rescue Instructor, MFRI
Department Chair, Emergency Medical Services
Aims Community College
Greeley, Colorado

Lieutenant Leonard E. Yox
Rescue Instructor, MFRI
Baltimore County Fire Department

Captain Chris Helminiak
Fire Training Academy
Prince George's County Fire Department

Ronald E. Moore
Specialty Rescue Instructor
Production Coordinator, American Heat
Carrollton, Texas

Secretarial Support:

Janie Filloramo
Institute Development Section

Nancy Cox
Institute Development Section

Graphic Design:

Dan Gross
Administrative Support Section

The Maryland Fire and Rescue Institute also acknowledges the professionalism, time, and effort put forth by the following external reviewers of the Rescue Technician Course. The comments, recommendations, and input from these experts in the rescue field have immeasurably enhanced both the content and delivery of this program statewide. They have the Institute's sincerest appreciation for a job well done.

Richard D. Butler
Rescue Instructor, MFRI
Firefighter/Paramedic
Annapolis City Fire Department

John W. Frank
Rescue Instructor, MFRI
Deputy Chief, Services Bureau
Howard County Department of Fire/Rescue Services

Ronald B. Graf
Rescue Instructor, MFRI
Riveria Beach Volunteer Fire Company
Anne Arundel County Fire Department

William R. Hamilton
Rescue Instructor, MFRI
Assistant Chief, Berwyn Heights Volunteer Fire Department
Prince George's County

Robert E. Knippenburg
Rescue Instructor, MFRI
Assistant Chief, Fire/Rescue
Midland Volunteer Fire Department

John E. Markey
Rescue Instructor, MFRI
Station #3, United Fire Company
Frederick, Maryland

Glenn E. Pearce
Rescue Instructor, MFRI
MIEMSS Office of Education/Certification

Robert C. Rhode, Jr.
Rescue Instructor, MFRI
Safety Technician, Town of Ocean City Waste Water Division

Micheal W. Robinson
Rescue Instructor, MFRI
Captain, Baltimore County Fire Department Training Academy
Chief Officer, Earleigh Heights Volunteer Fire Company

Lieutenant Robert L. Rose
Rescue Instructor, MFRI
Training/Research Division
Anne Arundel County Fire Department

Roger C. Simonds
Rescue Instructor, MFRI
Deputy Chief, Special Operations Division
Anne Arundel County Fire Department

Joseph C. Ward
Rescue Instructor, MFRI
Park Manager, James Island State Park

Clarence (Smiley) White, Jr.
Rescue Instructor, MFRI
Chair, Maryland State Firemen's Association Training Committee

Charles H. Wood
Rescue Instructor, MFRI
Facilitator, Western Maryland Regional Office
Maryland Fire and Rescue Institute

A WORD OF THANKS AND APPRECIATION

The Maryland Fire and Rescue Institute acknowledges the contribution made by the following organzations to its Rescue Technician's Training Program, by allowing the Institute to reproduce video segments for training purposes.

The success and acceptance of this program will be greatly enriched as a result of these training additions to the program. Our sincerest appreciation for a job well done is extended to Claire Merrick of Mosby–Year Book, Inc., Ron Moore, FETN, and General Counsel Susan Longley, ACTS Foundation, for making this happen.

Session Guide

Session 17	*Skills Proficiency Evaluation:* Passenger and Commercial Conveyance Rescue—Patient Packaging and Transfer *Practical* **Pass/Fail Point**	1 through 6 and 16
Session 18	Compliance Issues of Confined-Space Rescue Operations: First Responder Awareness	18
Session 19	Compliance Issues of Trench/Excavation Rescue Operations: First Responder Awareness	19
Session 20	Aquatic Emergency First Responder: Awareness **Pass/Fail Point** **Exam #3**	20, 16 through 20

Synopsis

Session 1 Rescue Operations: Compliance and Safety in Relation to the Incident Management System

This session introduces the rescue provider to the concept of operational readiness and its relationship to a macro approach to incident scene management. It encompasses baseline compliance and safety issues, the importance of personnel qualifications, interfacing of engines, squads, truck companies, and EMS on an incident with corresponding roles and responsibilities, and the importance of personnel accountability.

Session 2 Technical Aspects of Ropes, Hardware, and Harnesses

This session educates the student as to the different types of ropes and the associated software available for rescue operations, rescue hardware used in the mitigation of simple to complex scenarios, and the compliance and safety requirements related to the selection and use of rescue harnesses.

Session 3 Rescue Knots and Their Uses

This session expounds on the didactic materials learned in session 2 by using a practical format to teach the rescue provider the proper use of rescue knots for given scenarios and the terminology associated with rope rescue operations. It focuses on the premise that good knot skills application can mean the difference between a successful rescue and a failure.

Session 4 Principles of Rigging, Anchoring, and Mechanical Advantage Systems

This session builds sequentially on the contents of sessions 2 and 3, with information on natural and constructed anchors, block-and-tackle equipment, load computations, hauling, and picket holdfast systems. It also provides an overview on the importance of protecting anchor systems along with the safety rules applicable to the construction of these systems. Rescue providers will learn about the effectiveness of prusik cords when constructing mechanical advantage and hauling systems.

Session 5 Principles of Rigging, Anchoring, and Mechanical Advantage Systems

Rescue providers now apply the theories and applications presented in session 4 to practical scenarios involving the reeving of blocks and tackle, and construction of simple and compound anchoring and hauling systems.

Session 6 Incident Scene Approach to Patient Packaging and Transfer

This session enables the rescue provider to receive hands-on training to patient transfer devices currently used in lifting, packaging, and moving patients. This session addresses such topics as safety inspection procedures for transfer devices, patient packaging goals, and the triage process.

Session 7 Slope Evacuation

This session focuses on the challenges facing rescue providers when they encounter difficult terrain situations. Students, working in a team, will work with current technology and transfer devices that were introduced in session 6 and apply their use to litter rigging and litter bearer tie-ins, using vehicles as anchor points during roadside rigging scenarios, and the terminology associated with commands given during slope evaluation operations involving injured victims and patients. This session does not address high-angle rescue techniques.

Session 8 Skills Proficiency Evaluation: Rope Rescue Systems and Exam #1

This session is a practical skills application session requiring rescue providers to work as team members while addressing predetermined and randomly assigned skills. Students will be evaluated on overall proficiency in the materials presented in sessions 1 through 7, focusing on rescue knots, mechanical advantage and anchoring systems, and patient transfer devices. This is a pass/fail point in the program.

Session 9 Principles of Vehicular Construction and Associated Technology

This session introduces the student to basic types of vehicle construction, construction components, component reactions in collisions, vehicular fuel systems, and the challenges of new-age construction faced by rescue providers during extrication incidents.

Session 10 ABCs of Vehicular Rescue

Successful handling of a rescue incident is dependent on the development of a plan to effectively address the components of the incident. In this session students will be presented information on the decision-making process, preincident preparation, incident operational steps, and postincident evaluation. The ABCs concept allows a rescue provider to easily remember abbreviated steps to bring an incident to a successful conclusion.

Session 11 Vehicle Extrication Tools: Hand, Hydraulic, Electric, and Pneumatic

This session focuses on the realization that vehicle rescue and extrication scenarios involve more than the simple operation of various tools. Rescue providers must be familiar with the operational characteristics, limitations, maintenance, inspection, and safety aspects of all equipment utilized and supplied on their apparatus. Knowledge of operational characteristics and maintenance requirements will go a long way in preventing the catastrophic failure of various tools when they are needed the most.

Session 12 Vehicular Stabilization

One of the most overlooked phases of a vehicular extrication scenario is the stabilization requirements facing rescue providers. This session stresses the need for stabilzation at the earliest stage of the incident, the purposes, devices, and methodologies associated with the stabilization process, and the related safety concerns for rescue providers.

Session 13 Hand Tools and Vehicular Extrication

New space-age construction features of some vehicles dictate the need for rescue providers to be proficient in the use of hand tool technology. This session provides the rescue provider with an opportunity, during a practical format, to apply hand tool technology on entrapment and disentanglement situations and gain access through windows, doors, and alternative points on the body of a vehicle.

Session 14 Power Tools and Vehicular Extrication

The safe operation of power tools during vehicular extrication procedures requires knowledge, skill, and competence. This session provides practical skills in establishing safety perimeters, scene assessment, stabilization, and balancing techniques. It also shows how to gain access through roof and door areas and how to enlarge alternative access points.

Session 15 Skills Proficiency Evaluation: Vehicle Extrication and Exam #2

This sesion tests the retention of subject matter presented in sessions 9 through 14, and is a pass/fail point in the program. Students will be assigned to groups and perform skills as they relate to extrication problems involving vehicles on their sides, roofs, and resting on their wheels.

Session 16 Principles of Passenger and Commercial Conveyance Rescue—Buses and Trucks

This session examines the issues of truck and bus extrication as they relate to patients, vehicle size, mechanism of injuries, hazards associated with cargo, and the volume of cargo. Students will be presented with issues that pose serious challenges to their rescue skills and capabilities by determining workable solutions in extricating victims and occupants situated 10 ft. off the ground level.

Session 17 Skills Proficiency Evaluation: Passenger and Commercial Conveyance Rescue—Patient Packaging and Transfer

This session is a sequel to session 16 and provides a practical format whereby students can apply principles, theories, and techniques learned in sessions 1 through 6 and 16 to heavy rigs and buses. Students will be assigned to groups to perform patient packaging and transfer in a simulated incident involving trucks and buses. This is a pass/fail point in the program.

Session 18 Compliance Issues of Confined-Space Rescue Operations: First Responder Awareness

Confined-space rescue scenarios continue to claim the lives of would-be rescuers on a national basis. These types of situations pose a very serious threat to the life safety of all rescue providers involved in the incident. This session is designed to meet the training requirements set forth in 29 CFR 1910.146, governing "entrants" and "attendants," and provides awareness training for responders to confined space situations. It does not address "rescue" training from an operational standpoint.

Sesion 19 Compliance Issues of Trench/Evacuation Rescue Operations: First Responder Awareness

Trench/excavation rescue operations pose a serious life-safety hazard to emergency services personnel operating in and around this environment. Safety and compliance issues must be addressed in the interest of rescue provider safety and survival. Awareness of operational issues and the accompanying dangers involved as they relate to OSHA regulations is the first step towards understanding this process. This session addresses the inherent life-safety risks associated with the trench/excavation incidents and the appropriate levels of intervention expected of rescue providers from a first responder perspective.

Session 20 Aquatic Emergency First Responder: Awareness and Exam #3

This session defines the role of the rescue provider responding to an aquatic emergency and aspects of aquatic emergencies. It focuses on the contents of OSHA regulation 29 CFR 1926.21, which mandates that first responders be trained in the recognition and avoidance of unsafe conditions and the regulations applicable to their work environment to control and eliminate hazards. This session tests the retention of subject matter presented in sessions 16 through 20 and is a pass/fail point in the program.

Skills Card

This document identifies those sessions/objectives that require **demonstration** of skills. The contents of this document must be completed and signed off by the instructor of record prior to the participant receiving a satisfactory course completion certificate as specified by the AHJ.

RESCUE TECHNICIAN SKILLS PROFICIENCY EVALUATION

Objective/Skill

Rescue Knots and Harnesses (Individual Skill Evaluation)
Correctly tie the following family of figure-8's:
1. Figure-8
2. Figure-8 reweave
3. Figure-8 bend
4. Figure-8 bight

Correctly tie the following clove hitch knots:

5. Clove hitch *around* an object
6. Clove hitch *over* an object
7. Split clove hitch
8. Correctly *don and doff* harness specified by the evaluator.
9. Using the donned harness, correctly prepare for slope rappel.

Mechanical Advantage and Anchor Systems (Team Evaluation)

10. Correctly reeve a mechanical advantage block and tackle system specified by the evaluator.
11. Correctly reeve a "Z"-system.
12. Correctly reeve a piggyback system.
13. Correctly anchor the system using a natural anchor point.
14. Correctly anchor the system using an anchor point on vehicle.
15. Correctly anchor the system using a picket holdfast.

Patient Transfer Devices (Team Evaluation)

16. Correctly secure a patient in a Stokes basket.
17. Correctly secure a patient in a SKED stretcher.
18. Correctly prepare the transfer device for horizontal movement.

Vehicle on Its Side (Team Evaluation)

Correctly demonstrate the following:

19. Circle check
20. Stabilization
21. Gain access via removal of window glass using hand or power tools specified by the evaluator.
22. Gain access via through a roof flap using hand or power tools specified by the evaluator.
23. Safely remove all equipment.

Vehicle on Its Roof (Team Evolution)
Correctly demonstrate the following:
24. Circle check
25. Stabilization
26. Gain access via removal of window glass using hand or power tools specified by the evaluator.
27. Gain access via removal of doors using hand or power tools specified by the evaluator.
28. Gain access via removal of roof using hand or power tools specified by the evaluator.
29. Safely remove all equipment.

Vehicle on Its Wheels (Team Evaluation)
Correctly demonstrate the following:
30. Circle check
31. Stabilization
32. Gain access via removal of window glass using hand or power tools specified by the evaluator.
33. Gain access via removal of doors using hand or power tools specified by the evaluator.
34. Gain access via removal of roof using hand or power tools specified by the evaluator.
35. Dash displacement using hand or power tools specified by the evaluator.
36. Seat displacement using hand or power tools specified by the evaluator.
37. Safely remove all equipment.

Commercial Vehicle (Team Evaluation)
Correctly demonstrate the following:
38. Establishing incident command
39. Circle check
40. Stabilizing on wheels.
41. Constructing a safe platform to gain access.
42. Stabilizing the patient
43. Packaging and removing the patient to the ground (Evaluator will specify type of transfer device).

Buses (Commercial or School) (Team Evaluation)
Correctly demonstrate the following:
44. Establishing incident command.
45. Circle check
46. Stabilizing on wheels.
47. Constructing a safe platform to gain access.
48. Stabilizing the patient.
49. Packaging and removing the patient to the ground (Evaluator will specify type of transfer device).

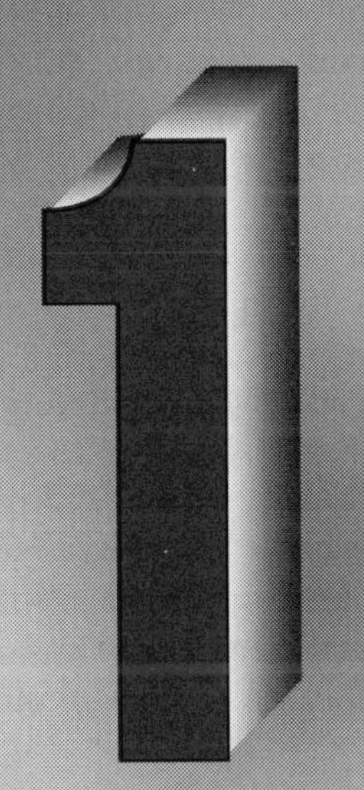

Rescue Operations: Compliance and Safety in Relation to the Incident Management System

OBJECTIVE

The student will be able to identify and describe the compliance and safety issues impacting the relationship between rescue/engine/truck/EMS companies operating on working incidents, along with the specific tasks of each, from memory, without assistance, to an accuracy of 70% and the satisfaction of the instructor.

OVERVIEW

Rescue Operations: Compliance and Safety in Relation to the Incident Management System

- Compliance and Safety Issues
- Qualifications of a Rescue Squad Team Member
- Role of the Engine Company
- Role of the Truck Company
- Rescue/Engine/Truck/EMS Company Interface
- Personal Protective Equipment
- Incident Safety and Accountability

ENABLING OBJECTIVES

1-1-1 Identify and describe the compliance and safety issues governing/impacting rescue incident operations.

1-1-2 Identify and describe the qualifications of a rescue squad team member and the accompanying mindset of professionalism necessary to carry out interrelated incident tasks.

1-1-3 Identify and describe the role of the engine company providing support operations on a rescue incident.

1-1-4 Identify and describe the multifaceted role of the truck company on the scene of a rescue incident.

1-1-5 Identify and describe how the rescue/engine/truck/EMS companies interface with specific task responsibilities under the incident management system or incident command system.

1-1-6 Identify and describe the appropriate personal protective equipment necessary for safety/survival at the scene of a working rescue incident.

1-1-7 Identify and describe the concept and purpose of establishing a safety perimeter at the scene of a working rescue incident and the importance of the rescue safety officer's role in managing accountability.

COMPLIANCE AND SAFETY ISSUES

General Perspective

Rescue/squad companies do not function in a vacuum. They are part of an integral approach towards addressing difficult situations where the potential for life-threatening injuries and victim entrapment exist. The concept of rescue first began during World War II when large groups of people had to be dug out and extricated from collapsed buildings resulting from massive bombing attacks.

Since that time, rescue training programs began to flourish internationally. The focus of these programs was on microjurisdictional scenarios rather than large-scale development, since the abatement of global conflict saw an end to the destruction of entire cities.

Each fire training agency/community identified their specific needs and requirements and developed rescue training programs to address the carnage that was occurring on highways across the nation. They also worked on programs that would provide response training for large-scale incidents involving earthquakes, floods, aircraft disasters, rail accidents, and private sector (industrial) scenarios.

With the incidence of injuries and death to emergency services personnel on the rise, it became apparent that the need for guidance by way of federal and National Fire Protection Association regulations and standards existed. The 20th century began an era of intervention on the part of federal and fire service organizations to address the safety and survival of field providers during rescue incidents.

As the complexity of rescue incidents grows, the level of training needed to bring an incident to successful conclusion rises proportionately. Hence, the introduction of key safety issues factored into these training equations ultimately results in regulations and standards to keep emergency services personnel out of harm's way.

This overview of OSHA/MOSH/NFPA regulations and standards is designed to provide a "wake-up call" for rescue providers and create an awareness for compliance/safety issues that shadow our daily response to working incidents. Safety and survival is a fire service issue that all participants have a personal and professional responsibility to maintain. *There is no compromise or viable alternative to safe practices whenever you are called on to provide a service. Safety is everyone's responsibility. It transcends personal agendas and the old philosophy of "We've been doing it like this for years, why change?"*

The end result of noncompliance to safety regulations and standards has three distinct outcomes that are universally unacceptable: injury, death, or liability to participants. When someone becomes injured or dies as a result of negligent acts during an incident, regulations and standards now make it very easy to identify where the responsibility lies. This is not an enviable position to be in when the investigations are concluded.

Safety, survival, and effective use of resources are first on the list of incident priorities. Rescue personnel, which include basic providers, officers, acting officers, and outside agency support, must be knowledgeable of regulations and standards targeted for specific rescue scenarios and other fire service incidents. The following is a sampling of the more prominent regulations and standards that influence the way in which rescue companies conduct business.

Permit-Required Confined Space (29 CFR 1910.146) Sets the requirements for practice and procedures designed to protect employees from hazards of entry into such things as tanks, vessels, silos, storage bins, hoppers, vaults, and pits.

Subpart P—Excavation (29 CFR 1926.650) Applies to all open excavations made in the earth's surface, which includes trenches.

Lockout/Tagout (29 CFR 1910.147) Addresses the servicing and maintenance of machines and equipment in which the unexpected energization or start-up of machines or equipment, or release of stored energy that would result in injuries or deaths to employees.

Personal Protective Equipment (29 CFR 1910.132) Applies to protective equipment for the eyes, face, head, and extremities; protective clothing, respiratory devices, and protective shields; barriers when necessary to protect against hazards of the environment; chemicals, radiological, and mechanical irritants impairing the function of any part of the body through absorption, inhalation, or physical contact.

Bloodborne Pathogens (29 CFR 1910.1030) Applies to all occupational exposure to blood or other potentially infectious materials that results from the performance of an employee's duties.

Hazard Communication (29 CFR 1910.1200) Addresses the issues of evaluating the potential hazards of chemicals and communicating information concerning hazards and appropriate protective measures to employees.

Hazardous Materials Response (29 CFR 1910.120) Addresses haz-mat training, Incident Management System (IMS), and operations, including emergency response.

Respiratory Protection (29 CFR 1910.134) Contains the requirements for type of respiratory protection, training of user, and maintenance.

Fire Brigade (29 CFR 1910.156) Contains requirements for the organization, training, and personal protective equipment of fire brigades whenever they are established by the employer.

NFPA 1500 Applies to organizations providing rescue, fire suppression, and other emergency services. It is the standard on fire department occupational safety and health programs and contains minimum requirements for a fire service-related occupational safety and health program.

NFPA 1521 Sets the standard for the fire department safety officer. It addresses the position of the safety officer which is required under NFPA 1500 and specifies minimum requirements for a fire department safety officer.

NFPA 1582 Contains medical requirements for firefighters and other organizations providing rescue, fire suppression, and other emergency services including public, military, private, and industrial fire departments.

Safety

The objective associated with safety is to eliminate, control, and neutralize existing hazards at the scene of a working incident. It is a very foolish rescue provider that places himself/herself in a position of trading lives or subjecting one's self to the potential of serious injury.

Safety considerations start with establishing priorities at the scene of the incident. The first priority is *you,* the rescuer. Your personal safety and welfare and that of your coproviders is first and foremost. The second priority is directed towards keeping onlookers, bystanders, motorists, etc., out of harm's way and inadvertently becoming involved in the incident. The third priority focuses on the safety of those victims already injured in the rescue scenario.

Safety hazards fall into two categories.

Category I: Hazards classified as visible or obvious. This means that they are easily detectable upon arrival. Vehicle fires, arcing wires, stabilization problems, and multiple entrapment readily present themselves during a visual size-up.

Category II: Hazards that are not readily visible or obvious upon arrival. This category can present extremely dangerous and deadly problems and requires perception and understanding of hazards and associated consequences on the part of rescue providers.

Hazards underestimated or not considered by rescuers on the scene can often lead to serious injuries and/or deaths. The lethal components contributing to this process are:

- Ignorance of scene management and policies
- Inexperience on the part of crew members
- Lack of preparation (training and preplanning)
- Poor attitudes ("I don't need training. I know how to do it!")
- Tunnel vision—failure to see the big picture
- Nonadherence to established safety practices
- Tasks may not be completed because a member of the team is removed from duty
- Overextending beyond your capability or training
- Failure to appoint an incident scene safety officer

QUALIFICATIONS OF A RESCUE SQUAD TEAM MEMBER

In order to function as a member of a rescue squad company, you must realize what it takes to function as a rescue squad team member. A person cannot perform a task without being qualified to do so.

Interest: An interest for, and a desire to do the job.

Enthusiasm for the job and related tasks: Keep a "spark" going. You must constantly be aware of changes in the subject. With an enthusiastic approach, you can stay on top of all new information and techniques.

Initiative: Be a go-getter. When you see a task that needs attention, do it! Do not wait for others, they may not have your initiative.

Must work as a team under supervision: Rescue work is not an individual endeavor. Many tasks require two or more people to perform. The squad needs supervision, someone to make the decisions, and take the guesswork out of your duties. Focus on the actual operation of equipment. The supervisor can stand back and observe the surroundings for any signs of danger and take action without any effect on the operational crew.

Mechanical aptitude: It helps to have a general knowledge of the way things operate, especially when the rescue squad functions as a "toolbox on wheels." With rescue operations not being an exact science, operations do not always work as planned. Tools can break; they can be too big, small, short, long. The rescuer should have this mechanical aptitude in order to overcome the problem and adapt to the situation.

Education and knowledge: There is a vast array of methods, tools, and problems that rescuers face. To maintain proficiency, you must train on both old and new equipment and methods. Read operating guides and manuals to save you from damaging costly equipment and embarrassing yourself on an incident. Read all information that you can on a given subject. Learn new terms that may be used when operating with other agencies (e.g., medical terms, haz-mat, and other technical support). Remember, the most significant step that a rescue organization and its members can take is training.

Confidence: In order for a rescue to be successfully concluded, tasks must be addressed properly. A confident crew is a successful crew. Have a "can do" attitude, know what you're doing and show it. If you don't have confidence in yourself, will your team members, officers, bystanders, and most of all your victims have confidence in you?

Competence: Know what is expected of you and strive to meet and exceed expectations. Realize what it takes to do your job and train accordingly. Learn all of the unit's equipment and its location. Keep updated on old skills. The scene is not the place to show your inadequacies due to a lack of competence.

Maturity: The rescue scene is often a very confusing and chaotic place. Your duty is to relieve the pain and suffering of the victims. During the various phases of rescue, you may encounter agonizing pain and accompanying screams, gruesome conditions involving people, and adverse environments. The rescue scene is a place that requires mature judgement, actions, and conversations.

Mindset and Professionalism

Discipline: The fire department is a para-military organization with accompanying rules, regulations and a chain-of-command that clearly defines *who* is in charge.

Rescuers must carry out orders from officers without delay. Failure to do so may result in loss of life to your victims, crew members, or yourself.

With discipline in place, your fire department has an efficiently run rescue scene, ultimately benefitting the citizens it serves.

Emotional stability: People have said, "I can't be in the fire department. I can't stand the gore involved. How can they do it?" They do it by having control of their emotions.

Reality sets the stage of your work. It's not a Hollywood "special effects" show; it's real, therefore you must be able to react. When you react to the factors thrown at you on the emergency scene, some emotional factors take control. You cannot allow your emotions to override your judgement and competence. You must maintain an air of emotional stability to protect your victims, their families, bystanders, and rescue personnel.

Emotions need to be vented, but should be done away from the emergency scene. Many times this can be effectively accomplished by expressing your feelings during post-incident analysis (critique) or simply around the firehouse table over coffee. In addition, there are critical stress debriefing teams and employee assistance programs that can help when a person has reached a saturation point.

Conversation: What you say and how you say it means different things to different people. Your tone of voice can mean a lot to people. People know when they are being talked down to. Don't raise your voice at victims or your co-workers. It usually results in animosity from all concerned. Use a normal tone of voice and speak the way you would want to be spoken to.

Use caution in your content and context as well. What you say may cause anxiety in patients. Do not discuss their injuries in front of them. You do not really know their extent. Focus on your task at hand and leave medical concerns to the EMS personnel.

Avoid telling them everything is fine or O.K. Why are they surrounded by rescue personnel, tangled metal, or in an ambulance if this is the case?

Victim's medical conditions and information are confidential. Use due caution with information you disclose. Improper disclosure may result in legal action against you!

Professional conduct: A *professional* is defined as one conforming to technical or ethical standards of a profession or occupation. Professionalism is achieved not by a paycheck, but by the way individuals present themselves.

Part of being a professional includes a neat and clean appearance. Not only does this inspire confidence on the part of victims, but it has its sanitary purposes as well. Many times you are in close contact with your victims and your appearance is carefully monitored.

A clean uniform or appropriate turnout gear is another sign of a professional. Uniforms and turnout gear allow you to stand out in a group as well. Wear uniforms and gear properly, appropriately, and proudly. Remember, *you* represent a fire service organization.

A professional should remain calm in a crisis situation. One of the rescuer's tasks is to calm and reassure the victims involved. How are you going to calm a victim if you are not calm and reassuring yourself?

A professional is efficient. Make proper use of your time on an incident. A professional is confident. He/she is confident in the fact that what is being accomplished is an effective rescue practice. Confidence is knowing that you and your crew are doing the job properly. A professional needs to lend a sympathetic ear, yet needs to be firm in dealing with the victim, family, and bystanders.

A professional needs to be a team player. Virtually every aspect of the fire/rescue/EMS service dictates that you work in teams of two or more. A rescue operation requires the discipline of working together as a team. There is no room in the fire/rescue/EMS service for freelancing or going solo. This is an unacceptable and dangerous practice.

Attitude: Attitude is a persistent disposition to act either positively or negatively toward a person, group, object, situation, or value. More easily stated, it is the way you present yourself and the manner in which you carry out your duties. Attitudes can be developed, either good or bad.

A rescuer with a good attitude is courteous, pleasant, and considerate to others in their surroundings. Your attitude towards others can provide a reassuring, positive outcome not only to the victim, but the overall rescue operation as well.

Attitudes can change over time. Response "burnout" can negatively impact one's attitude. You may need a break from burnout to prevent a bad attitude being presented to the citizens you serve. There are professionals who can assist fire/rescue/EMS personnel with burnout attitudes. Check your local jurisdiction/department options.

ROLE OF THE ENGINE COMPANY

In many jurisdictions it is standard practice to dispatch an engine company on all rescue assignments. This is in addition to the medical and rescue/squad units assigned to the initial response.

Generally, an engine company is defined as a "Class A" pumper that is equipped to carry and supply water in varying quantities for use on a working incident. An engine company is often the first to be dispatched and the first to arrive at the scene of a rescue incident. Consequently, it will set the stage for the management of the entire scenario. Part and parcel to this is the realization that the first arriving engine company will be charged with the responsibility of incident size-up and assessment.

As a member of an engine company dispatched/assigned to a rescue incident, your role is distinctly separate from that of the rescue company. Some overlap may be required in certain circumstances. It is often difficult to maintain this perspective, especially when the urge to be involved is strong. You must allow the rescue company to perform its task(s). While rescue is a task-specific function, yours is limited to providing support activities.

In certain circumstances, however, the engine company may be involved in the following activities as the first arriving unit:

- Vehicle stabilization
- Establishing scene security
- Initiating/maintaining hazard control
- Providing first responder/EMT medical care to victims
- Victim extrication when faced with imminent danger to life requiring prompt action

As the scene unfolds there may be additional responsibilities delegated to the engine company at the direction of the incident commander (IC). These include:

- Application of foam agents against flammable/hazardous vapors
- Fire suppression activities with charged attack lines in place
- Damming/diking of hazardous liquid runoff
- Clean-up of vehicle glass and other nonhazardous components from roadway surfaces

- Traffic and crowd control
- Providing enhanced availability of staffing resources for other tasks (option of the IC)

Multitask Vehicles/Rescue Pumpers

Those organizations with rescue pumpers have the best of both worlds. These units provide a multipurpose role in serving the interests of rescue/extrication and structural/conventional fire suppression. They are usually equipped with the same firefighting tools and equipment as that of a Class A pumper along with water and tank configuration.

Rescue pumpers are very flexible because they carry a combination of firefighting and rescue equipment and tools. Once on location they are able to address whatever situation arises for the most part. The main disadvantage to running a rescue pumper, however, is that a company must determine qualifications criteria for its members riding this vehicle. Officers are faced with the task of splitting crews into those with, and those without, rescue/extrication training. If equipped to handle an 8- to 10-person crew, it is often difficult to preselect those members that will respond to various incidents.

Rescue pumpers are generally equipped to carry all the essentials and tools for light- to heavy-rescue scenarios. Complex and/or larger incidents may require additional resources.

ROLE OF THE TRUCK COMPANY

Truck Company Duties

A truck company is a fire department company that is equipped with an aerial ladder or elevated platform. The truck company's normal fire ground duties are:

- Perform obvious rescues
- Search and rescue
- Forcible entry/gaining access
- Ventilation
- Ground ladders
- Elevated streams
- Aerial ladder
- Salvage and overhaul
- Utility control
- Perform vehicle extrication

Truck Company Assistance on Rescue Incidents

In some jurisdictions, aerial/ladder/tower companies carry out extrication duties due to the limited number of heavy-duty rescue squads.

The truck company and heavy-duty rescue squads carry virtually the same tools with the exception of the obvious aerial or ground ladder supply. However, the squads tend to carry a larger amount of heavy extrication hydraulic, pneumatic, electrical, mechanical, and gasoline tools.

Sometimes a truck company is dispatched on a primary rescue assignment or as a specialty request. What can a truck company do on a rescue? Although a truck carries many rescue tools, its most important component is the crew itself. Many members of the fire service are cross trained in the various sectors (EMS, Truck Co., Engine Co., Rescue Squad, and Haz-Mat), lending a myriad of experience to the rescue operation. The crew can be of assistance just in numbers of personnel alone.

Many trucks carry both on-board and portable generators. These can be used as additional or back-up power supplies for the rescue operation. With the amount of energy drawn from portable power supplies by rescue tools, it never hurts to have several available.

Numerous rescues are performed at night or in light-deficient environments. Truck companies can assist rescue companies by providing additional lighting as required.

Truck companies may be called on to assist in ventilating a rescue scene. This may include but is not limited to:

- Smoke removal.
- Fresh air induction in confined space rescue (many of these circumstances present oxygen-deficient atmospheres).
- Hazardous materials may produce vapors detrimental to the health of victims and rescuers. Ventilating may displace vapors.
- Gas leaks—gas settles into low areas or pockets creating an explosive atmosphere. Ventilating pockets may make for a more habitable atmosphere.

Uses of Ladders: Another important and invaluable tool on a truck company is its complement of ladders. The uses of ladders on rescue incidents are innumerable. The following constitutes a sampling:

Vertical access: Up or down, not all rescues are on ground level.

Ice rescue: Ladders evenly distribute rescuers' weight over ice, making a safer rescue platform. The ladder, even if it should fall into the water, will act as a handhold for victims enabling them to pull themselves along, or allow the rescuers to pull the ladder and victims to safety.

Horizontal access or bridging: This method can be used if rescuers need to cross openings without going in them. Check OSHA standards, if applicable, for ladder use that may require fall protection. Such instances might be:

- Crossing ravines
- Rock crevices
- Small streams
- Across buildings

These are only a few. With imagination and aptitude many more options can be devised.

Bridging fences: When a fence does not have a nearby gate or opening, it may be more efficient to climb over the fence using a ladder on each side.

Ladder gin-pole or A-frame: With the introduction of "A-frames" on heavy-duty squads, the "gin-pole" boom method is outdated. It may still be beneficial to practice this method, however, in case no A-frames are available. Remember, this is a noncompliant system and must only be used as a last resort, not as a substitute for approved hoisting or lifting devices and anchoring systems.

The A-frame is a more justifiable method than the gin-pole. The purpose of a tripod is to hoist or lower a line directly in the center of an underground opening, enabling true vertical lifting or lowering. To achieve the tripod effect, two ladders are fastened at the top where a block and tackle is attached. The two bottom ends are separated and straddled over the opening. The ends are then secured to prevent collapsing, therefore achieving the tripod effect.

Tower ladders: Towers offer a safer and quicker means of moving people and tools than ground ladders. They are more stable than ground ladders, enabling rescue crews to bring tools and equipment with them in a safer method. A tower also provides capabilities of elevated water streams when necessary.

Salvage and Overhaul Duties: Truck companies also perform salvage and overhaul duties. Examples where these duties may fit into a rescue operation or scenario include:

Water removal: Truck companies may be called on to clear drains of water, open floors to create new drainage, and if necessary, introduce portable pumps to remove water. These methods may be necessary due to water accumulation threatening the well-being of the victims.

Debris transfer: Ladder trucks come equipped with salvage buckets and shovels. An example of their usage would be a cave-in situation where the substance can only be cleared by handful or shovelful at a time. The substance is placed in buckets and hauled out of the excavation and disposed of.

Scene protection: Rescuers may be called on to protect the scene and victims from elements and debris.

Such methods may be salvage covers protecting victims from snow, wind, mud, rain, ash, or debris resulting from the rescue operation. It may also be beneficial to protect the victim and scene from public view by using salvage covers as curtains.

On long-term incidents it may also be necessary to cover the scene to protect it from the elements.

Scene stabilization: The last step in a rescue is to restore and safeguard the area. This can be accomplished by simply backfilling an excavation, or applying bracing methodologies to an unstable structure. The purpose in restoring and stabilizing a scene is to prevent injuries to rescuers and spectators during and after the fact.

Stabilizing structures: A structure can be stabilized using carpentry tools, commonly found on trucks, and wood found or provided on the scene to prevent any further danger of collapse. Structures may need temporary bracing during or after an incident to render them safe to enter or just to prevent them from falling. Rescuers should call the building office or public works for supplies and personnel if appropriate.

Utility Control: Utility control is another important duty of the truck company, not only on fire incidents, but rescue incidents as well. Many collapse incidents can disable any or all of a building's utilities. The importance of each utility is described below.

Electricity: The thought of electrocution raises awareness on the emergency scene. The possibility of water and electricity both being uncontrolled on a scene create an even more hazardous scenario. The truck company's ability to gain control of the electrical system can be vital to firefighter safety and survival. *Do not be led into a false sense of security with electricity. When in doubt deenergize!*

Water: Water is beneficial in fire suppression, but it can also be very dangerous on a rescue. Quantities can be hazardous because of weight, depth, and proximity to electrical hazards. Water weighs approximately 8.34 lbs. per gallon. In a structure already weakened, water in small quantities may cause a collapse. Buildings have collapsed with rainwater on the roof, adding just enough weight to break structural elements. Therefore, it is imperative that you keep water from accumulating at the scene. With skills and proper tools, the truck company can control the water problem or hazard.

Gas: Natural gas or propane is used for heating, cooking, and processing. The two most common means of storing gas are piping and tanks. Propane is more commonly found in above-ground storage tanks, either large mounted or portable tanks. In either case, uncontrolled gas can produce explosive results if exposed to an ignition source. All gas supplies on an appliance, tank, or meter have control valves. Many times adjusting these controls is all that is needed to remedy the situation.

As with all utilities, your job is to control and prevent them from inflicting harm. It is the utility company's responsibility, not the fire department's, to reenergize when the appropriate time arrives.

RESCUE/ENGINE/TRUCK/EMS COMPANY INTERFACE

Rescue involves a delivery process whereby a trapped or stranded victim is freed and safely removed from a hazardous condition that may or may not pose a serious threat to life. Rescue scenarios involve multitask functions and the utilization of jurisdictional resources.

It is now becoming the rule, rather than the exception, to find EMS, specialty units, engine/truck/rescue companies, and law enforcement working together in various roles on the scene of a rescue incident. This is neither the time nor the place for turf battles. The success or failure of a rescue scenario is predicated on the ability of the participants involved to carry out an informational exchange, along with the expeditious assignment of tasks and responsibilities.

Response personnel must recognize the diversity in staffing and the associated levels of training of all participants. When an incident escalates from simple to complex, the right people with the proper credentials should be assigned to perform the tasks needed to successfully conclude an incident. This may necessitate separating the higher trained individuals from the lesser experienced.

Engine Company and EMS Interface

Engine companies work in conjunction with EMS companies/personnel by providing these services:

- Transport mechanism to deliver first responders and/or EMTs to the scene.
- Administer patient care on the scene when no suppression hazards exist.
- Assist in providing ingress and egress points for basic life support (BLS) and/or advanced life support (ALS) personnel during the phase of gaining access.
- Provide security for other personnel operating on location of an incident.
- Engine companies carrying ALS/Paramedic-level personnel may be used to coordinate on-scene communications with a hospital facility and/or a helicopter responding to a landing site.

These levels of activities require constant communication between engine company and EMS crews. This will ensure complete informational exchange thereby reducing potential safety hazards.

Rescue/Engine/Truck/EMS Company Interface

Rescue operations focus on the activities of all of the emergency services units and accompanying personnel on location, and the protection of individuals involved in life-safety situations. Interface activities may involve a combined service effort. Crews, tools, equipment sharing, and vehicles all contribute to this process.

Truck companies often double as rescue companies on various incidents. When a truck company performs the primary rescue function, it must coordinate its activity level with the engine company(ies) and EMS unit(s) on location. The truck company may be used in a support capacity to the rescue pumper if this unit happens to be the designated rescue unit at the scene.

Truck company and rescue pumper personnel will be charged with the responsibility of gaining access for the EMS personnel on location. In the interest of safety, EMS personnel not wearing personal protective equipment (PPE) should be kept away from hazard exposure in a designated staging area of the cold zone until this process is completed. This is necessary because EMTs only receive vehicle extrication awareness exposure in the EMT course. Both groups are aware of their primary tasks and associated equipment requirements.

EMS personnel in general are a group of trained BLS or ALS providers whose purpose is to provide:

- Patient assessment and monitoring
- Treatment regimens
- Packaging protocols
- Removal of occupants on EMS devices
- Transport to a medical/trauma facility

PPE is crucial to safety, especially for those EMS companies that provide rescue functions with multipurpose units. What PPE policy is in place in your jurisdiction for EMS personnel?

Rescue Squad Functions: Squads differ from rescue vehicles according to task descriptions by jurisdiction. The term *squad* generally refers to heavy-equipped vehicles for multipurpose role assignments. Rescue vehicles, on the other hand, are generally recognized as smaller specialty units for extrication tasks. Many jurisdictions use the terms *squad* and *rescue* interchangeably. What may be called a squad in Anne Arundel County may be referred to as a rescue truck in the far reaches of Allegany County. Terminology is based on preference, mission, size, cost, geographical area, and/or the jurisdiction's policies and procedures.

Some jurisdictions dispatch units on a rescue incident using the terminology *Rescue 14* or *Squad 12*. Again, terminology is not important. The mission of the company using this apparatus and its designed intent is really what matters the most. The bottom line is very simple: Squad/rescue personnel are all on the same team. Regardless of the type, designation, and task performed by numerous units working on an incident, everyone functions under some form of incident command with a formal/informal incident management or incident command system in place.

Professionalism, teamwork, competence, and safety are key to the success of any rescue mission. There is no place on a rescue incident for interpersonal conflicts. Personnel should maintain the proper focus on why they are there: for the victims that requested their assistance!

Incident Management System

Incident Management System Characteristics

a. Bring order to confusion and chaos

b. Accomplished through command and control

c. Affords the delegation of functional responsibilities to officers who manage smaller teams/groups

d. Chain-of-command is well defined to all participants

e. Enables the person in charge to take size-up information, training and experience, and available resources and develop incident objectives

f. Results oriented, with focus on efficiency and safety

g. Designed for modular expansion based on incident size, complexity, and required resources

h. Effective command established from the earliest moments of an incident yields the greatest potential for success

i. The senior-most member of a first arriving EMS/suppression unit on the scene should establish initial command, gather size-up information, and begin to develop the necessary strategies

j. Divisions or groups address effective "span of control"—five to seven individuals per officer/supervisor

k. Engine companies, truck/ladder companies, rescue/squad companies, and EMS are usually deployed as single resources within the emergency management system

Rescue incidents basically fall into two categories: simple and complex. Small-scale incidents are generally in the simple category. These incidents typically have a chief officer in charge if he/she responds on the assignment. The senior lieutenant or captain on the engine/squad/truck company may end up being the designated IC. Command structure is based on whether or not an incident requires a full rescue assignment or a reduced response to a motor vehicle accident with or without entrapment. Any unit on location could be designated by the senior officer in charge as the field communications unit during the entire rescue or extrication process. Keep in mind that even simple incidents should have someone assigned as a safety officer to monitor activities.

There is a mindset that "routine" motor vehicle accidents and noncomplicated entrapment or extrication activities do not require protective measures by standby or rapid intervention teams. This constitutes "old school" thinking and ways of doing things in the past. The "new age" approach is:

> Engine companies on location should be supporting the rescue function with a designated crew, staffing a charged 1½ in.–1¾ in. attack line, for purposes of fire suppression and/or rapid intervention, in the event some unforeseen or sudden problem occurs that threatens the life or safety of the rescue participants. This crew should be appropriately attired inclusive of self-contained breathing apparatus (SCBA) with face masks donned if deemed appropriate by the IC and/or standard operating procedures (SOPs).

All too often squad/engine companies are dispatched to a landing site to provide safety for medivac helicopters. Upon further analysis, it is not uncommon to observe rescue participants standing by with an SCBA bottle on their back, a 10 lb. dry chemical extinguisher in their hand, no

INCIDENT COMMANDER			
OPERATIONS OFFICER	PLANNING OFFICER	LOGISTICS OFFICER	FINANCE OFFICER

Figure 1–1 Incident command structure.

face mask donned, and no attack line with a water source extended. *What's wrong with this picture?* The point here is obvious. What good will a 10 lb. dry chemical extinguisher do on 300 gals. of JP4? What protection is afforded to the rescue provider or engine company crew member(s) if they are not appropriately attired and something goes wrong? Is a charged attack line, which does not include a booster line, more desirable for the intended purpose than a dry chemical extinguisher? Whose responsibility is it to see that this assignment is conducted in the proper way? *Answer: The person in charge and/or the safety officer.*

Large-scale incidents (complex) will generally have a chief officer in charge. There may be a shared responsibility if box areas or running assignments overlap. On larger-scale incidents the management structure may involve the delegation of multitask assignments. These tasks are typically addressed using the incident command structure (ICS) shown in Figure 1–1.

The size of the incident will dictate the extent and involvement of the ICS/IMS needed to manage the overall operation. Small-scale incidents may only require an operations officer to oversee a rescue process, while a building collapse will require implementation of a full-scale management system. The components of this system are:

Incident Commander/Command Post Responsible for the entire rescue incident and all associated functions. Usually the chief officer of a company, district, or battalion. Safety officer, liaison officer, and public information officer (PIO) assigned here for immediate disposal of inquiries and problems.

Operations Officer Designated/appointed by the on-scene IC to manage the actual rescue operations sector and support staff.

Planning Officer Works under the IC to track resources and technical specialists that may be required on the scene in the event of an unplanned escalation.

Logistics Officer Oversees facilities, services, and equipment for the working units on location. Ensures proper staging of additional resource units responding to the incident.

Finance Officer Responsible for all the financial aspects associated with the incident (e.g., private contractors or vendors required for specific or specialized functions).

Complex incidents generally require additional responsibilities that are delegated in this format:

Staging Officer Works under the operations officer to manage/assign tasks to on-scene or additional units responding. (May also be assigned to the logistics officer as the need dictates.)

Rescue Sector Managed by a chief officer or senior officer. Comprised of a fire suppression team and accompanying safety officer.

- **Extrication Sector** Comprised of a rescue officer and accompanying safety officer.
- **Specialty Extrication Resource Sector** Comprised of bus/truck/big rig/aircraft/train officer in charge with accompanying safety officer.

Emergency Medical Services Sector Overseen by an EMS chief officer or senior EMS control officer on location.

- **Triage Sector/Group** Comprised of an EMS officer (Paramedic) and medical units assigned.
- **Patient Treatment Sector Group I** Comprised of BLS crews and EMS supervisor.
- **Patient Treatment Group II** Comprised of ALS/EMT-P crews and EMS supervisor.
- **Patient Treatment Sector Group** Comprised of an EMS officer or supervisor and a liaison from the outside agency(ies) involved.
- **Medical Unit Staging Sector Group** Comprised of an EMS chief officer or senior EMS officer and medical units responding to the incident on the first or subsequent alarm(s).

Question: Why is it necessary to have in place an IMS/ICS at the scene of a rescue incident?

Response: The answer is *because:*

Because: The inherent benefits of a formally or informally structured incident management process will expedite the entire rescue process and bring it to a successful conclusion.

Because: It will bring order to confusion and chaos.

Because: Order is accomplished through command and control.

Because: It allows the delegation of functional and operational responsibilities to officers and acting officers who manage smaller teams.

Because: The chain of command is well defined for all incident participants.

Because: It enables the person in charge to take size-up information, training, experience, and available resources, and develop incident objectives.

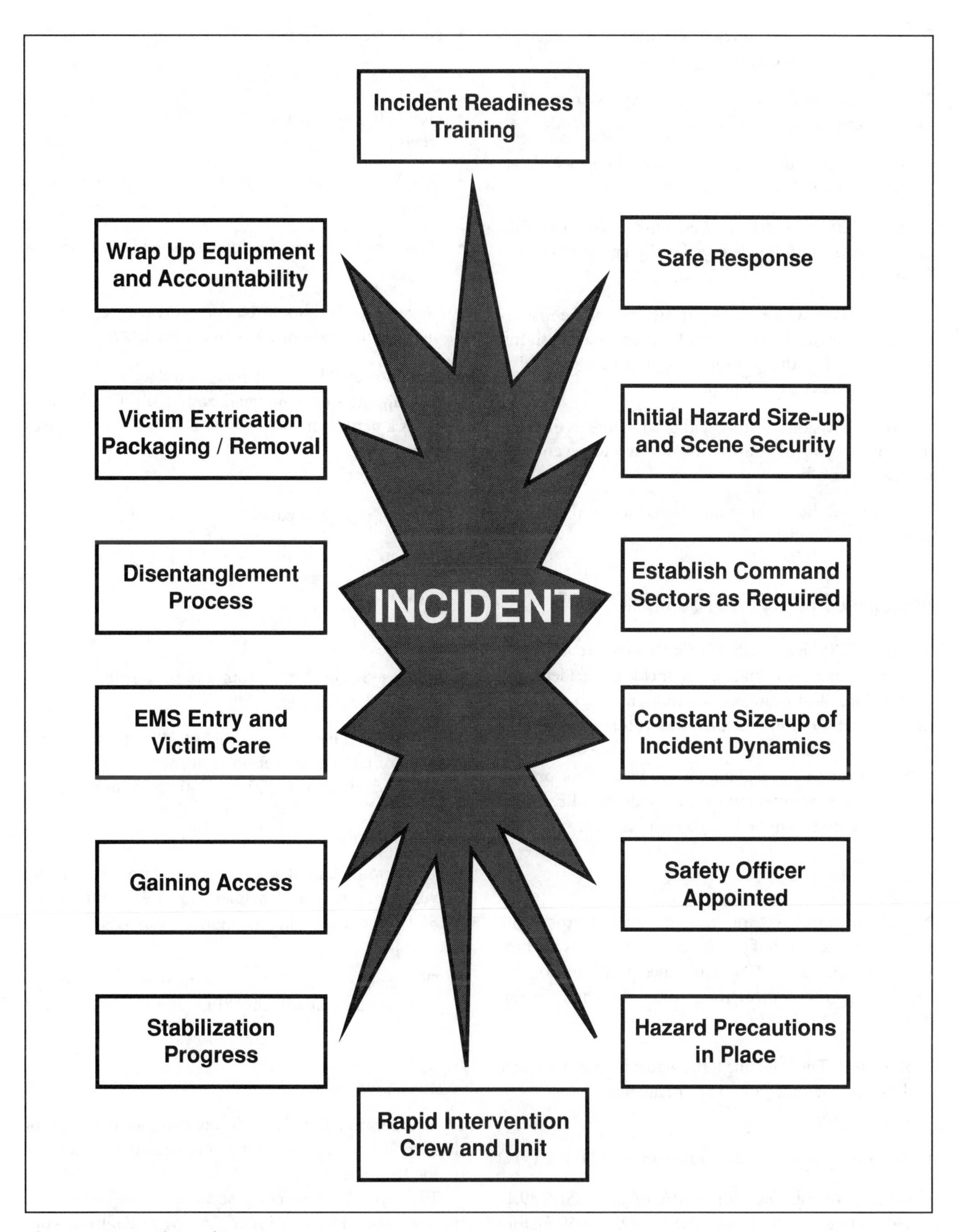

Figure 1–2 Incident tasking.

Because: This process is results oriented with a keen focus on efficiency and safety.

Because: It is designed for modular expansion based on incident size, complexity, and required resources.

Because: It provides a "toolbox" containing a wide array of options and systems components.

Because: Effective command established from the earliest moments of an incident yields the greatest potential for success.

Because: It allows for the senior member of the first-arriving fire/rescue/EMS unit on location to establish initial command, gather size-up information, and begin to develop the necessary strategies.

Because: Divisions, sectors, and groups address effective supervisory span of control, usually five to seven team members per officer.

Figure 1–2 shows the components that need to be addressed in an incident.

PERSONAL PROTECTIVE EQUIPMENT (PPE)

The use of PPE is an absolute safety/survival requirement on the scene of a working rescue incident. Incidents can escalate into life-threatening situations for rescue personnel in a matter of minutes, therefore you need to be protected. Even though NFPA 1971–74 sets the standard for PPE for structural firefighting, it can be used for protective measures on working rescue incidents. PPE should be selected based on the hazards encountered.

Zones

Not all situations require the same level of protection. For this course, level of protection requirements are broken down into zones. The zones used in this section coincide with the control zones used elsewhere in this course.

Hot Zone: The hot zone is the actual involvement area with the rescue, out to a 100 ft. perimeter.

PPE required:

- Turnout coats and pants (compliant with NFPA 1971)
- Helmets (compliant with NFPA 1972, ANSI Z89.1-1986 after 7/5/94, and ANSI Z89.1-1969 before 7/5/94)
- Gloves (compliant with NFPA 1973)
- Footwear (compliant with NFPA 1974)
- Hoods (compliant with NFPA 1971, for suppression crews)
- SCBA (compliant with NFPA 1981, for suppression crews)
- Wrap-around eye protection (face shields alone are not adequate)
- EMS personnel should be equipped with emergency medical PPE (compliant with NFPA 1999)

Warm Zone: The warm zone includes the equipment (tools) support area, command post, and PIO. This area includes a perimeter of 100 ft. to 200 ft. from the actual incident.

PPE required:

- Turnout coats and pants
- Helmets
- Gloves
- Footwear
- Hoods—SCBA (wrap-around eye protection are optional at the discretion of the IC)

Cold Zone: The cold zone includes the apparatus staging area for rapid intervention group access. This area includes the perimeter of 200 ft. to 500 ft. from the actual incident.

PPE required:

- All personnel in staging with apparatus should be wearing coats, pants, helmets, footwear, and gloves. (SCBA is optional unless assigned to rapid intervention crew.)
- The staging officer/IC has the final authority to upgrade or downgrade the PPE requirements on the scene.

Equipment Advisory

Rescue personnel should seriously consider the laxity of dress code requirements and its subsequent enforcement on the rescue scene.

When you become complacent and elect not to don the required PPE, you invite hazards to confront you. Most rescue personnel injuries occur due to carelessness and complacent acts that show disregard for established SOPs and guidelines.

Is it worth losing your eyesight because a metal fragment from a cutting tool became embedded in your eye—an action you could have prevented? Work smart, work safe!

INCIDENT SAFETY AND ACCOUNTABILITY

Safety Perimeter

A perimeter is a line or a definitive designation surrounding an object. Simply stated, a circle with the focus in the middle.

A safety perimeter on a rescue scene is a circle around the accident or incident. Its purpose is to reduce congestion and confusion, limit ingress and egresses, and provide organization to potential chaos. The safety perimeter is broken down into four zones: operational perimeter, hot zone, warm zone, and cold zone.

Operational Perimeter (inner circle): A 25 ft. radius from the center of the incident. It is the actual rescue operation zone. The only permissible personnel in the operational perimeter are those attending directly to the victims and the extrication process.

Hot Zone (outer circle): An area encompassing the operational perimeter extending 100 ft. out from the center of the incident. This area may contain the power plant for rescue tools and a rescuer to operate it. Lighting equipment for the operational perimeter and a standby suppression crew with a charged hoseline are also located here. Personnel in the hot zone are support personnel for those in the operational perimeter.

Warm Zone: An area 100 ft. to 200 ft. from the center of the incident. The warm zone is an organizational area used for support, not actual engagement in operations. Located here are staging areas for tools used in the operations, additional support personnel, the command post, and the PIO. The outside of this perimeter should be cordoned off to the public and nonessential rescue personnel.

Cold Zone: An area 200 ft. to 500 ft. from the center of the incident. This area is used as a staging area for apparatus and nonessential personnel. The rapid intervention team is also staged in the cold zone and in a high state of readiness.

Note: These zone designations provide a basic overview for scene management. Check with your own jurisdiction for differing SOPs and/or operational directives.

The Rapid Intervention Team

The rapid intervention team is a fairly new concept derived from NFPA 1500. Its purpose is for the rescue of emergency rescue workers in the event of a sudden and/or rapid escalation of the incident. Like the IMS/ICS, the rapid intervention team concept can be scaled up or down to fit the needs of the incident.

Rapid intervention teams may be composed of engine, truck, squad, and EMS with an additional officer assigned, usually a chief. The composition is designated by the IC. For example: a simple one- or two-vehicle accident may only require a single engine company, where a Level III hazardous materials incident may require all units. Rapid intervention teams are uncommitted, on-scene units, designated for rapid intervention assignments. These teams are staged in the cold zone with clear access to the operational perimeter.

Personnel on the designated units are to be in a "battle-ready" state, meaning fully dressed in PPE, SCBA on and ready (facepieces and regulators are ready to be donned if needed). Members shall also have any specialized rescue equipment ready to operate. While in the staging, the rapid intervention team shall ensure that if the need should occur, the suppression force has an established water supply.

Being prepared or battle ready does not mean sitting on the back step, undressed, drinking soda, and smoking cigarettes. It means being prepared! Your co-workers and fellow rescue team members may be depending on you to save their lives.

The Safety Officers' Role in Accountability

The IC is ultimately responsible for personnel safety and accountability. The amount of responsibility placed on the IC's shoulders nearly makes the job impossible at times. To alleviate the workload, some tasks must be delegated to subordinate personnel. One of those delegated positions is that of the safety officer. The safety officer oversees scene safety issues and advises the IC of those issues. Among the primary safety issues is accountability. Accountability is having an awareness of the location and function of all units and personnel on the incident.

The safety officer can designate an accountability sector officer to handle the jurisdiction's accountability procedure. Accountability must be maintained on *all incidents*. Every person on the incident should be able to be tracked by using the accountability system.

Table 1–1
Level III Accountability Entry Control Chart

Name	*Unit*	*Assigned Location*	*Air Supply 30 Min/60 Min/4 Hr*			*Time*	
						In	*Out*

Some of the terms used in this section are:

Accountability chart: A form or board used by the accountability sector to record operating units, personnel, and assignments.

Collector ring: A ring used to collect personnel accountability tags (PATs) of personnel assigned to a piece of apparatus.

Entry control chart: A form used to account for Level III accountability. (See example in the "Level III" section.)

Personnel accountability tag: A tag that each fire department member carries which identifies him/her by picture and/or barcode and is attached to the units or apparatus collector ring.

Point of entry/exit control: An officer is assigned this position on Level III accountability. The officer records an individuals entry/exit on the entry control chart.

Levels of Accountability: Accountability is based on three levels. The example used in this text represents a system used in a typical fire department. The concept is the same wherever your department is located. However, the actual components and structure may vary slightly.

Level I Accountability: Used during the response mode. All personnel attach their PATs to their riding position or on the vehicle's collector ring. Some jurisdictions mandate that the officer riding the right seat collect them. Normally once all PATs are collected by the officer or acting officer on the apparatus, they are either brought to the command post and given to the accountability officer or retained by the officer in charge of the crew.

Level II Accountability: Used during an operation where conditions exist or may develop into a dangerous situation. The collector ring with PATs attached are then brought to the command post and affixed to the accountability board. This level is maintained by the accountability sector or officer along with coordination of unit and other sector officers. Once command has been terminated, the collector rings are returned to their respective units.

Level III Accountability: This level is used when strict control of entry must be observed. Examples of situations requiring Level III accountability include:

- Metro or subway tunnel incident
- Confined space excavation rescue incidents
- Hazardous materials incidents

When the need for Level III is determined, an officer is located at all entry and exit points with an entry control chart. The entry control chart records the person's name, unit assigned, assigned location, duration of air supply, time entered, and time exit made. (See Table 1–1)

As individuals exit the area, they report their exit to the entry/exit control officer, and pick up their PAT. (PATs on Level III are maintained at the point of entry or as determined by the IC.) When members exit from a point that is distant from their entry, notification must be made to the original point of entry officer to keep personnel from being listed as engaged in the rescue activity inside.

Accountability Responsibility: Every unit, company, and sector officer is responsible for the accountability of all personnel under his/her command at all times. The company officer or senior member in charge shall be responsible for all personnel riding on the apparatus.

Company-level officers must know the exact number of personnel under their command. Sector officers must know the exact number and identification of all companies under their command.

Each crew member also has a personal and professional responsibility to ensure the presence and location of other crew members. Whenever a member cannot be accounted for, an immediate search shall be initiated.

SUMMARY

This session should help you gain the understanding that a rescue operation involves more than a heavy-duty squad company. There are many multifaceted units in the fire service that can be utilized on a rescue incident such as the truck company previously discussed. Do not let the name "Truckee" stop you from using this service. Use your head, think logistically, and use your ingenuity to solve the crisis at hand with the tools you have.

REFERENCES

Anne Arundel County EMS/Fire/Rescue Department, 1996. *Operational Procedures Manual:* 81-Rapid Intervention. Anne Arundel County, MD.

Moore, R.E. 1991. *Vehicle Rescue and Extrication.* St. Louis: Mosby Yearbook, Inc.

NFPA 1500: *Standard on Fire Department Occupational Safety and Health Program,* 1992 edition, American National Standards Institute, National Fire Codes, Volume 8, Revised 11/96.

NFPA 1521: *Standard on Fire Department Safety Officer,* 1992 edition, American National Standards Institute, National Fire Codes, Volume 8, Revised 1/97.

NFPA 1582: *Standard on Medical Requirements for Firefighters,* 1992 edition, American National Standards Institute, National Fire Codes, Volume 8, Revised 11/96.

OSHA 29–Labor, Code of Federal Regulation

Permit-Required Confined Spaces, 1910.146
Excavation Requirements, 1926.650
The Control of Hazardous Energy
(Lockout/Tagout), 1910.147
Personal Protective Equipment, 1910.132
Bloodborne Pathogens, 1910.1030
Hazardous Communication 1910.1200
Hazardous Materials Response, 1910.120
Respiratory Protection, 1910.134
Fire Brigade, 1910.156

Published by: The Office of the Federal Register, National Archives and Records Administration, as a special edition of the Federal Register. 1997. Washington, DC: US Government Printing Office.

Prince George's County Fire Department. 1995. *General Order 3-10 Accountability.* Prince George's County, MD.

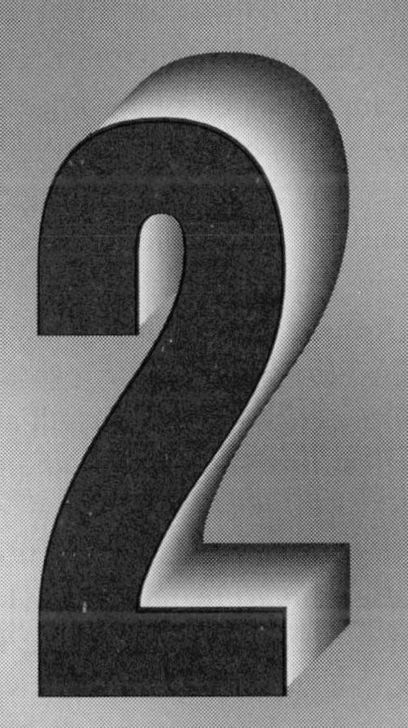

Technical Aspects of Ropes, Hardware, and Harnesses

OBJECTIVE

The student will be able to identify and demonstrate the use and care of various types of rescue rope, hardware, and harnesses, from memory, without assistance, to an accuracy of 70% and the satisfaction of the instructor.

OVERVIEW

Technical Aspects of Ropes, Hardware, and Harnesses

- Types of Rope and Software
- Rope Strengths and Classifications
- Care and Storage of Software
- Types and Care of Rescue Rope Hardware
- Uses, Classifications, and Care of Rescue Harnesses

ENABLING OBJECTIVES

2-1-1 Identify the types of rescue rope and software and their methods of construction.

2-1-2 Describe the strength classification of rescue ropes/software, and factors that affect the rope strength.

2-1-3 Describe the care, maintenance, and storage of rescue rope and software.

2-1-4 Describe the use and care of the various types of rescue rope hardware, including carabiners, descenders, ascenders, and edge protection.

2-1-5 Describe the uses, classification system, and care of rescue harnesses, including emergency harnesses, and demonstrate the appropriate use of rescue harnesses.

TYPES OF ROPE AND SOFTWARE

Vines were the first material used for rope. Animal parts were also used as rope as this material was freely at hand. When these natural ropes were found to be too short, or lacked sufficient strength to perform their intended task, people began tying them together for length and weaving them together for strength. By combining tying and weaving, early rope makers were able to make ropes of any length or strength necessary to accomplish the tasks of the period. These early ropes were not very flexible and were very bulky and heavy. Thus began the manufacturing of rope, first from vines and animal parts, then from the fibers of various plants.

In most instances, using plants which were naturally at hand, proved to be not much better than the original vines or animal parts. Later, as trade grew among various tribes, the stronger more flexible ropes, some woven from spun animal hair while others were made from natural fibers, became a trade item. The use of water transportation expanded the availability of exotic fibers for the making of rope. Maritime trade also increased the need for stronger, more flexible ropes as the need for bigger and better sailing ships grew.

Before the introduction of nylon, and later other synthetic fibers, manila rope, made from the natural fibers of the abaca plant, was the standard of the maritime and rigging trades. Manila was the only acceptable rope used for rigging and consequently rescue work. Today it is difficult, if not impossible, to find a number-one grade manila rope. Manila fibers were preferred in making rope because of their long length (13 ft. to 14 ft. long). The hemp plant provides the fibers for another widely-used rope. Hemp fibers are 11 ft. to 12 ft. long, but are more brittle than manila; thus they are easily broken when tied into knots or used in rigging. The most common rope is made from a plant called *sisal* and its fibers are from 5 ft. to 9 ft. long. Cotton rope, often found in clothesline, is the weakest rope and of little or no value to the rescuer.

Rope made of synthetic materials, in general, has a higher strength for its size, consists of single fibers run continuously through the rope, withstands minor shock loading, ages slower, and does not rot. Nylon rope is the most common for rescue. It has a high tensile strength but loses strength when wet and can be damaged by corrosives. Polypropylene and polyethylene ropes are used for water rescue throw rope. They have a low tensile strength and float on water. Because they are high-stretch ropes, they are not used for rappelling or rescue systems. Polyester rope has a moderate tensile strength and is resistant to some acids. It is used in industrial and confined space incidents.

It is important for rescue rope to have long fibers. Figure 2–1 depicts what occurs to manila and nylon ropes when loaded to within 50% of their breaking strengths and allowed to sustain that load for up to five hours. Manila rope creeps or what appears at first to be stretching. The fibers first tighten up their twist, then they start

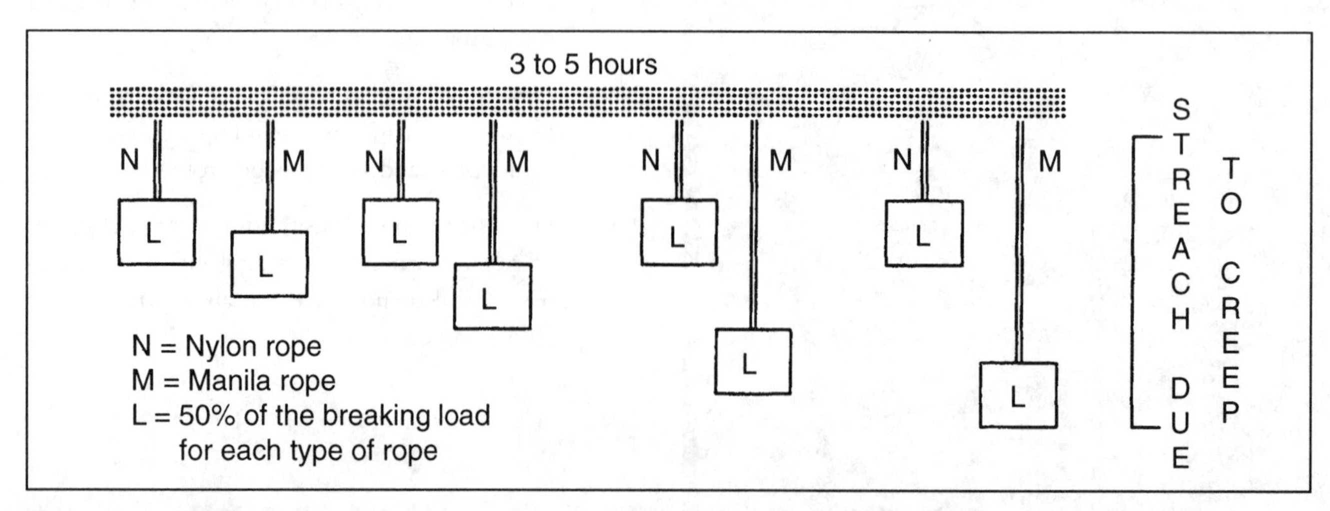

Figure 2–1 Manila v. nylon rope.

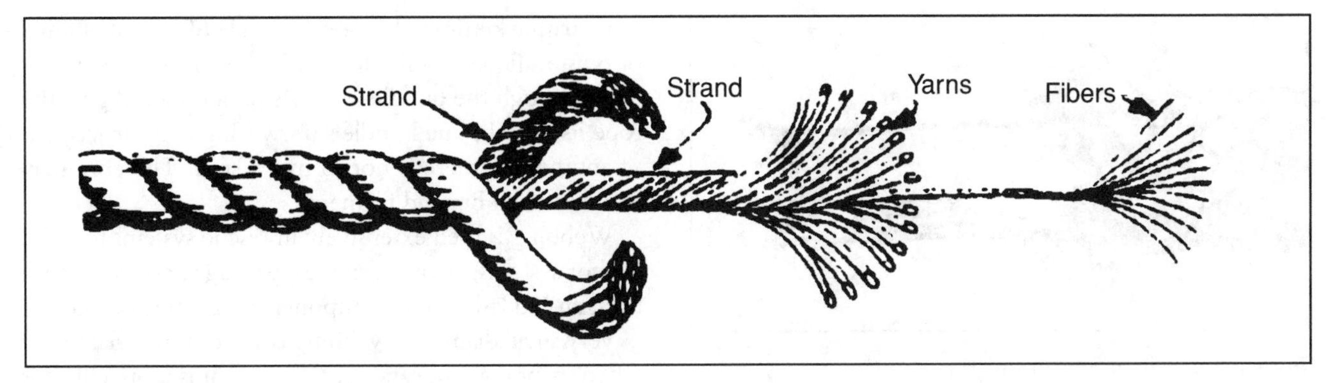

Figure 2–2 Hawser-laid rope.

slipping or sliding apart. At some point in time, the rope will fail as the fibers slip completely apart. Of course, the shorter the fibers, the quicker the rope will fail; the heavier the load, the quicker the failure. A reduction of the load will lengthen, if not eliminate, the slippage failure potential. As shown in the figure, the nylon rope has not stretched or slipped at all. Fiber slippage such as occurs in manila rope can occur in rope (such as nylon) if the fibers do not run the full length of the rope. For this reason, MFRI recommends that all rescue ropes be constructed of continuous-run or full-length fibers. Because of the probable failure of natural material rope, they are no longer used in rescue operations.

Rescue ropes made with fiber materials were hawser-laid ropes. Regardless of the type of material from which the rope is constructed, the method of manufacturing hawser-laid rope is still basically the same. First the fibers are twisted into yarns. These yarns are next twisted together into a strand. This twisting into a strand is done in the opposite direction to the twist of the fibers. The strands are then twisted together into the rope, again twisting in opposite direction to the twist of the strands. This reversal of twist in each segment gives the rope a balance or set and eliminates the tendency to unwind. The twisting can be done either tight or loose, making the rope either a "hard-laid" or "soft-laid" rope. Hard-laid rope is stiffer and more resistant to abrasion, whereas soft-laid rope is stronger. Figure 2–2 depicts a hawser-laid rope.

Cotton rope is constructed by braiding the fibers together. This type of construction has followed into the synthetic rope manufacturing process. Figure 2–3 depicts a braided rope.

The introduction of braid-on-braid rope came with the advent of synthetic rope. Braid-on-braid rope has found wide acceptance in the marine trade. As Figure 2–4 indicates, the core of the braid-on-braid rope is hollow.

Selecting the types and sizes of rope to be used for rescue work is of utmost importance. Properly selected rope ensures the well-being of those who must use it—the rescuer as well as the victim.

Today's rescue ropes are made from synthetic materials. These ropes should have fibers that are continuous from one end of the rope to the other end, regardless of length. They should be of a straight, central core with an abrasive, resistant-woven covering around the complete rope. Rescue ropes purchased for utility purposes, however, may have some fibers that do not run the full length of the rope. These fibers may be tied to another fiber if a break should occur or if the spool runs out before the rope's full length is reached. Purchased utility ropes are normally of the hawser-laid type.

With the advent of synthetic ropes, the emergency services (along with those involved in mountain climbing and associated high-altitude work) pressed manufacturers to develop a rope that would meet its requirements.

To meet this demand, the industry developed kern-

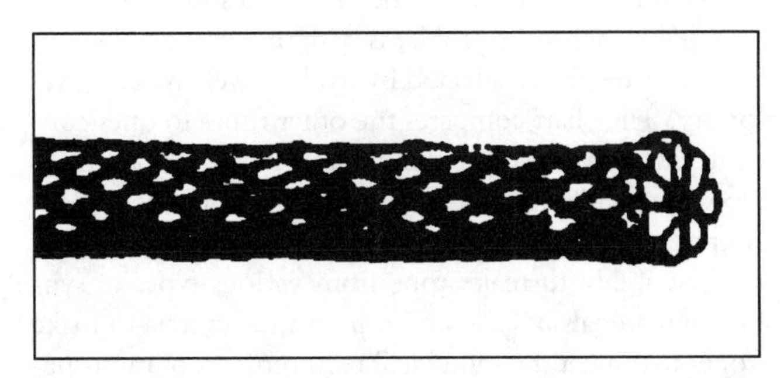

Figure 2–3 Braided rope.

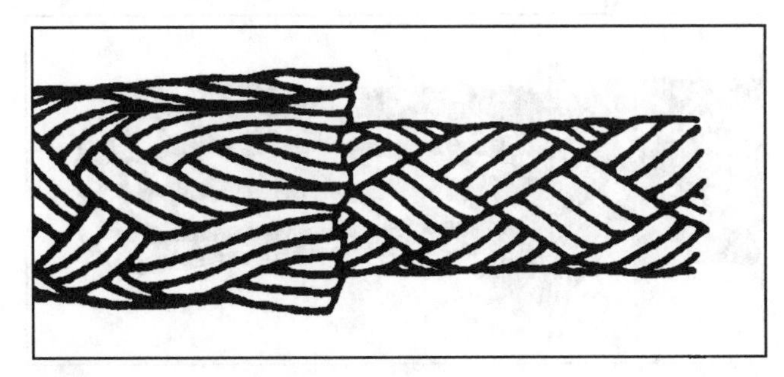

Figure 2–4 Braid-on-braid rope.

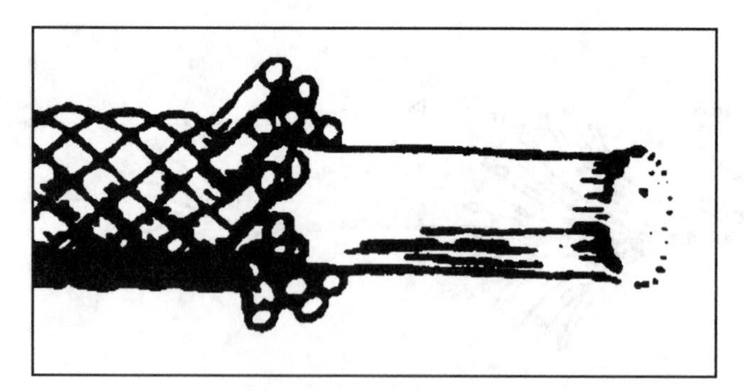

Figure 2–5 Static kernmantle rope.

mantle ropes. Kernmantle rope is a European, two-component design. The *kern,* a high-strength inner core, is covered by an outer, braided protective sheath called the *mantle* (or mantel). Figures 2–5 and 2–6 depict kernmantle ropes.

Kernmantle ropes have different kinds of sheaths for different purposes. Some have sheaths that are loosely woven and loose on the core. This type of rope is good because it is flexible and easy to handle. It works best in situations requiring it to be handled often and having knots changed frequently. The disadvantages are that the loose weave lets dirt and grit into the core easily, the sheath is less abrasion resistant, and a parted sheath will slip along the core for a great distance.

More tightly woven sheaths are manufactured for static ropes. Such ropes are not as flexible and knots are harder to tie, but the sheath is more grit and abrasion resistant and will not slip as far if parted.

The core can be made of parallel filaments or filaments spiraled into cords. Each bundle of woven fibers in the core usually runs the entire length of the rope. The core of this rope is about 75% of the total strength of the rope. The way the rope is made also determines whether the rope is *dynamic* (elastic; stretches 20% to 40% in use) or *static* (not so elastic; stretches 2% to 3% in use). Use only static kernmantle as rescue rope. Figure 2–5 depicts a static kernmantle rope, while Figure 2–6 depicts a dynamic kernmantle rope.

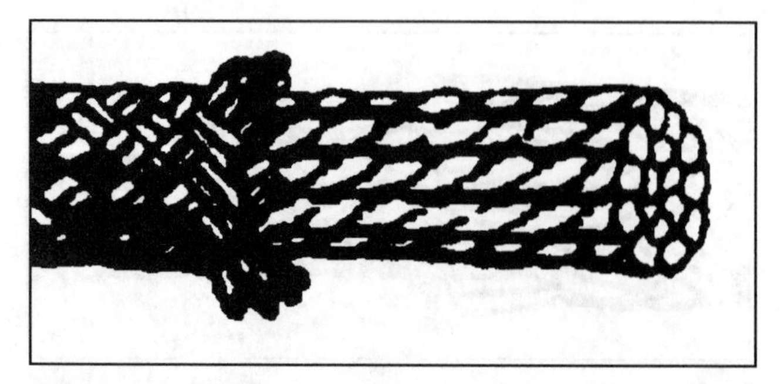

Figure 2–6 Dynamic kernmantle rope.

Dynamic kernmantle cores are made of several bundles of twisted fibers, similar to a laid rope. The difference is that although the bundle untwists under load to give the rope its stretch, one bundle's untwisting counteracts that of another, so there is not so much spin. The core may also consist of braided filaments.

Webbing is used extensively in rescue systems to build anchor systems, create harnesses, package and secure victims, and to lash rescue components together. Because of its very small diameter, webbing is a better material to use when snapping into carabiners because it is more efficient in maintaining its strength. It is relatively inexpensive, and can be cut to lengths for various uses.

Webbing can be purchased in either flat or tubular styles. Flat webbing (such as car seatbelts) provides high strength, but is very stiff. Tubular webbing (generally looks like a flat tube) is softer and easier to work with, but is slightly less resistant to abrasion. Only webbing from reputable manufacturers/suppliers with strength data supplied should be used for rescue.

ROPE STRENGTHS AND CLASSIFICATIONS

Rope Strengths

Although kernmantle rope has very high strengths, it does have limitations. In general, 7/16 in. static kernmantle rope has a minimum strength of approximately 6,000 lbs.; 1/2 in. rope, a minimum breaking strength of approximately 9,000 lbs.; and 5/8 in. rope, a minimum breaking strength of approximately 13,000 lbs. A single strap of 1 in. tubular webbing can hold about 4,500 lbs. and 2 in. about 6,000 lbs. All of these strengths represent new, unused materials, with no knot losses, bends, hardware, or other strength losses. Therefore, they represent the best case scenario, and one not achieved in the field.

Factors that Affect Strength

Do not become complacent with the use of synthetic material ropes and believe they have no shortfalls. Table 2–1 points out some problems with these ropes. The different materials are affected by loads as well as being wet or dry. The chart compares the other ropes to ones constructed of nylon. Note the nylon rope absorbs water, as does the manila, and both lose strength because of this absorption.

The ability to make rope from various types of synthetic materials has allowed rope manufacturers to make ropes that meet the individual requirements of most specialized applications. This includes a rope that floats, or

Table 2–1
How Rope Materials are Affected by Loads and Wetness

Relative Strength of Fiber Rope (Dry) Strength		% Change of Rope When Wet
Type of Rope	*Relative Capacity (%)*	*% Change in Strength*
Nylon	100%	−10%
Polyester	87	No change
Polypropylene	60	+5
Polyethylene	52	+5
Manila	37	−5

one that is resistant to a specific chemical, or perhaps one that withstands constant exposure to saltwater.

Table 2–2 indicates some of the effects of extreme temperatures on different types of rope. Temperatures much higher than those listed in the chart can readily be found on the fireground or in rescue operations, even those not involving fire.

The final effect, that of daily usage, must be considered. Tying knots, running the rope over pulleys, lashing timbers and stretchers, and just generally applying loads to the rope causes it to work. This work is also known as *flexing*. Flexing of any material eventually will cause it to fail. Some materials fail quicker than others, depending on the material and if the basic material is mixed with other materials. For instance, nylon rubbing against nylon in the same spot will generate heat, and has caused kernmantle rope to fail. Any material will eventually fail.

Another common enemy to rope endurance is *abrasion*. Approximately 90% of all rope failures are due to inadequate edge or abrasion protection. Abrasion is most often caused by the rope rubbing against some other object or edge. That object can be another rope or most frequently a sharp edge where a rope runs across between the anchor point to the load. This may be a window sill, a roof edge, a parapet wall, etc. By providing protection to the rope at these points, most abrasion can be eliminated. A hose roller works well on parapet edges and window sills. A blanket, piece of hose, or some other pliable substance that also offers a somewhat rounded surface will go far to eliminate abrasion. There are occasions where the rescuer needs the friction to control the lowering of loads. In these cases, where possible, smooth rounded surfaces provide both the friction desired to control the load as well as abrasion protection to the rope. When selecting these rounded surfaces, realize that small diameter objects cause abrasion to the rope by overbending it. This overbending is almost as damaging as bending the rope around a sharp-edged object. Therefore, within reason, the larger the diameter of the friction point, the less damage to the rope.

Table 2–2
Strength Loss v. High Temperatures

	Temperature (°F)				
Type of Rope	*68*	*105*	*140*	*175*	*212*
Manila	0	−3%	−8%	−20%	−30%
Nylon	0	−2%	−7%	−14%	−20%
Polypropylene	0	−7%	−18%	−30%	−40%

Safe Working Load

Knowing that rope can fail, how do we make allowances for normal wear and tear of rope? A formula has been developed that takes into consideration the usage factors. When this formula is applied to the manufacturer's specifications, the answer dictates the safe loads applicable to that particular rope. Understand, such mathematical information does not preclude the responsibility each rescuer has to inspect every rope before he/she uses it. Such inspection is to determine if the rope has been damaged by previous users. Whenever a rope is suspect, it must *immediately be removed from service*. The formula discussed here provides the safe working load (SWL), or the amount of weight that can be safely applied to a specific type and size of rope. Each rope manufacturer provides the breaking/tensile strength of its ropes. Divide this number by 15 to determine the SWL:

$$\frac{\text{BREAKING STRENGTH}}{\text{SAFETY FACTOR (15)}} = \text{SWL}$$

NFPA Rope Classification System

4-1.1.1 Rope designed to have a maximum safe working load of at least 300 lbs. shall be designated as class one-person life-safety rope.

4-1.1.2 Rope designed to have a maximum safe working load of at least 600 lbs. shall be designated as class two-person life safety rope.

4-1.2.1 The maximum working load ... shall be calculated by dividing the new rope minimum breaking strength . . . by a factor of not less than 15.

CARE AND STORAGE OF SOFTWARE

The traditional criticism of kernmantle is that it is very difficult to define core damage through the sheath. This concern has been found to be erroneous. In fact, it is very difficult to damage the core without obviously disrupting the sheath weave. One possible exception is localized tensile stress and compression at a knot or over an edge producing a shear component. However, hawser-laid ropes are equally unlikely to experience this sort of injury. The possibility of hidden core injury is still a controversial subject and open to much discussion. The braided nature of the sheath makes a kernmantle rope much easier to use than most other types. It has a softer feel than some types and, for the most part, makes tighter, therefore potentially safer, knots.

MFRI, as does OSHA, requires the *immediate removal from service* of any lifeline that has sustained the load of a person falling with such fall being arrested by that rope. While this may seem to be an expensive requirement, especially after inspection of the rope has shown no visible damage, it is the only positive way of being assured a rope is safe for lifelines. Even though Figure 2–1 indicated no damage to nylon rope from load, remember the figure uses nylon as the standard. Standards can fail when subjected to conditions of greater magnitude than their design criteria. With this safety regulation, and the common-sense rule it dictates, there should never be an accident due to lifeline failure in Maryland. All lifelines should be marked as such (by insertion of a continuous water-resistant identification tape) and when removed from service, such identification must be immediately removed. Also lifeline rope must be stored in special containers away from other ropes, as they may otherwise be used for lashing, rigging, etc.

At the conclusion of each rescue operation, all ropes used in the operation should be uncoiled and visually inspected for damage from overstress or exposure to harmful substances. *Immediately remove from service* any lifeline that has sustained the load of a person falling with such fall being arrested by that rope. Any rope that has been knowingly subjected to chemical exposure should be immediately flushed with water and removed from service until the harmful effects of that chemical on the rope can be ascertained.

Inspection can be best accomplished by running the rope through the hands and looking at each segment, as well as feeling for change in the normal rope structure. Inspect the *pic* (single square of mantle) for wear. If any pic has greater than 50% wear, or if the core fibers are exposed, downgrade the rope to utility. Feel the kern for lumps or narrow sections, indicating internal failure. Hard parts in the rope may indicate overstress or exposure to heat or chemicals as well as discoloration or a bad smell. Other irregularities in the shape or weave of the rope, lumps, or depressions including roughness and fuzziness, may spell trouble and require a more critical inspection. Gloves should be worn by the inspector(s) while performing this examination to reduce the danger of cutting their hands from foreign materials that may have become embedded in the rope. Hawser-laid ropes should be opened every 3 or 4 ft. to determine if foreign substances have entered the inside of the rope. With kernmantle or braided rope, however, it is impossible to look inside the rope, therefore the feeling and looking inspection is more critical.

Rope should be inspected about every three months even if it is not used. Dirty synthetic ropes can be washed by running them through a rope washer or hose washer. If such a machine is not available, a washtub or front-loading washer can be used, provided the machine can hold the weight of the rope and wash it without damaging it. Where the rope manufacturer has not provided cleaning information, cold water with mild soap (e.g., Woolite, Ivory, or other "safe for all synthetics" soap) can be used. While most synthetic ropes may be stored away wet, it is best to hang them in a hose tower or lay them out on a hose rack to dry first. Always remember that ultraviolet light (sunlight and some fluorescents) is harmful to rope. Therefore, rope should not be laid out in the sun to dry or exposed to excessive heat. Rope should be visually inspected only; it should never be subjected to a load test as part of an inspection program.

The rope history log (Table 2–3) is an important part of using a lifeline for rescue purposes. This log allows you to track the uses (and misuses) of a rope, along with information like age, manufacturer, and construction. This log should be maintained for each rescue rope, with specific ID numbers on the rope and log. ID numbers can be put on ropes using plastic shrink tubes, some clear tapes, or "whip dip."

When storing rope on the apparatus, it should either be properly coiled and hung up, or "flaked" in a rope bag and hung up. It should never be thrown into a compartment on top of, beside, or under any equipment, or thrown on the vehicle floor where it can be walked on. Also rope should not be stored in a compartment that contains gasoline, diesel fuel, or any other hydrocarbon-type materials as they and/or their vapors may adversely affect the rope.

TYPES AND CARE OF RESCUE ROPE HARDWARE

Rescue hardware is essentially rope components that are hard, and usually made out of steel or aluminum. They are used to permit connections, cause friction, change di-

Table 2–3
Rescue Rope Log

Serial Number	*ID Marking*	*Length*	*Diameter*

Date of Mfgr	*Date of Issue*	*Date in Service*

Fiber Material	*Color/Stripe*	*Construction*	*Mfgr's Lot Number*

Date Used	*Incident Location*	*Type of Use*	*Rope Exposure*	*Date Inspected*	*Inspector Initials*	*Rope Condition and Comments*

Purchased from	
Purchase Date	
Purchase Order	

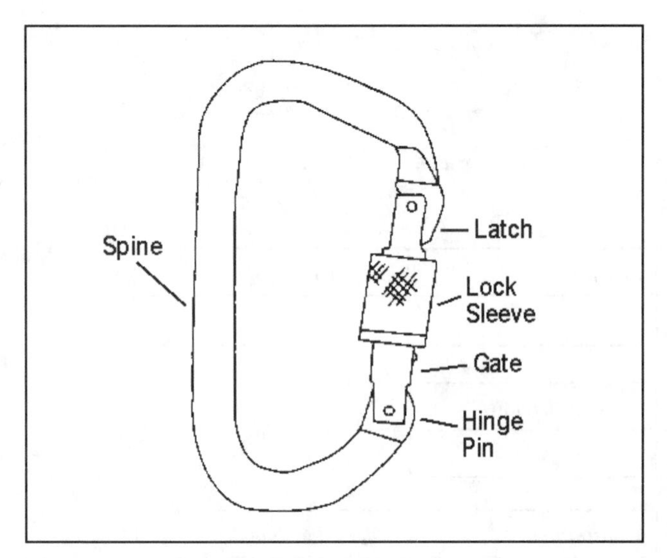

Figure 2–7 Basic parts of a carabiner.

rections, and build systems. Rescue hardware includes such devices as carabiners, descent control devices, ascenders, pulleys, and edge protectors.

Carabiners

Carabiners, sometimes called snap links, crabs, or biners, are metal connectors that link the different components of a rescue system together. There are five basic parts of a carabiner (Figure 2–7):

- Spine
- Latch
- Gate
- Lock sleeve
- Hinge pin

Carabiners for rescue work should be locking carabiners to prevent unwanted gate openings. Locking carabiners are at full strength when the gate is closed and locked. A locking carabiner should not be unlocked and opened when under load.

Most carabiners are between 10% and 90% weaker when unlocked. Gates could be self-locking/spring loaded.

Carabiners come in a variety of shapes and sizes. Standard oval carabiners are used for recreational climbing. D-shaped carabiners are preferred for rescue work because their shape takes advantage of the strongest portion of a carabiner, which is the spine. The D shape of the carabiner directs the majority of the load's forces to the spine when loaded. Large locking D carabiners are available and will fit over most rescue litter rails; some will fit over ladder rungs.

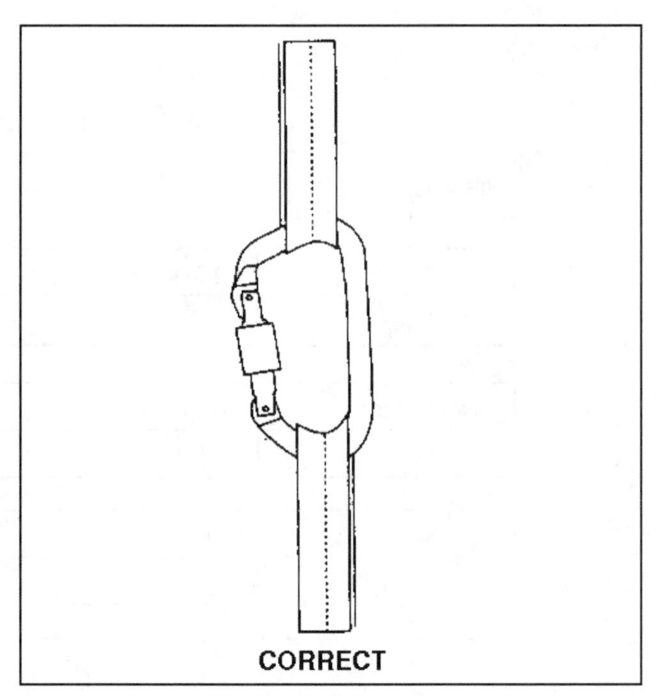

Figure 2–8 Carabiners are designed to be loaded end to end.

Standard locking rescue carabiners that meet the NFPA standard are strong enough to stand alone. Some rescue systems advocate doubling up carabiners and turning them so the gates are opposed and opposite. This is to prevent accidental opening of a gate during a rescue and the loss of the connection. With locking carabiners this is unnecessary, and in fact, has led to side loading of carabiners and damage to carabiner gates and locking mechanisms. Carabiners are designed to be loaded end to end (Figure 2–8); they should never be side loaded (Figure 2–9).

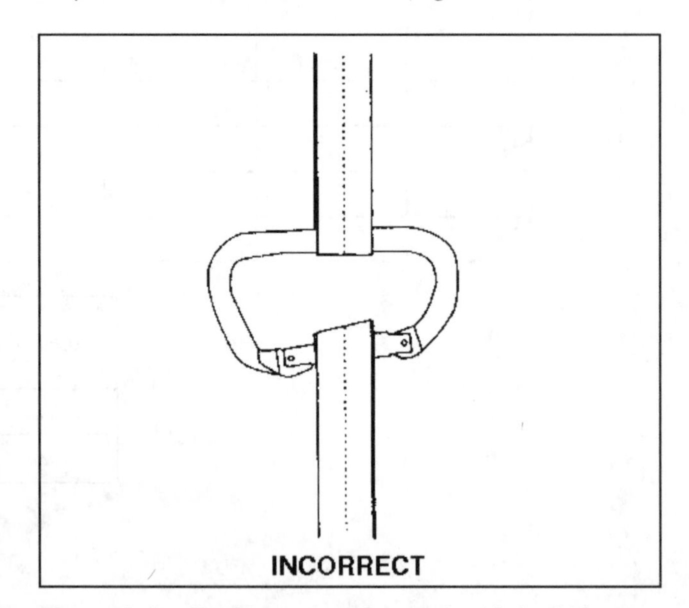

Figure 2–9 Carabiners should never be side loaded.

Carabiners are made of aluminum or steel. Rescue teams which must carry their equipment long distances, such as mountain rescue teams, tend to use the lighter weight aluminum variety. Rescue teams which are not as concerned about portability tend to use the stronger but heavier steel variety.

Aluminum carabiners:

- Are lighter
- Do not rust
- Are usually less expensive
- Wear out faster
- Are not as strong
- May be damaged by dropping and shock loading

Steel carabiners:

- Are stronger
- Are less susceptible to abrasion and wear
- Are heavier
- Are more expensive
- Tend to rust
- Require more maintenance

Carabiners' strengths vary depending on the manufacturer, but aluminum carabiners can be found with up to 6,000 lb. breaking strength. Steel carabiners run between 9,000 lb. and 13,000 lb. breaking strengths.

Under some circumstances a locking carabiner can come unlocked on its own while in a system. This can happen if the locking mechanism is rolled across the face of a cliff or building. It can be overcome by making sure the gate is turned away from the face. Another way gates have come open is from vibration, which can cause the lock to unscrew. This can be overcome by turning the gate down so gravity is working against the gate to keep it closed.

Carabiners used in industrial fall protection equipment are covered under ANSI Z359.1, "Safety Requirements for Personal Fall Arrest Systems, Subsystems, and Components." Carabiners which must meet this standard are required to be both automatic closing and automatic locking. As such, screw-locking carabiners are not permitted in these applications.

A common mistake is locking a carabiner while it is loaded. When the weight is taken off the system, the carabiner shrinks and the locking mechanism will not come undone. This can potentially damage the locking mechanism, so do not fully tighten down a loaded carabiner.

Carabiners must be kept clean of dirt and oil. Wipe them down with a clean rag and keep them off the ground to prevent dirt from entering the gate and locking mechanisms. Use a ground cloth, coat, or other object to lay out hardware when setting up systems. This will not only keep everything clean, but will prevent the loss of equipment as well.

Sharp burrs and nicks in carabiners and other hardware are damaging to software (ropes and webbing). If they are small they can be gently filed or sanded off. Carabiners with gates that stick or will not close should be discarded if they cannot be fixed by blowing out the latch and hinge with an air hose. Do not use oil or grease to lubricate because it will collect dirt and dust, which will act as an abrasive compound and wear out or jam the mechanism.

Descent Control Devices

Descent Control Devices (DCDs) provide control of a moving rope by providing a variable level of friction. Commonly used DCDs include the figure-8 and the rappel rack.

Figure-8s (Figure 2–10) were designed as descent or rappelling devices. Figure-8s can be used in a rescue set-

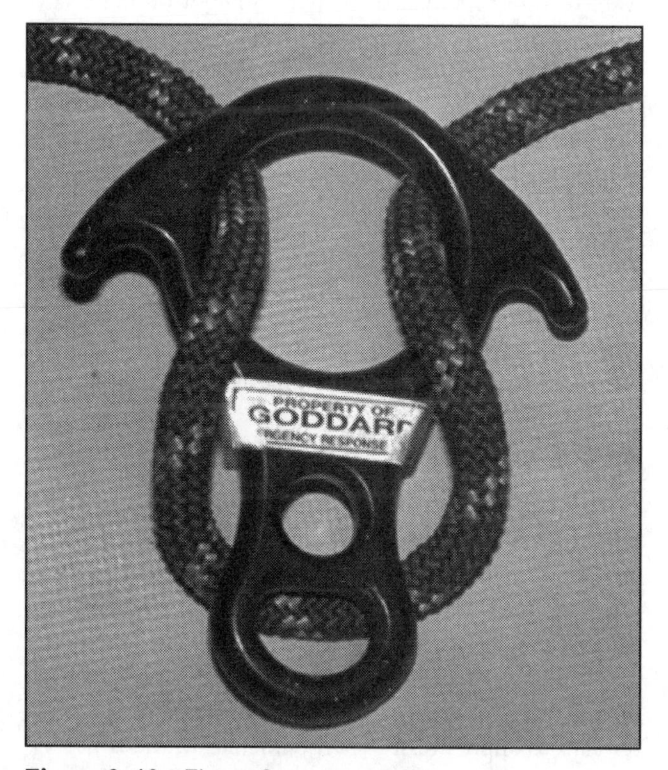

Figure 2–10 Figure-8.

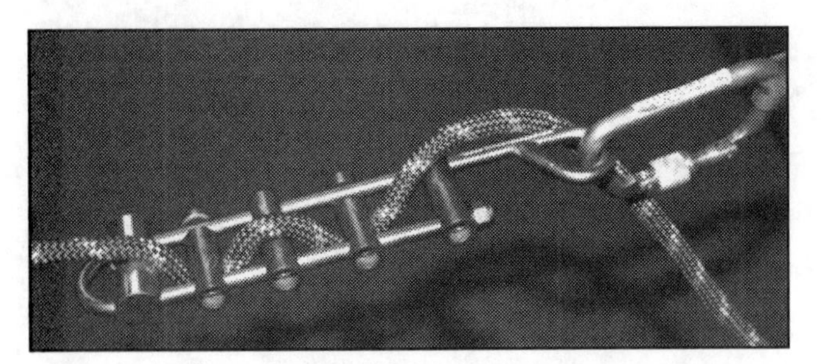

Figure 2–11 Rappel rack.

ting in rappels of 100 ft. or less. Greater distances are difficult, as the weight of the descending rope will create its own "belay" with the figure-8, requiring the rescuer to "push" the rope through the figure-8. Figure-8s are available with and without ears. Figure-8s with ears should be used in rescue work to ensure the rope does not slip up and create a girth hitch. It also helps in locking off.

The rappel rack (Figure 2–11) consists of several steel or aluminum bars mounted on a U-shaped rack. Rope is threaded back and forth through the bars. The turns in the rope, along with the ability to variably space the bars, can create a wide variety of frictional loads on the rope. Since the rope runs "straight" in the device, the "spin" of a figure-8 is eliminated. As such, the rappel rack is the preferred device for frictional-lowering systems in technical rescue.

The rappel rack can also be a complex piece of hardware to rig properly. Bars may be straight or angle slotted, and may not "pop loose" when loaded incorrectly. However, once weight is applied to the device, incorrect bar loading will result in the rack coming loose from the rope. As such, it is critically important to load-check the rappel rack prior to the rescuer using the rack in a descent or system.

NFPA 1983 requires that general-use DCDs withstand a 2,400 lb. load without damaging the rope or the device. In addition, the device must withstand a 5,000 lb. load without failure. Keep the device clean and dry. Check for burrs and rough edges and bent hardware.

Ascending Devices

Ascending devices are used to provide a "one-way" movement on a rope for climbing. They are also used to provide a positive form of attachment to a rope in systems, such as hoisting rigs. Examples of ascenders include cam ascenders, handled ascenders, and prusik ascenders.

Mechanical ascenders, whether closed shell or handled, generally secure to the rope by turning an off-center cam to apply pressure perpendicular to the rope. Increased forces provide greater pressure. Since they are designed not to slip on the rope when loaded, excessive forces may cause the mechanical ascender to damage the rope (most often "desheathing"), with catastrophic results. While there is no shock load test, NFPA 1983 requires that all mechanical ascenders support a static load of 2,400 lbs. without damage to the rope or device.

Cam ascenders (such as Gibbs or Rescuecenders) are generally used in hauling systems (Figure 2–12). They consist of a curved shell with the cam enclosed. As such, they must be disassembled to attach to a rope. While this may be inconvenient, it provides positive assurance that, once attached, the ascender will not come off the rope. These ascenders are designed for specific rope sizes, and can be found in both spring-loaded and free-running varieties. Cam ascenders can damage a rope with a static load of about 3,000 lbs. However, most manufacturers and rescue teams do not allow cam ascenders to be used in systems over 1,000 lbs. In addition, any shock loading which can exceed 1,000 lbs. must be protected by tear-apart shock absorbers (e.g., Screamers) to prevent catastrophic rope damage.

Handled ascenders (such as Jumar or Petzl) are specifically designed for personal climbing (Figure 2–13). Their cams have small conical teeth for better grip under adverse conditions. As they were designed for the loading of the weight of a single person, they are not

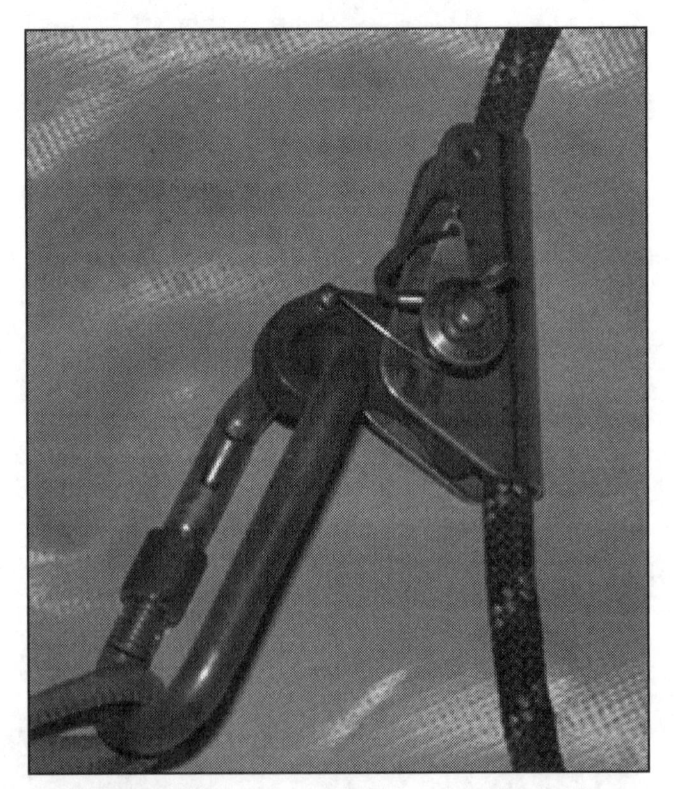

Figure 2–12 Cam ascenders.

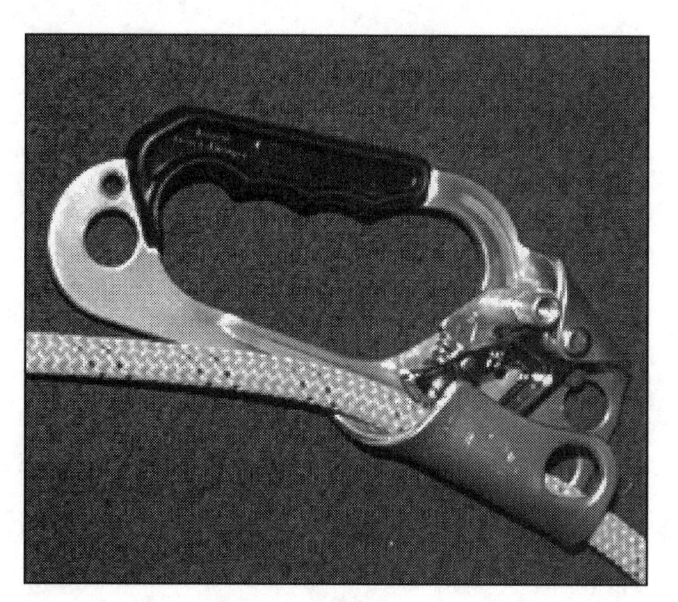

Figure 2–13 Handled ascenders.

permitted to be installed in *any* rope system. Desheathing may occur with as little as 1,000 lbs. Handled ascenders can also be attached or removed without disassembly to aid in ascending over ledges and similar obstacles.

Prusik ascenders can also be used as ascenders, as a "soft" rope grab knot. While they take some effort and technique to slide and set, they will support between 2,700 lbs. and 3,000 lbs. of force (8 mm prusik on ½ in. line) and can be used in shock-loaded systems. The method of failure of a prusik is that it slides on the rope until enough friction heat is generated to melt the prusik. While this can also cause glazing on the lifeline, many rescuers feel that this method of failure is preferrable to rope desheathing. As such, the prusik is many times the ascender of choice for safety and belay systems subject to high or shock loading. Care and maintenance is same as for other hardware.

Pulleys

In technical rope rescue, rescue pulleys are used to:

- Change direction of force on a running rope
- Reduce rope friction
- Create mechanical advantage for hauling systems

There are many types of pulleys on the market for use in high-angle situations. The lightweight type used by climbers to haul loads and perform self-rescue is not strong enough for rescue work.

Rescue pulleys are made of all metal for maximum strength. The *sheave* or the area that the rope runs on should be metal, and should be the proper width for the diameter of rope used. Not only should it be wide enough, but its diameter should be large enough for minimum loss of rope strength as the rope bends around the wheel. Traditionally, pulley size has been recommended as four times the rope diameter, however, some manufacturers indicate that synthetic ropes can be used on pulleys as small as 2.5 diameters.

The *side plates* must be moveable so they can be placed on the rope anywhere in the system.

The *axles* should be firmly attached with rounded bolt heads to prevent damage to other rescue system components.

The *bearing* should be a sealed ball-bearing type so it turns freely and will not get contaminated with dirt and debris (Figure 2–14).

As with other hardware, pulleys should be inspected for any type of deformities, especially bent load-bearing structures such as pulley axles. If the integrity of any rescue hardware is in question, it should be destroyed and discarded.

Pulleys must be kept clean and free of sharp edges, nicks, and burrs. These can be lightly filed or sanded off. Make sure the axle bolts are tight, and that the sheave and side plates rotate freely. The attachment should be

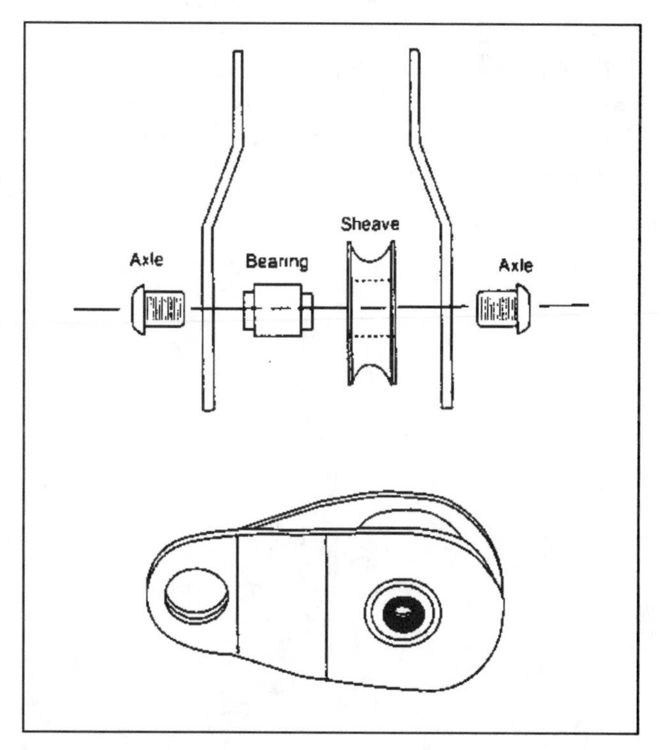

Figure 2–14 The pulley's bearing should be a sealed ball-bearing type.

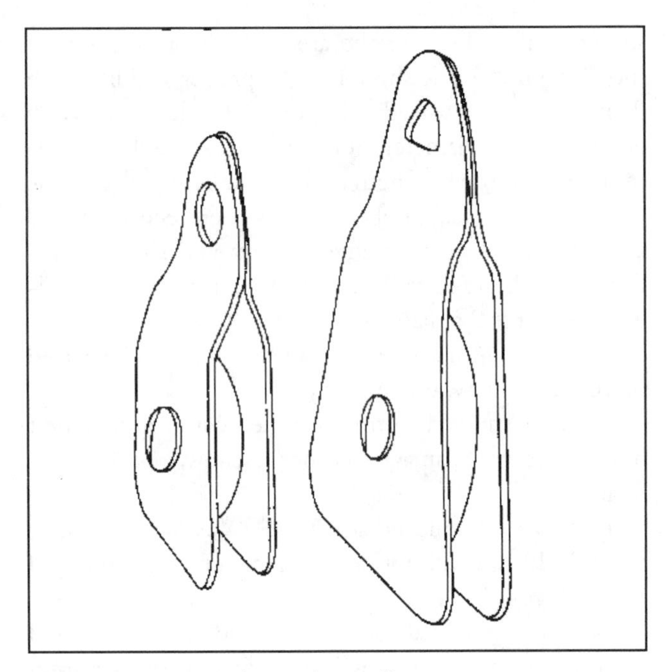

Figure 2–15 Prusik-minding pulleys.

checked for wear and elongation which indicates excessive loading. Discard the pulley if such defects are found.

NFPA 1983 requires that general-use pulleys withstand a static test loading of 5,000 lbs. without distortion, and 8,000 lbs. without failure.

Special Pulleys: There are special pulleys manufactured to meet technical rope rescue problems.

Prusik-minding pulleys (Figure 2–15) work with prusiks to make a self-tending brake system for safety lines and ratchets for mechanical advantage pulley systems.

Knot-passing pulleys (Figure 2–16) allow a knot to pass through. This is important when two lines need to be tied together in order to reach a victim. This type of pulley allows the knot to pass right through the mechanical advantage system, which would not be practical with standard pulleys.

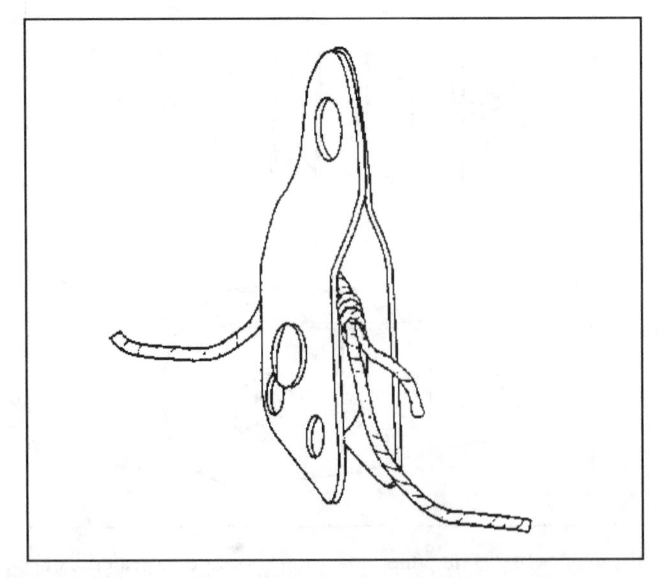

Figure 2–16 Knot-passing pulleys.

Double-sheave or triple-sheave pulleys have multiple pulleys within a single unit. The are valuable for setting up parallel systems or for increasing mechanical advantage (e.g., block and tackle).

Edge Protectors

Edge protectors are used to reduce abrasion on the rope, since 90% of all rope failures are due to inadequate rope protection.

Static protectors are used for nonmoving ropes, such as rappel lines over an edge. These protectors include canvas pads, turnout coats, commercial rope covers, and even the jute backing of carpet squares.

Dynamic protectors are used for systems where the rope is moving across a surface, such as hoisting rigs. Since all of these devices incorporate some type of rolling wheel, they can also greatly reduce the friction caused by the edge being crossed. Dynamic protectors include devices such as roof rollers and edge rollers.

USES, CLASSIFICATIONS, AND CARE OF RESCUE HARNESSES

Uses of Harnesses

Rescue harnesses provide the means to attach the rescuer to the rope systems. They can be used for access in rappelling, hoisting, and lowering systems. They are used for the removal of conscious and unconscious patients or victims. They are used in rescue and industry to provide work positioning (e.g., limiting how close to a roof edge a worker can get) or fall protection. They are also used to provide emergency egress, such as a firefighter trapped in a high-rise fire.

Classifications of Harnesses

NFPA 1983 provides classification and construction specifications for harnesses used in rescue. All NFPA harnesses require permanent labeling with harness class, date of manufacture, and sizing. Specific NFPA harness classes include:

NFPA Class I: Seat-style harness for emergency escape or one-person loads—*not for rescue.*

NFPA Class II: Seat-style harness for rescue and other two-person loads (Figure 2–17).

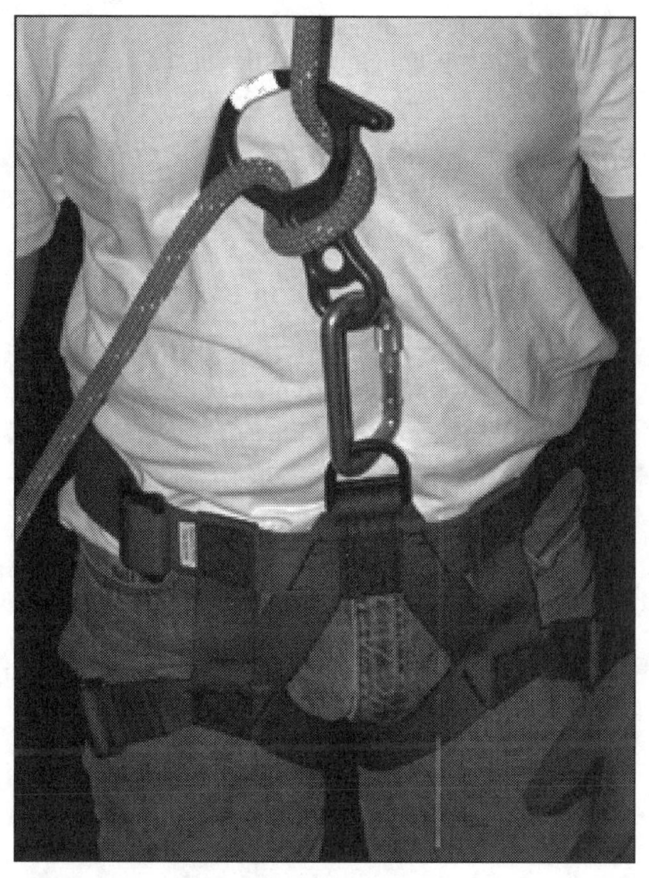

Figure 2–17 NFPA Class II harness.

NFPA Class III: Full-body harness for rescue and other two-person loads where inverting may occur. It may be a one- or two-part harness. It is practically the only effective harness for victims/patients, and it requires no skill or knowledge on the patient's part once in the harness (Figure 2–18).

NFPA Ladder/Escape Belt: Waist belt that can be used for a positioning device or as an emergency self-rescue device (Figure 2–19).

While not NFPA-compliant, some instances may require the use of "site-made" harnesses (Figures 2–20 and 2–21). These are harnesses made of rope or webbing, and are to be used for emergency self-rescue and egress *only*. They are not to be a part of a planned rescue system or attempt.

ANSI Harness Ratings: Industrial harness ratings are specified by ANSI. An ANSI rating or class is *not* equal to an NFPA rating or class. For reference, these harness uses are classified by ANSI:

Class I: Positioning belt

Class II: Chest harness

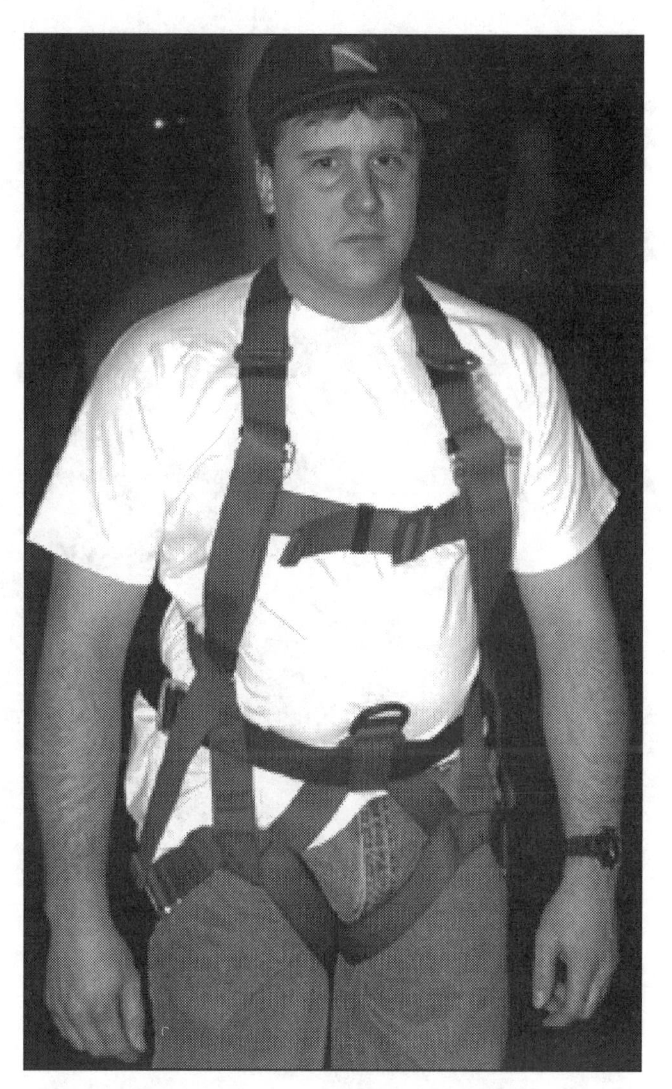

Figure 2–18 NFPA Class III harness.

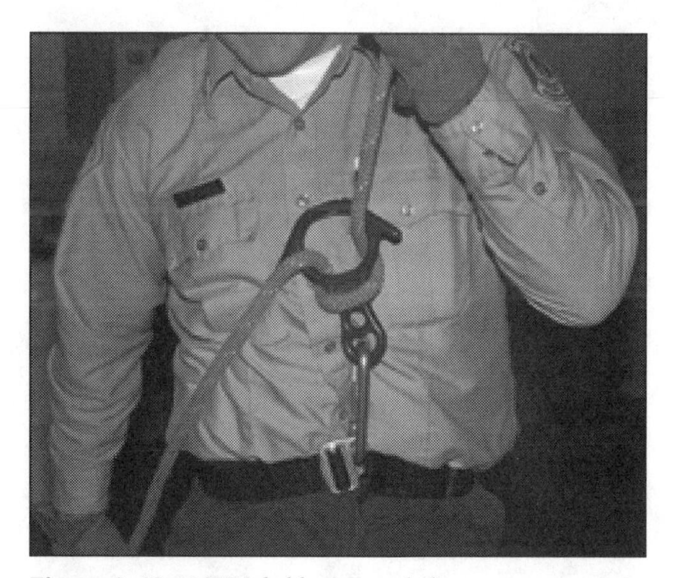

Figure 2–19 NFPA ladder/escape belt.

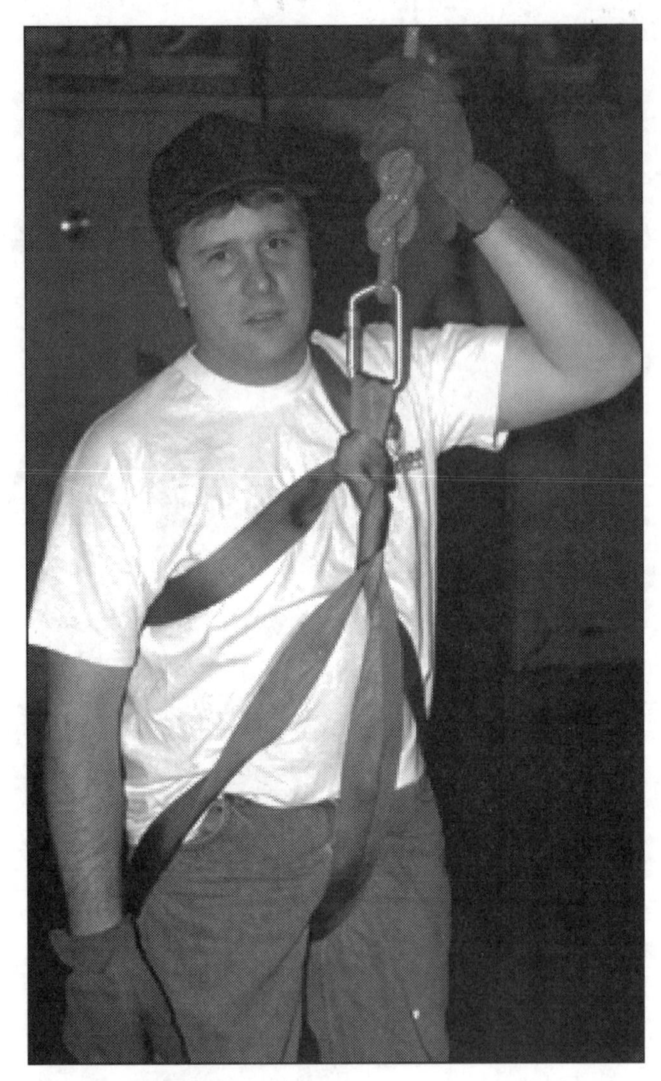

Figure 2–20 Site-made harness.

Class III: Full-body harness

Class IV: Seat harness

The following instructions are included for general guidelines on the donning of rescue harnesses. However, specific manufacturer's guidelines and instructions should always be followed. Questions regarding harness use should be directed to the company safety officer or the harness manufacturer.

NFPA Class I, II Harnesses

1. Select proper size.
2. Shake out and inspect harness.
3. Step through harness, adjust buckles. Fit high and tight; check by squatting.
4. If possible, free ends should be backed up with safety knot.
5. Metal connector ring is for metal connectors (e.g., carabiners). If tying on rope directly, tie to harness strap.

Note: Rope to harness ring forms very sharp bend in the rope, and sometimes the ring has casting burrs.

NFPA Class III Harnesses

1. Select proper size.
2. Shake out from back lifting ring and inspect harness.
3. With all buckles open except shoulder straps, put on harness like you would a jacket.
4. Fasten waist strap. Adjust shoulder straps.
5. Fasten leg straps.
6. Fit should be high and tight; check by squatting.
7. If possible, free ends should be backed up with safety knot.

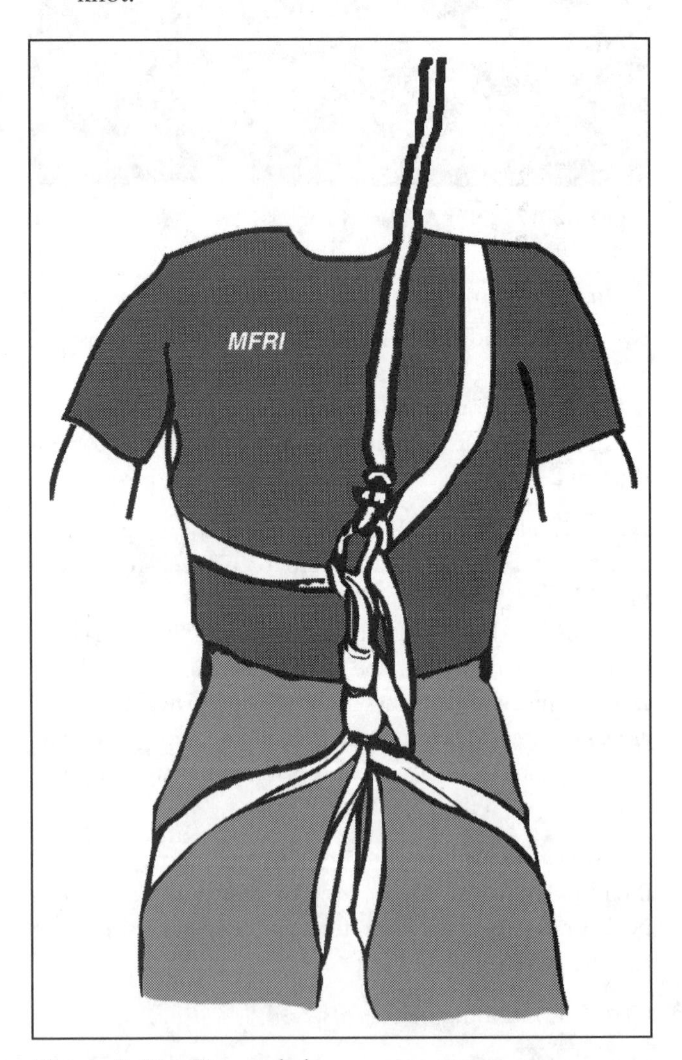

Figure 2–21 Site-made harness.

8. Metal connector ring is for metal connectors (e.g., carabiners). If tying on rope directly, tie to harness strap.

NFPA Ladder/Escape Belt

1. Select proper size.
2. Inspect belt.
3. Put on as belt. If possible, put through belt loops.
4. Connect only to rated points; use carabiner.

Site-Made Harnesses (Hasty Hitch) (Figure 2–21)

1. Start with 14 ft. or longer loop of 2 in. webbing, with water knot and safeties.
2. Drape loop over left shoulder.
3. Reach behind on right and pull section of loop around waist on right side. Gather in hand with front descending strap.
4. Reach between legs and bring bight of webbing up to chest. Wrap bight around gathered descending straps until all slack is removed.
5. Overhand knot the bight end around one of the "leg straps."
6. Insert a carabiner in the remainder of the bight end, and clip to both "shoulder straps." This will also serve as the connection point for the hoist line/carabiner.

Care of Harnesses

Since harnesses are essentially webbing and hardware, care and maintenance is similar. Harnesses can be soaked in cool water and mild soap (such as Woolite, Ivory, or other "safe for all synthetics" soap). To avoid impact on hardware, do not machine wash. Hardware on harnesses should be inspected and maintained as with other rescue hardware. Damage to hardware, webbing, or stitching immediately places the harness out of service. Damaged harnesses must be recertified by the manufacturer before reuse.

REFERENCES

American National Standard Institute. 1992. *Safety requirement for personal fall arrest systems, subsystems, and components: ANSI Z359.1.* New York: American National Standard Institute.

Brown, M.G. 1992. *Rope rescue manuals 1–3.* Virginia Beach, VA: Virginia Beach Fire Department.

Frank, J.A., and J.B. Smith. 1992. *Rope rescue manual.* 2d ed. Santa Barbara, CA: CMC Rescue, Inc.

National Fire Academy. 1993. *Rescue systems I.* Washington, DC: United States Fire Administraiton and California State Fire Marshal's Office, Fire Service Training and Education System.

NFPA 1500: *Standard on Fire Department Occupational Safety and Health Program,* 1992 edition, American National Standards Institute, National Fire Codes, Volume 8, Revised 11/96.

NFPA 1983: *Standard on Fire Service Life Safety Rope and System Components,* 1995 edition, American National Standards Institute, National Fire Codes, Volume 9, Revised 11/96.

Setnicka, T.J. 1980. *Wilderness search and rescue.* Boston: Appalachian Mountain Club.

Vines, T., and S. Hudson. 1989. *High angle rescue techniques.* Dubuque, IO: Kendall/Hunt Publishing Co.

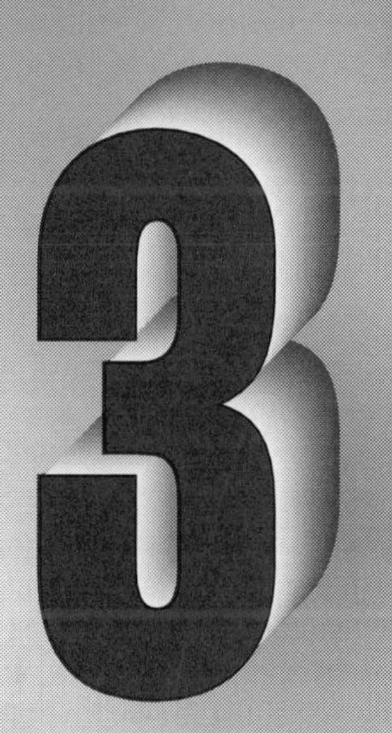

Rescue Knots and Their Uses

OBJECTIVE

The student will be able to identify and demonstrate the proper use of various types of rescue knots, from memory, without assistance, to an accuracy of 70% and the satisfaction of the instructor.

OVERVIEW

Rescue Knots and Their Uses

- Types of Knots in Rescue
- Strength of Knots
- Rescue Knot Terms
- How to Tie Rescue Knots

ENABLING OBJECTIVES

3-1-1 Identify types of knots used in rescue.

3-1-2 Describe the effect of knot strength in rescue.

3-1-3 Define common knot terms in rescue.

3-1-4 Demonstrate knots used in rescue work.

TYPES OF KNOTS IN RESCUE

In rescue, a "knot" is the tool used to harness the tremendous strength of rescue rope. It allows you to effectively connect rope to hardware, anchors, personnel, or other objects. Good rescue knots help make operations easier, while lesser knots may cause difficulties or even failures.

Knot Characteristics

There are many types of knots used in rescue, but all rescue knots have the same general characteristics:

Ease of Use A rescue knot must be relatively easy to tie under adverse conditions. The knot must allow simple visual inspection for correctness. Finally, the knot should be easy to untie after operational use during the incident termination phase.

Knot Strength The effective rescue knot must not excessively reduce the strength of the rope system. In doing so, you eliminate the need for "overengineering" of rope systems. As such, critical rescue resources (e.g., rope or hardware) can be more effectively used.

Safety Knot You've probably already heard the phrase, "A knot isn't a rescue knot without a safety." Safety knots control the loose ends of rescue knots, reducing the possibility of untying during operations. Unless both ends are controlled (e.g., tied to something else), safety knots are generally required.

Rescue Knots

The knots used in rescue fall into five broad categories, based on their uses:

Stopper/Safety Knots Stopper knots are used to control the rope ends, but normally bear no load. Examples of this include safety knots and the stopper knot at the end of a rappel line to prevent rappelling off the end. Stopper knots include the overhand knot and the basic figure-8 knot.

Bends Bends are knots which join two ropes together. This may be for the purpose of extending lifelines where one will be too short, or joining the ends of a prusik cord or webbing. Examples of bends include the figure-8 bend, the double fisherman's knot, and the water (or waterman's) knot.

Loops Loops provide the capability to attach carabiners and other hardware to the rope. They allow you to attach the rope to personnel or anchors. "Loop" knots include the figure-8 on a bight, as well as the figure-8 reweave.

Hitches Hitches are used to connect a rope to a "standing object," such as a post or bar. Uses of hitches include tying guylines to stakes, or putting a patient into a Stokes basket. Hitches used in rescue include the clove hitch and the split clove hitch.

Ascender Knots Some knots, such as the prusik, will slide freely on the rope until loaded. Once loaded, they maintain their position, much like a mechanical ascender. These knots can be used for ascending (climbing) a vertical rope. More importantly, these knots are used in safety backup systems in rope rescue.

STRENGTH OF KNOTS

The bends in a rope, whether caused by a knot, pulley, or other device, are of particular concern to the rescue technician. Bends in a rope produce unequal stresses in the rope (tensile stress on the "outside" curve of the bend, and compressive stress on the "inside"). These stresses reduce the effective strength of any rescue rope. Tighter bends (e.g., over a carabiner) produce more stress and weakness than wide bends (e.g., over a 4-in. pulley).

Knots contain bends which stress the rope as well. However, some knots, such as the figure-8, utilize less tight bends than others. For that reason, the "Family of 8s" knots are preferred for rescue, primarily due to their strength (80% to 85% of rope strength) and simplicity. Most other common knots vary between 60% and 70% of rope strength. Of note is the square knot, which reduces rope strength to less than half.

Over the years, there has been much time, energy, and paper dedicated to the research of knot strength/losses. We must realize, however, that knot strength is a minimal part of the actual rescue. Setnicka said:

> While it is of interest how strong one knot is versus another, it is important to realize that knots do not *break,* at least not on the testing machines in laboratories. Climbers simply are not found at the bottom of crevasses and caves with broken knots protruding from their harnesses.[1]

Setnicka was right; a good rescue knot won't fail you. Ropes will fail when you don't provide edge protection, without a safety knot, when knots untie during use, and when bad knots are used, they may not work at all. These failures should be the focus of the rescue technician's efforts.

RESCUE KNOT TERMS

It is necessary to know the nomenclature of the tools you are working with. Rope is a tool and has nomenclatures for its parts as you begin to form it into knots and later into various configurations for rigging.

The "running part" of the rope is used for work such as hoisting, pulling, or belaying.

The "working end" of the rope is used to tie the knot.

The "standing part" of the rope is between the working end and the running part.

A "bight" is formed by making a U-shaped curve in the rope without crossing the ends of the U.

A "round turn" is made when the ends of the bight's U are crossed.

A "bend" is a knot whose purpose is to join two ropes together.

A "hitch" is a knot used to fasten a rope to an object.

A "splice" is a method of weaving together two ropes or the strands of two parts of the same rope to form an eye.

An "anchor" is an immovable object.

A safety knot is a knot, such as the overhand or Fisherman's, used to control the running end of knot to reduce the chance of accidental untying. The half-hitch is not acceptable for a safety.

A "whip" is a special wrap done on the end of a rope to keep it from unraveling.

Figure 3–1 depicts one of the ways to whip the end of a rope. With most synthetic ropes, a hot blade is applied to melt the ends together. Usually the same hot blade is also used to cut the rope.

There are so many knots that it would take a lifetime to learn them all. All of these knots had a purpose and have served that purpose well in most instances. With the advent of synthetic ropes, however, it rapidly became apparent that a large portion of the basic knots that were previously "safe to use" (because they never failed) were failing. The slipperiness of synthetics causes some of the knots to slip apart. New techniques had to be learned to ensure the safety of the rescuers and those that they were helping. These new methods can also be safely applied when using natural fiber ropes.

HOW TO TIE RESCUE KNOTS

This section provides diagrams (Figures 3–2 to 3–8) showing how certain rescue knots are tied. While studying these diagrams, remember that they are shown loosen for clarity. All knots require "dressing", or tightening and flattening them. In addition, safety knots need to be set and tightened as close to the original knot as possible.

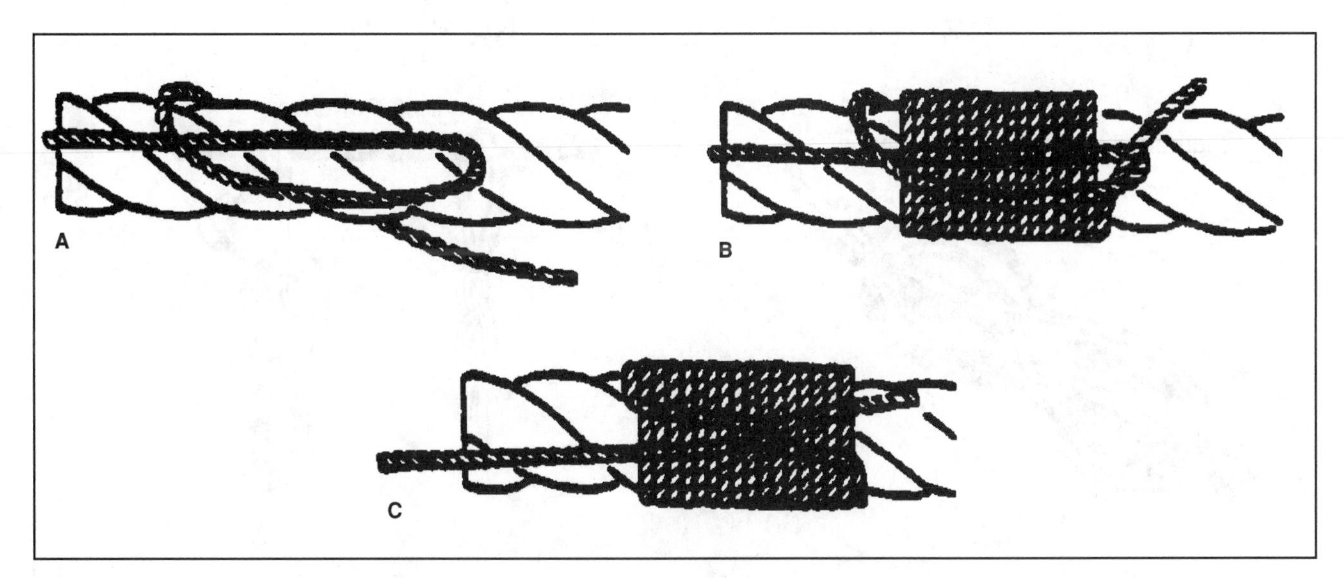

Figure 3–1 Whip the end of a rope.

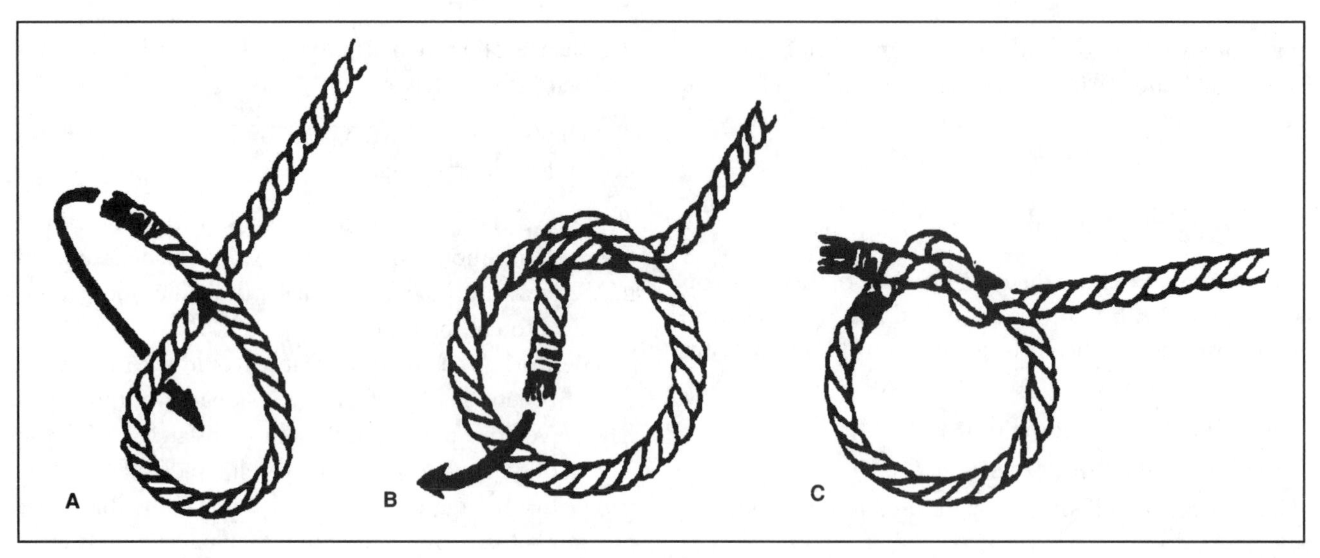

Figure 3–2 The overhand knot.

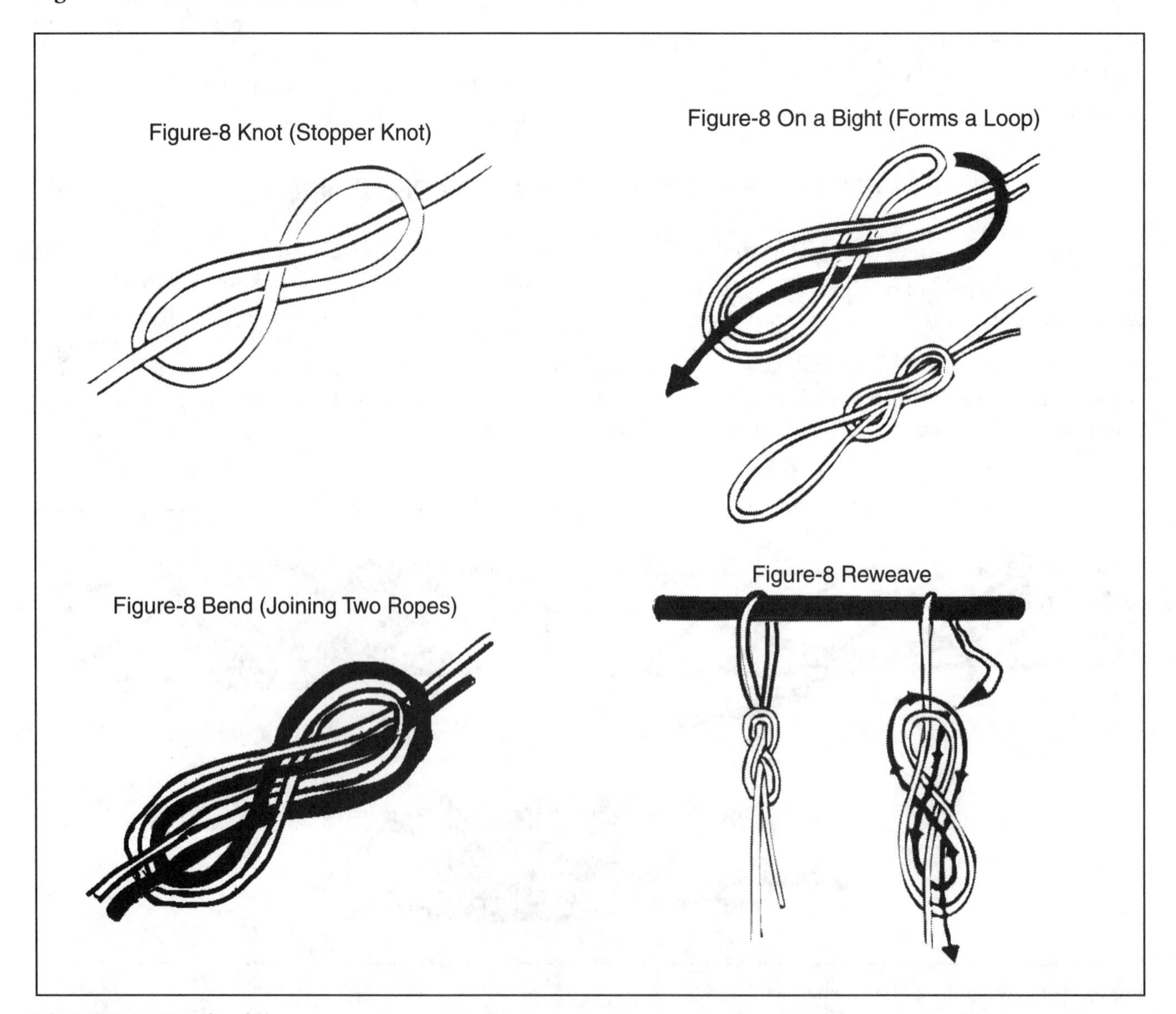

Figure 3–3 Family of 8's.

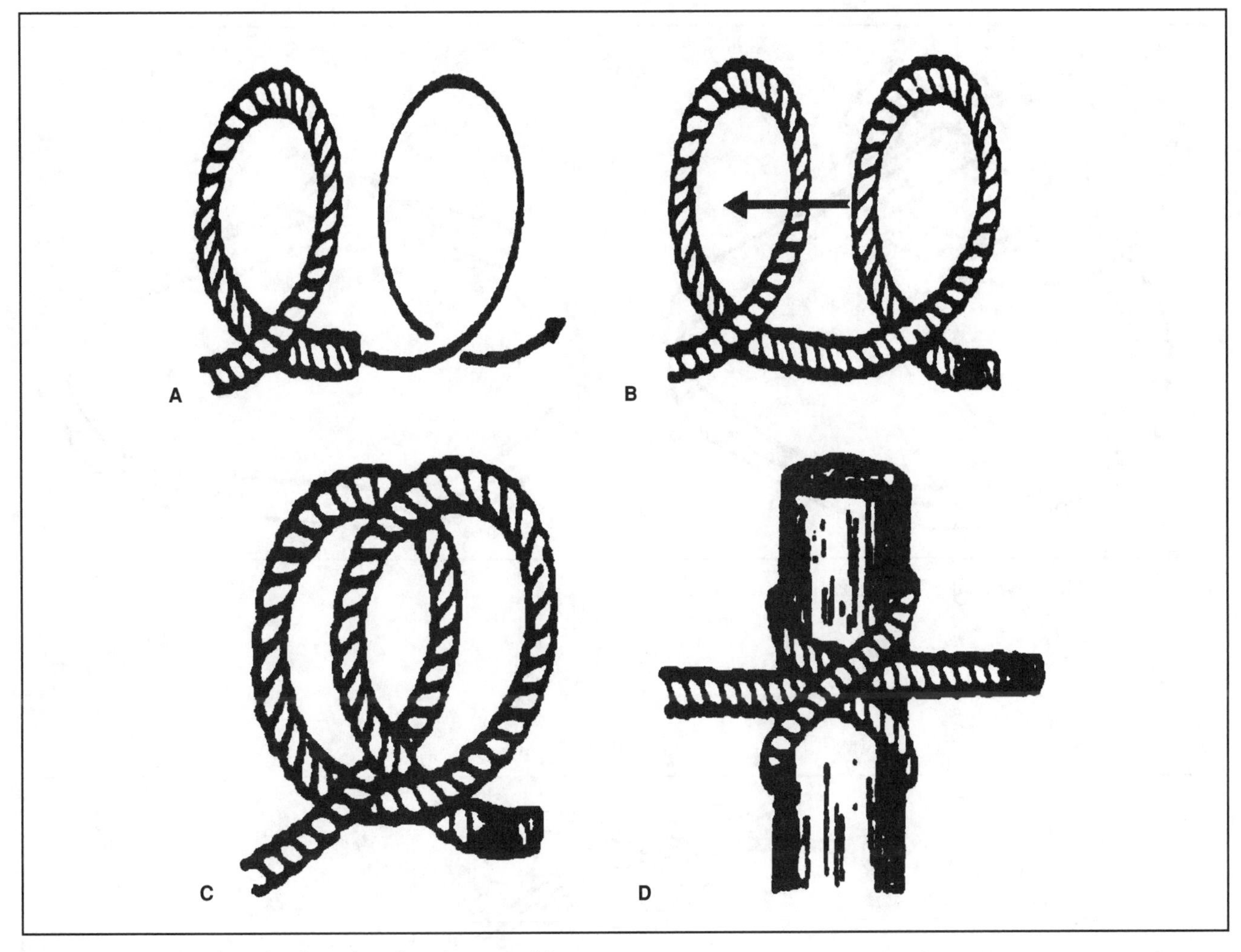

Figure 3–4 The clove hitch tied to drop over an object.

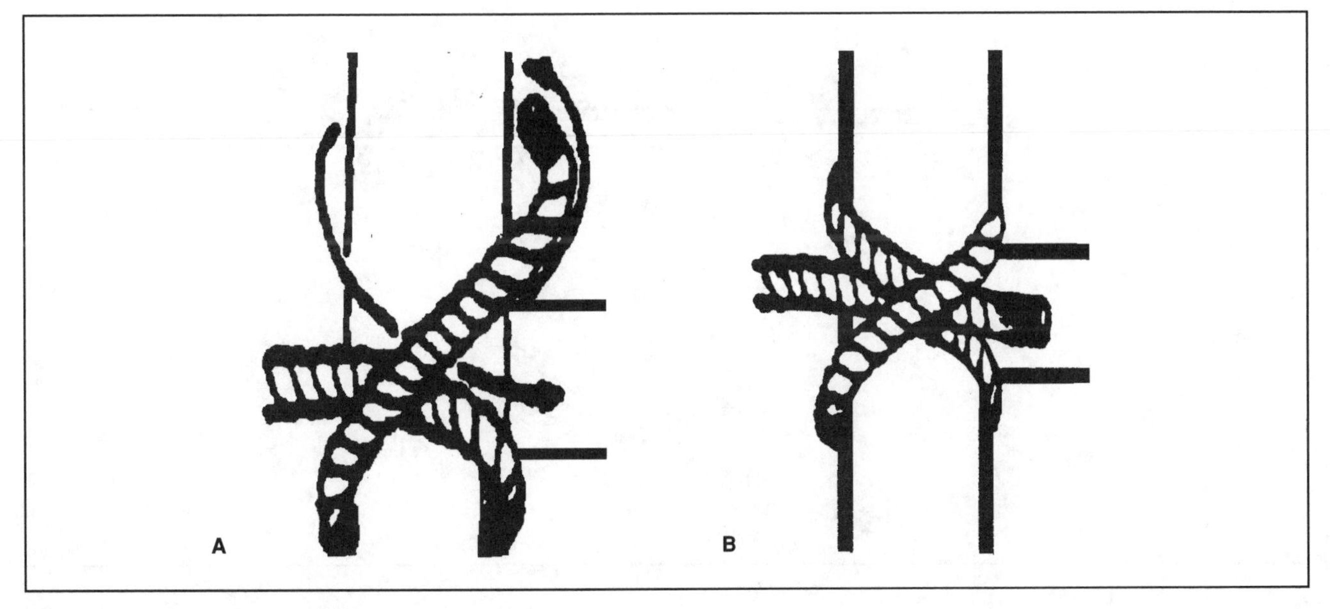

Figure 3–5 Split clove hitch.

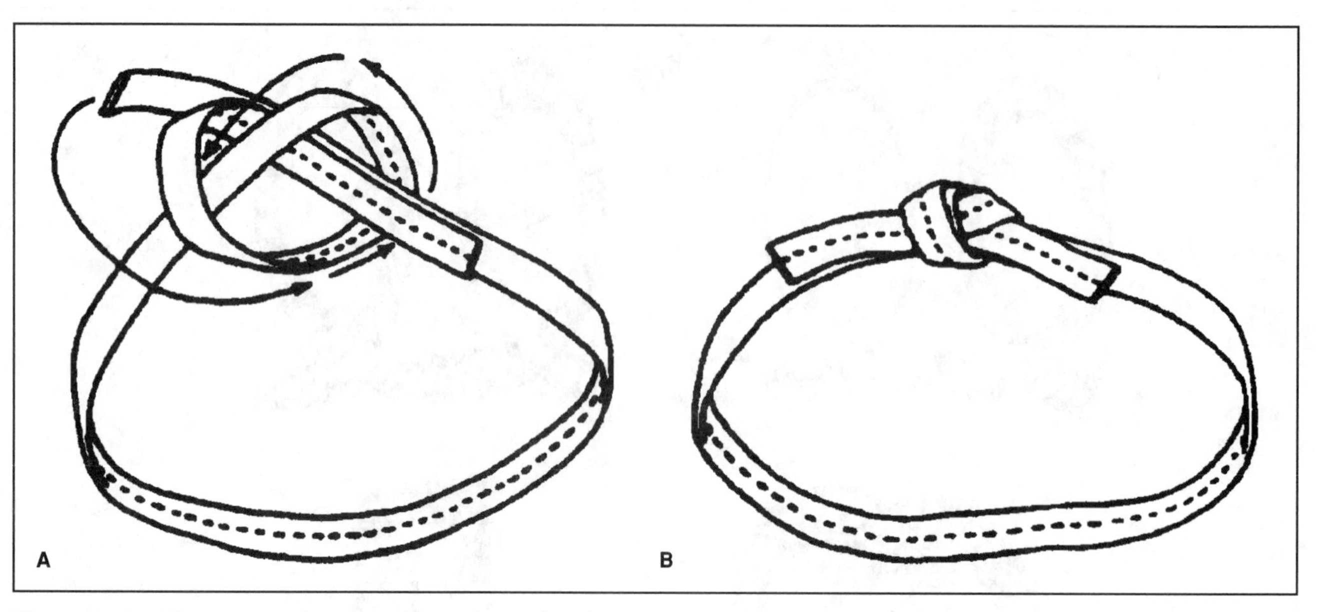

Figure 3–6 The reweaved overhand knot (water knot).

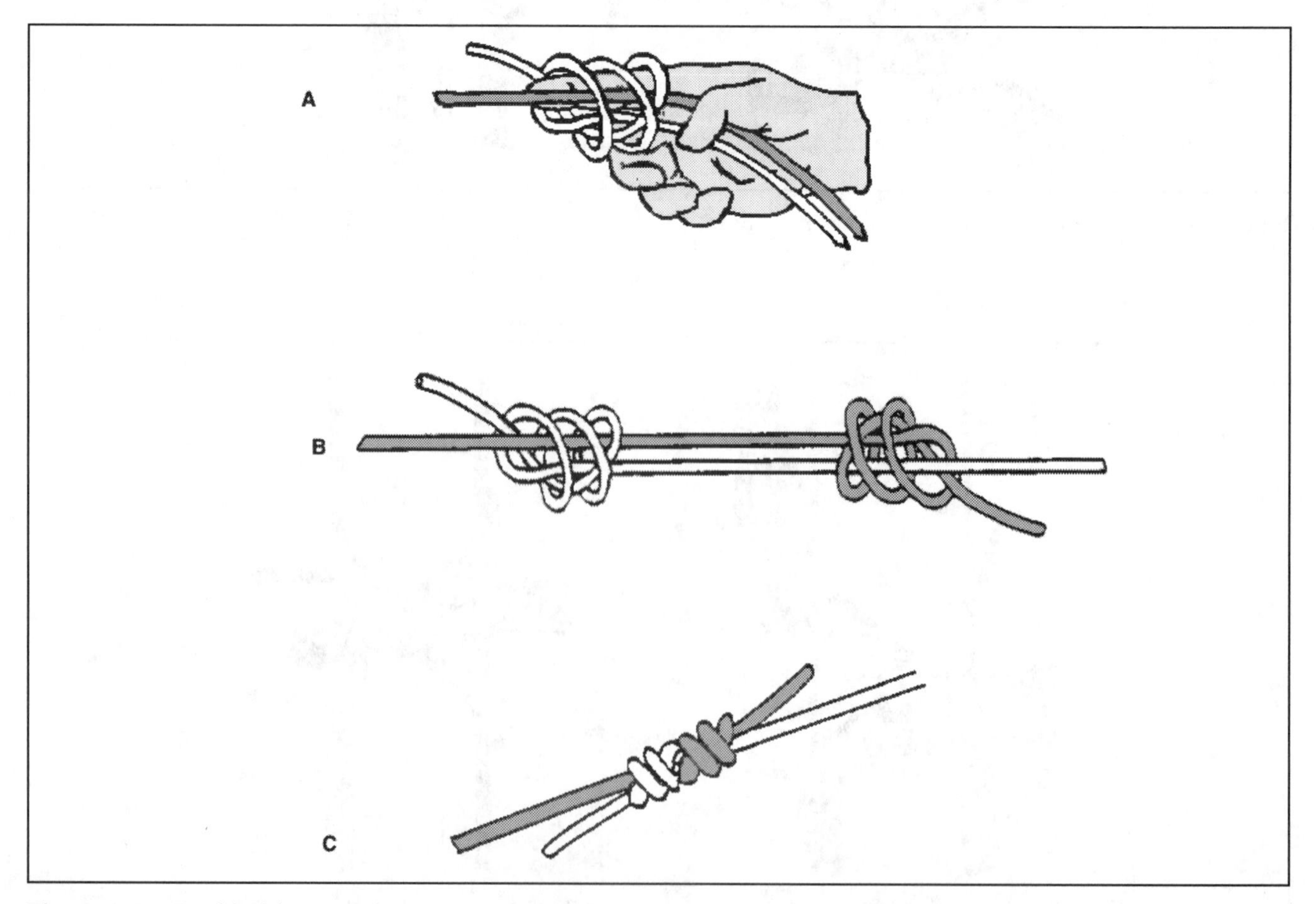

Figure 3–7 Double fisherman's bend.

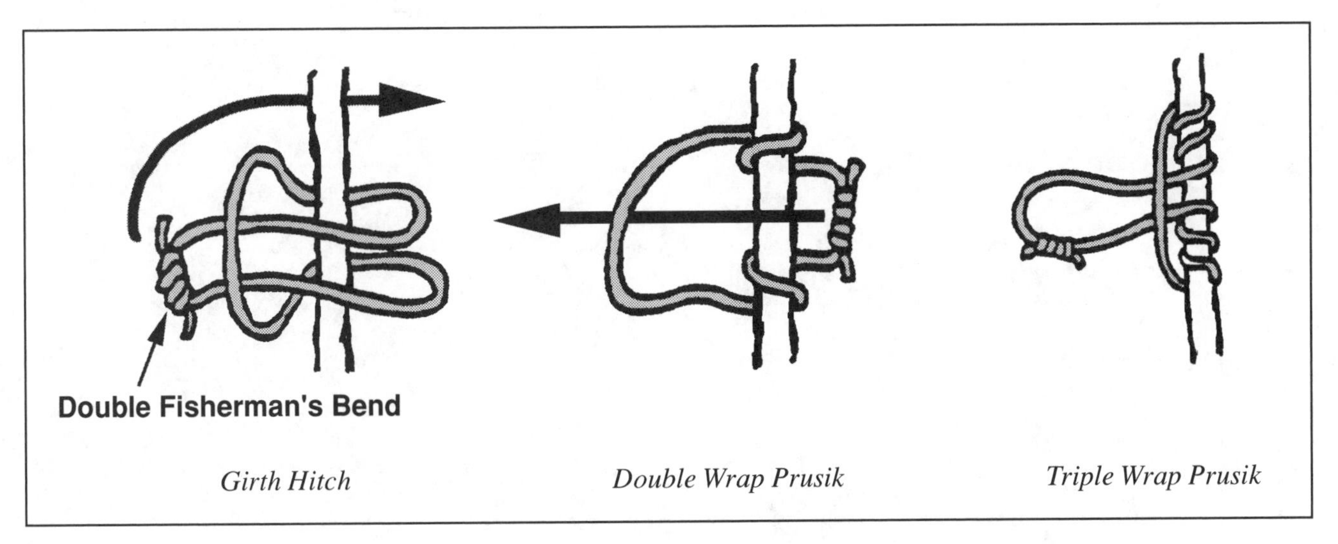

Figure 3–8 Prusik knot.

Endnote

1. Setnicka, Tim. *Wilderness Search and Rescue,* Appalachian Mountain Club, 1980, p. 195.

REFERENCES

Brown, M.G. 1992. *Rope rescue manuals 1–3.* Virginia Beach, VA: Virginia Beach Fire Department.

Frank, J.A., and J.B. Smith. 1992. *Rope rescue manual.* 2d ed. Santa Barbara, CA: CMC Rescue, Inc.

National Fire Academy. 1993. *Rescue systems I.* Washington, DC: United States Fire Administraiton and California State Fire Marshal's Office, Fire Service Training and Education System.

Setnicka, T.J. 1980. *Wilderness search and rescue.* Boston: Appalachian Mountain Club.

Vines, T., and S. Hudson. 1989. *High angle rescue techniques.* Dubuque, IO: Kendall/Hunt Publishing Co.

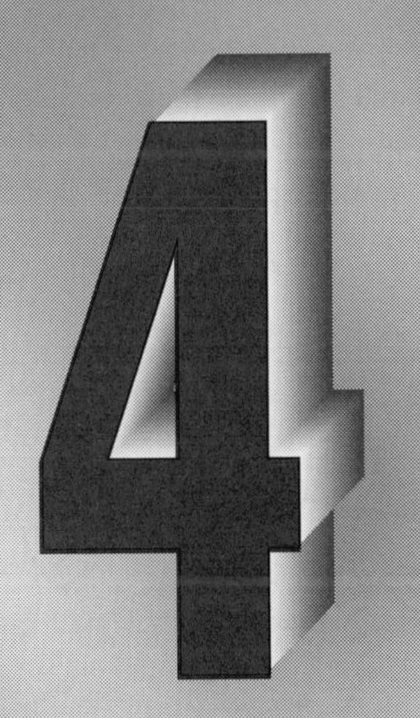

Principles of Rigging, Anchoring, and Mechanical Advantage Systems

OBJECTIVE

The student will be able to explain and demonstrate various selected anchors and anchor systems, given the appropriate materials, and be able to explain and identify various mechanical advantage systems, from memory, without assistance, to an accuracy of 70% and the satisfaction of the instructor.

OVERVIEW

Principles of Rigging, Anchoring, and Mechanical Advantage Systems

- Types of Anchors
- Anchoring Safety Rules
- Anchor Attachment
- Protecting Anchor and Equipment Integrity
- Rigging
- Block and Tackle
- Reeving Block and Tackle
- Computing Rope Length and Mechanical Advantages
- Hauling Systems
- Securing to a Fixed Object
- Holdfasts and Pickets

ENABLING OBJECTIVES

4-1-1 Identify types of natural and human-made anchors.

4-1-2 Select anchor points following prescribed safety rules.

4-1-3 Describe how to set up a single-point anchor and describe a tensionless anchor (with and without a backup).

4-1-4 Determine if hardware, ropes, and slings are being properly used, and describe appropriate padding for edge protection.

4-1-5 Identify the uses of block and tackle and the parts of a common block (double or triple).

4-1-6 Describe the safety points, duties, measurement, and care of a block-and-tackle system.

4-1-7 Describe reeving a block-and-tackle system.

4-1-8 Compute the length of rope required and determine the mechanical advantage for a block-and-tackle system.

4-1-9 Describe a Z-rig and piggyback hauling system.

4-1-10 Describe how to secure a block and tackle to a fixed object.

4-1-11 Recognize and explain a picket-and-holdfast system.

TYPES OF ANCHORS

You cannot expect any rope system assembled for a rescue or recovery to work if it does not have an adequate *anchor.* An anchor is something that serves to hold an object firmly.

To assemble a system, you must first be able to recognize types of anchors. You must also be able to evaluate an individual anchor depending on the intended use, and what you are attaching to the anchor (e.g., haul system, rappel point, etc.).

There are two basic types of anchors: natural and human-made.

Type I. Natural Anchors

- Trees
- Boulders
- Brush/undergrowth
- Root systems
- Rock outcroppings

Type II. Human-Made Anchors

- Vehicles (tow eyes, frame members, etc.)
- Guard rails (be sure to pad the rail)
- Utility poles
- Fire escapes/fixed ladders
- Structural members

Each type of anchor contains many possibilities. As in any other facet of rescue, you must evaluate each intended anchor separately. This ensures your safety as well as the safety of any victim(s) involved.

ANCHORING SAFETY RULES

The intended anchor could be rusted, rotten, broken, etc. *Never assume!!!*

After closely evaluating and selecting your intended anchor, follow these anchoring safety rules as a double-check.

1. How much is my anticipated load? 300 lbs., 500 lbs., more?
2. Is the anchor suitable, given the direction of the load?
3. Does the anchor have sharp edges?

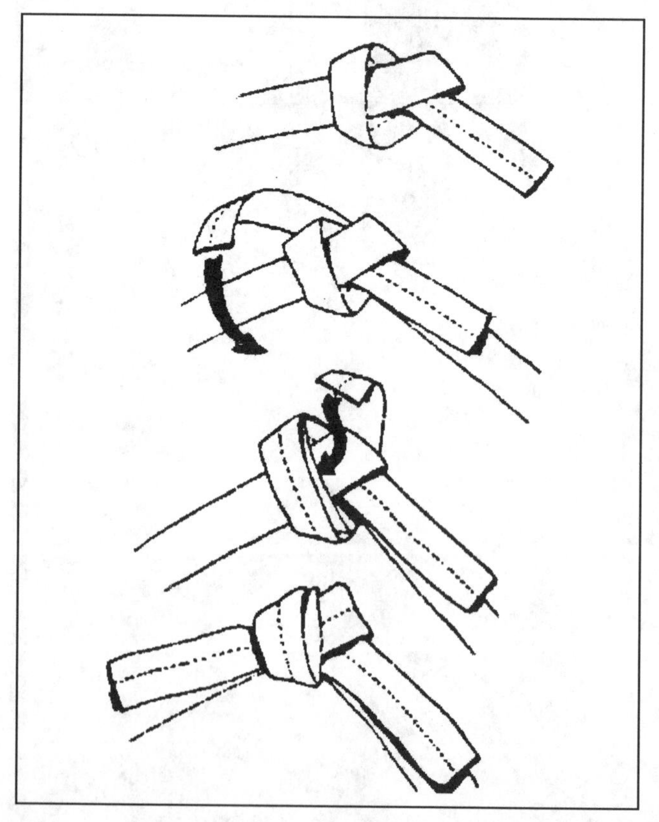

Figure 4–1 A doubled section of 1 in. tubular webbing is used to attach to the anchor.

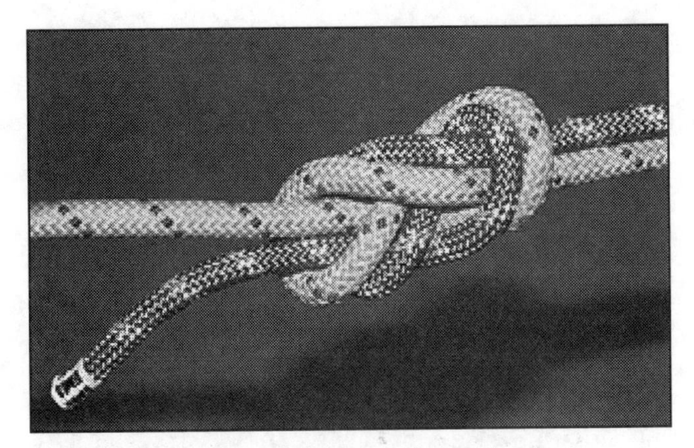

Figure 4–2 Rope joined with a figure-8 bend.

4. Where does the sling go?
5. Does the anchor have sufficient mass?

If all of the safety concerns are answered, the anchor then needs to have the system attached to it. There are many ways to attach a system to an anchor or construct an anchor. This session describes several.

A single-point anchor is suitable when you have a "bomb proof"—absolutely solid—anchor available (e.g., utility pole).

ANCHOR ATTACHMENT

The single-point anchor is very simple and is frequently used in urban settings. You can attach to the anchor with a doubled section of 1 in. tubular web, joining the web with a water bend. You must use at least 1 in. doubled (Figure 4–1) tubular web to maintain adequate breaking strength.

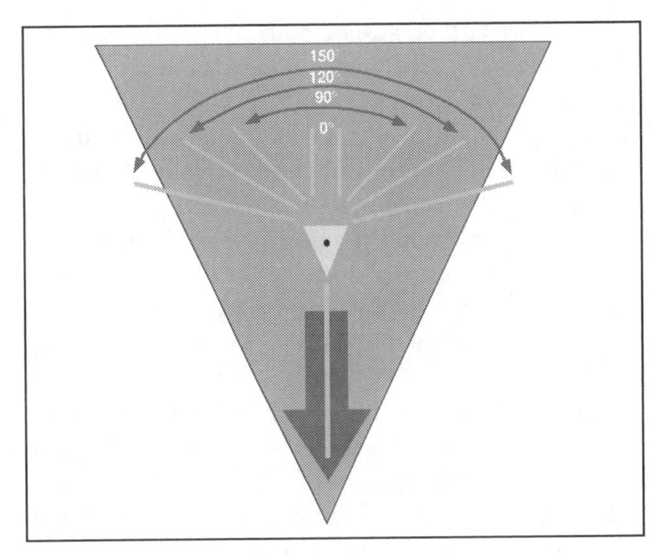

Figure 4–3 Optimal angles for field use.

You can also form a fixed loop of rope around the anchor, joining the rope with a figure-8 bend. If the rope is not strong enough, double the rope (Figure 4–2).

When attaching to an anchor, attention must be given to the angles the rope or web approaches the anchor. If the angle exceeds 120°, the loading on the anchor strap increases significantly.

While an angle of 0° is best, a realistic angle of 90° is optimal for field use (Figure 4–3).

Another preferred way of attaching a line to an anchor is by using a tensionless anchor. This is accomplished by wrapping the main line around the anchor five or six times, then connecting the rope back into itself. The connection can be a carabiner or a rewoven figure-8 (Figure 4–4).

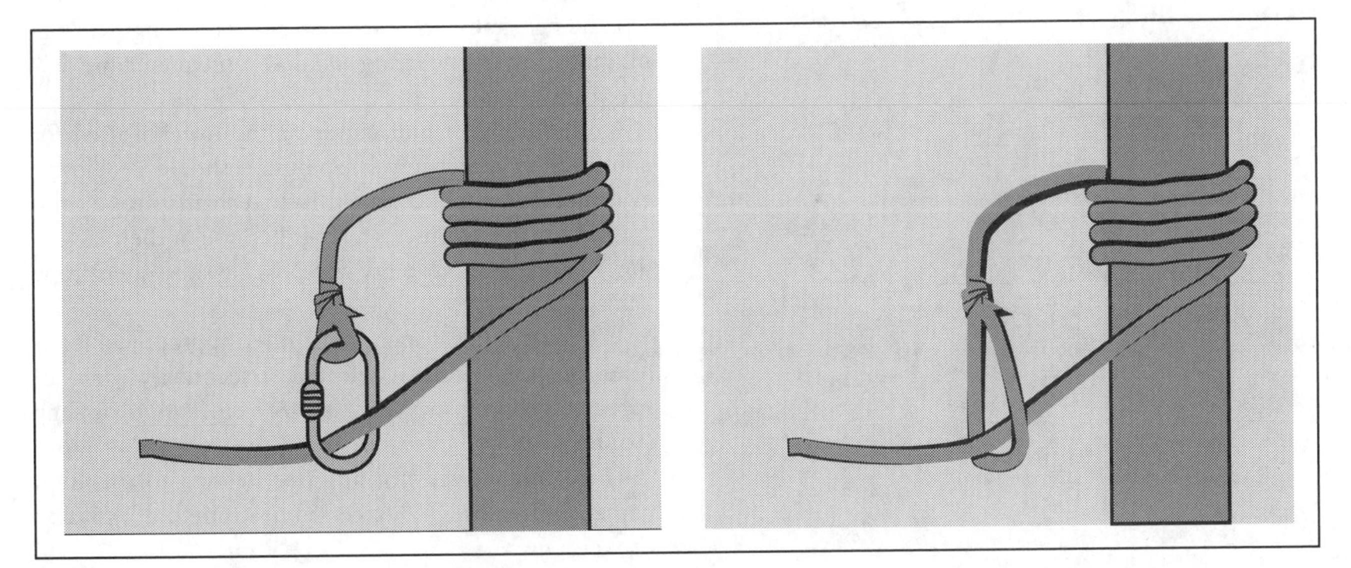

Figure 4–4 Line attached to a tensionless anchor.

When two anchors are near each other, and one anchor by itself does not seem quite enough, an anchor can be backed up. One acceptable way is to use a tensionless anchor, then take the rope around a second anchor, finishing on the second anchor with another tensionless anchor.

If no available anchors are nearby, and stakes can be driven into the ground, a picket line can be used as an anchor. Three pickets are needed for the anchor point. Tie off to the bottom of the last picket and run the support line to the top of the picket in front as shown in Figure 4–5.

Additional information on pickets is provided in the "Rigging" section. A picket system will also work in snow if proper precautions are taken.

If anchors are present, but none are considered bomb proof, an equalizing anchor can be used (Figure 4–6). This anchor is multidirectional, while sharing the load between two or more points. Use a web sling or prusik loop to form a figure-8. Connect the carabiner across the waist of the figure-8, not around it.

Although for our lesson a two-point self-equalizing system is discussed, three or more points may be used. Systems can also be stacked. For example, two, two-point self-equalizing anchors are rigged together, providing four-point protection.

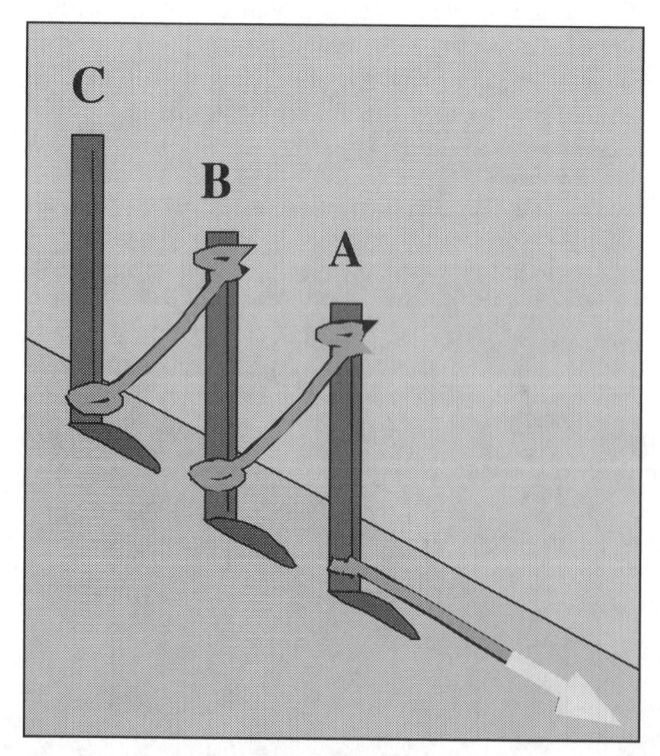

Figure 4–5 Picket line used as an anchor.

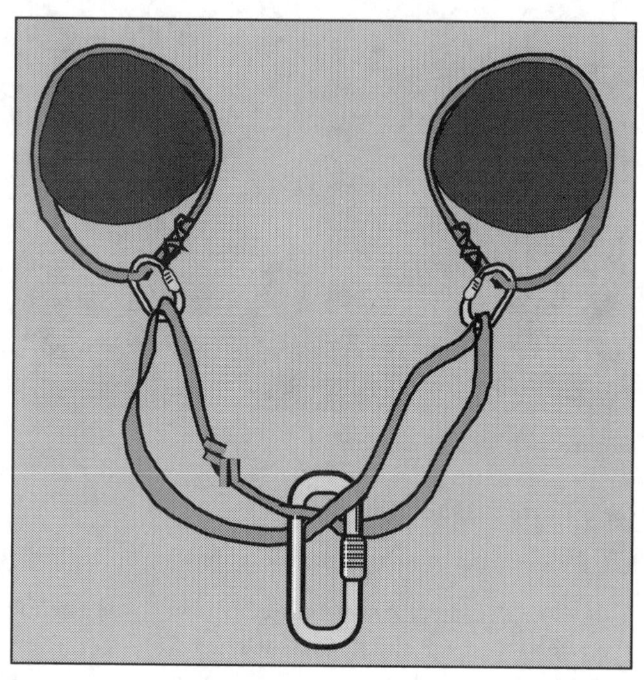

Figure 4–6 Equalizing anchor.

PROTECTING ANCHOR AND EQUIPMENT INTEGRITY

After selecting your anchor and deciding on the method of attachment, the next concern is protecting the integrity of the anchor and the equipment attached to it.

One major concern is the proper loading of carabiners (Figure 4–7). Carabiners are designed, regardless of material, to be loaded only along the long axis. How you tie your anchor point also affects the working strength of your carabiners.

Loading carabiners other than along the long axis, significantly lowers the rating and may cause premature failure (Figure 4–8).

Regardless of manufacturer or the material used for construction, mechanical rope grabs should be closely evaluated before being used. Most mechanical rope grabs are not suitable for use as safeties because of their lack of shock-absorbing capability and possible subsequent rope damage.

While tensionless anchors are often appropriate, if another anchor system is selected, a secondary piece of rope or webbing may be used to form a loop or sling (Figure 4–9).

Girth hitches are not appropriate due to the high percentage of loss (70% to 80%) of strength of the rope or webbing.

Another concern regarding anchors is their padding.

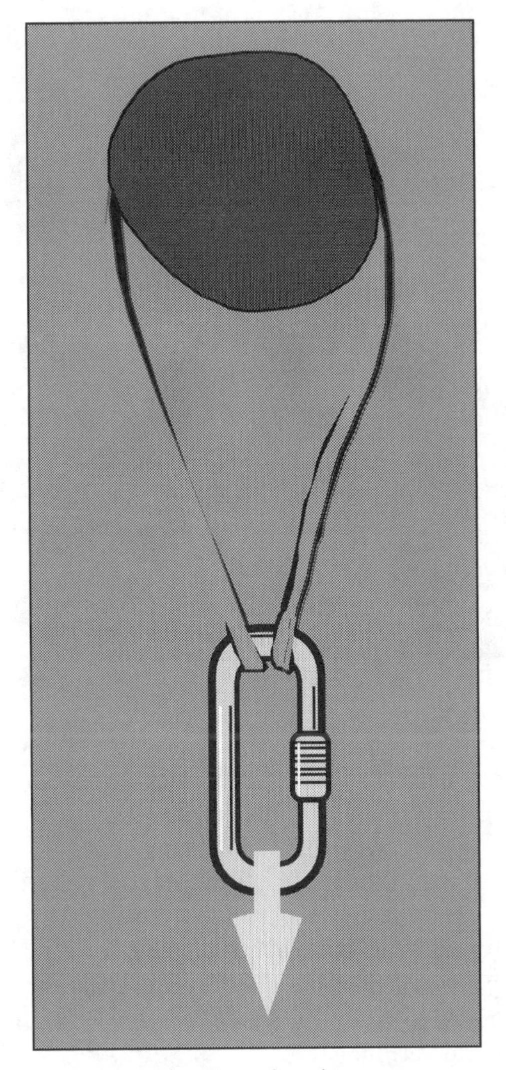

Figure 4–7 Proper loading of carabiners.

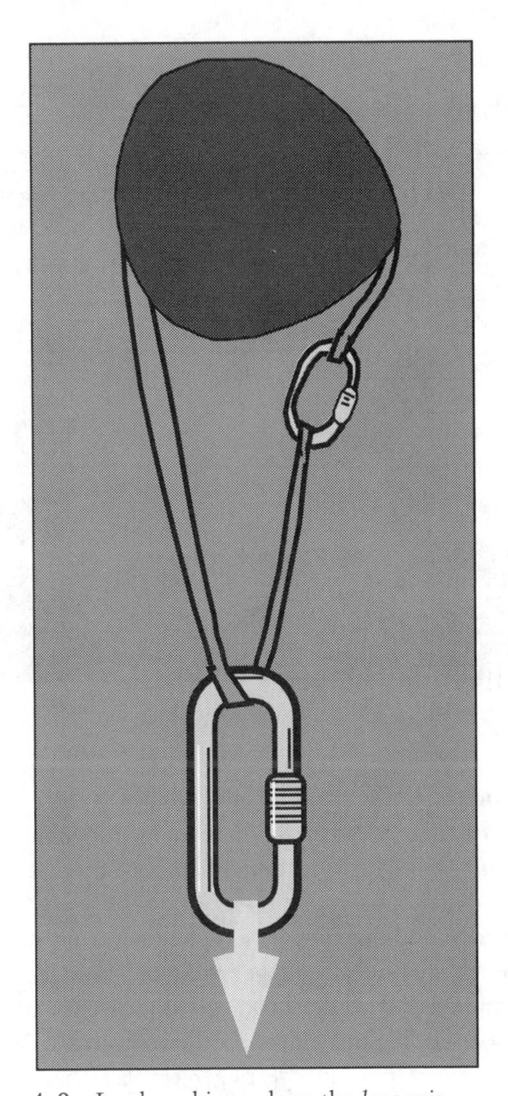

Figure 4–8 Load carabiners along the *long* axis.

Padding protects the sling material, rope, or webbing that is used (Figure 4–10).

In addition to padding the anchor, remember to pad any edges or protrusions that the rope runs over or next to. Although the webbing and ropes used are extremely strong, with a good safety factor (15:1), catastrophic and sudden accidents may occur if padding is not used properly.

RIGGING

Rigging may be defined as the use of rope in a variety of applications wherein objects are secured against movement, or they are moved under controlled conditions with reduced effort. The tall ships of yesteryear saw the art of rigging reach its apogee in the securing of the great masts and the long spars and the raising, lowering, and trimming of the massive sails. The movement of cargo

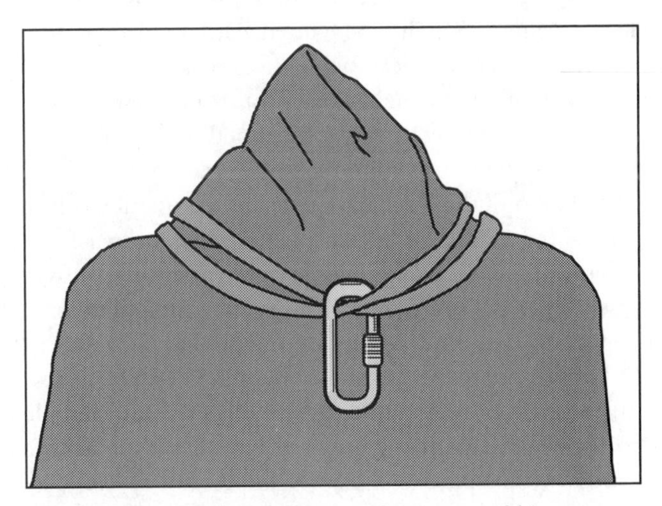

Figure 4–9 A secondary piece of rope or webbing may be used to form a loop or sling.

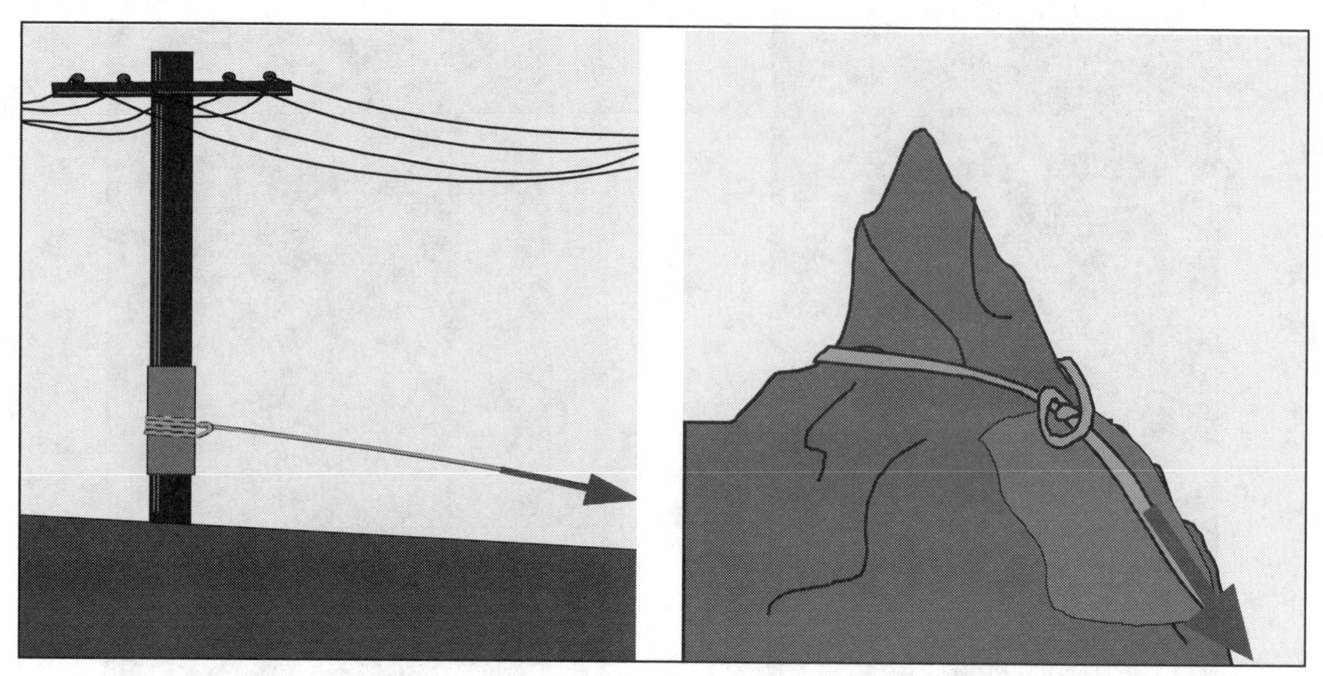

Figure 4–10 Padding protects the sling material, rope, or webbing.

into and out of the holds and the control of the cannons, both in adverse weather and in reducing movement during firing, were both accomplished with the use of rigging.

The addition of pulleys to a rope system will either develop a mechanical advantage system or allow the rope to change direction without damage to itself or nearby objects. The lashing of timbers or other objects into specific configurations permits the rigger to place his/her lifting/lowering device (ropes and pulleys) into a position over the object to be moved and to safely move that object up or down and/or from side to side.

Rigging is used to move rescuers and victims from one level to another often where fire department ladders will not reach or are not accessible. It is also used in conjunction with fire department ladders for various rescue tasks.

Mechanical advantage (MA) is defined as the advantage gained by the use of a mechanism in transmitting force, or the ratio of the force that performs the useful work of a machine to the force that is applied to the machine. Simply put, it is the difference between work in to power out or, the amount by which a machine multiplies force applied to it in order to lift or move a load.

How can rescuers equate the definition of MA to rescue work and more particularly to rigging? An example to show MA involves an injured *individual* lying on the ground with a pipe weighing 30 lbs. on top of *him*. The rescuer could just lean over and pick it up. If the weight was raised to 300 pounds, 2 rescuers could pick it up, depending on the available room around the pipe. To make sure no one gets hurt, 4 rescuers will pick it up. With four rescuers lifting, each one is only lifting 75 lbs.

$$4 \times 75 = 300$$

This was an MA of 4 lifters (people) to one load (pipe). If the pipe weighed 3,000 and 40 people were used, the amount each person would lift remains at 75 lbs., and the MA would become 40:1.

Four people could not lift the 300 lb. pipe if it were placed in a ditch so narrow they could not gather around it. By attaching ropes to four equally distant points on the pipe, and with each person standing on the edge of the ditch and pulling on a rope, each would still be lifting only 75 lbs. If that's the case, then each rope is lifting 75 lbs.

Terminology

Special blocks may also be used to redirect the lead line to a point where it can be more easily handled. These blocks are called *snatch blocks* and can be reeved onto the line at any desired point without passing the end of the lead line through it. Figure 4–11 depicts a snatch block.

Mountain climbers have developed single-sheave blocks that perform as both standard blocks and snatch blocks (Figures 4–12 and 13).

These blocks may also be rigged as single-, double-, or triple-sheave blocks. In reality all of the standing blocks are attached to the anchor point while all of the running

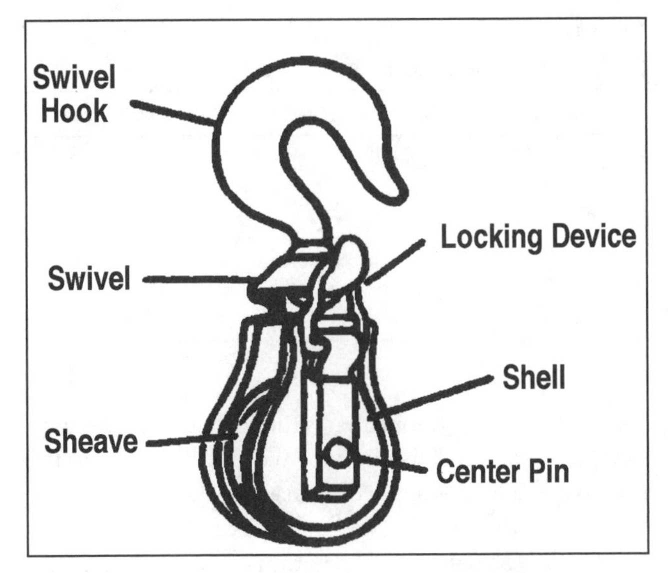

Figure 4–11 Snatch block.

blocks are attached to the load. In most instances carabiners are used to make the attachments.

These special blocks offer several advantages. They may be loaded into the center of a line without the standard reeving procedure. They are also compact and lightweight. When used as multiple-sheave blocks, remember the additional spacing of the sheaves will increase the chock-a-block to well over the traditional 4 ft.

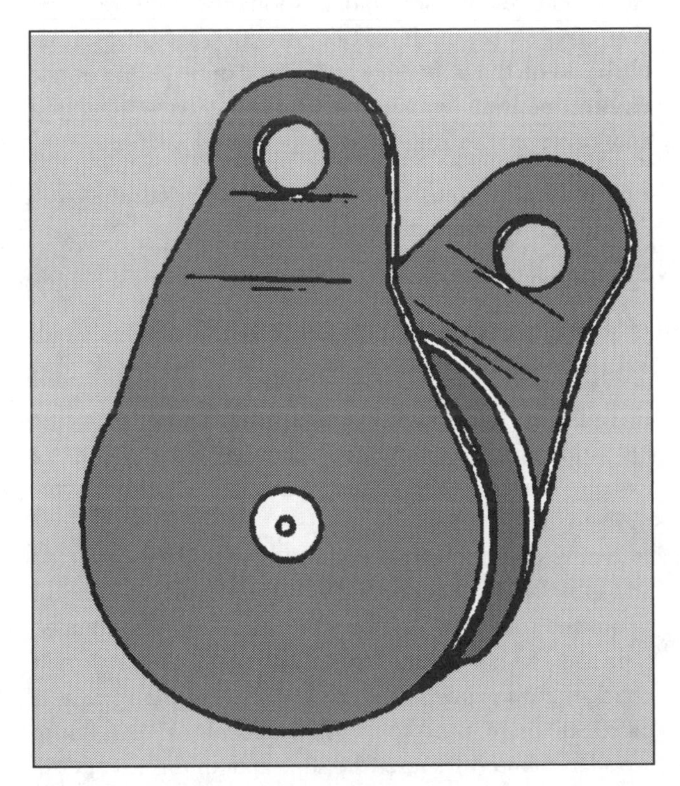

Figure 4–12 Single-sheaved block.

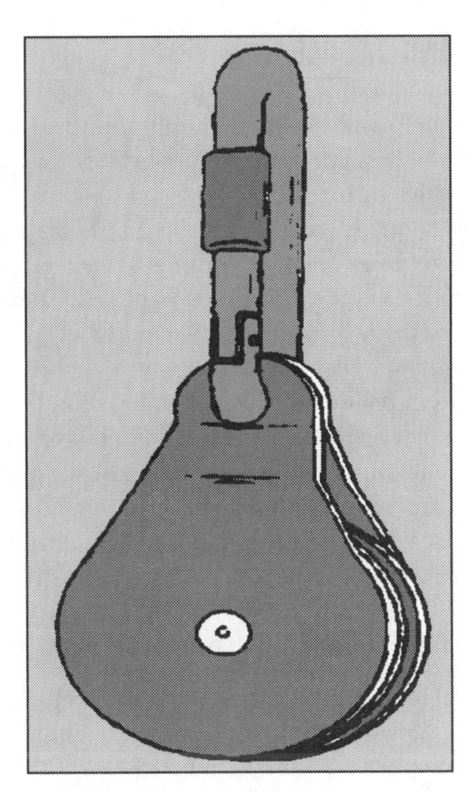

Figure 4–13 Single-sheaved block.

A carabiner is also a multifunctional device. It is a mainstay in mountain climbing equipment because it can join together various pieces of equipment. The rescue technician also will find this device very useful. Always position a carabiner so that the load is applied to the ends. Never allow a load to be applied to either the side or gate of a carabiner (Figure 4–14).

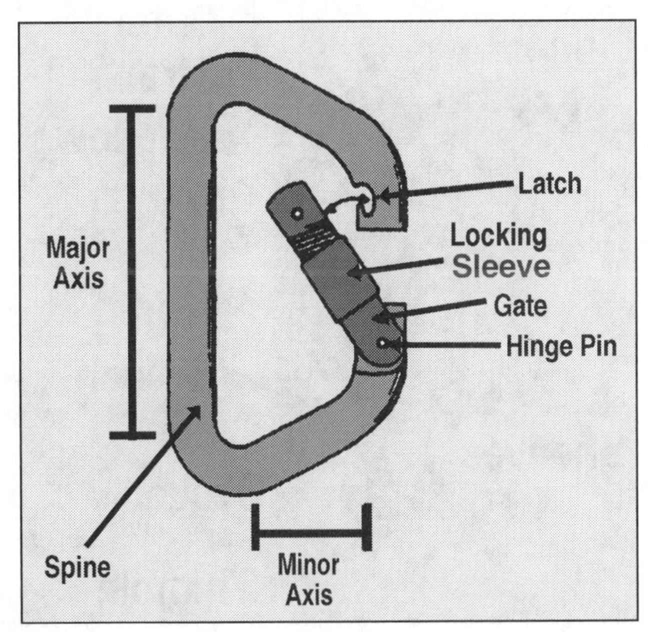

Figure 4–14 Carabiner.

BLOCK AND TACKLE

The use of blocks is an asset in gaining MA when moving objects with rope. Figure 4–15 depicts a block and identifies its parts.

Blocks come in various sizes; from little ones used to raise and lower awnings, to enormous crane blocks 8 ft. tall, and from single sheaves to as high as 20 sheaves per block. Blocks are measured by the length of the cheeks or shell.

Blocks can be used in either a tension or pull manner. In using a block, make certain it is not subjected to a side load that will cause an additional or unknown loading to the block and to the total system.

To reduce damage to rope, it is important that the rope size, regardless of its type, be matched to the sheave size.

Measure Shell of Block

This matching of sizes applies to both fiber rope and wire rope. Too small a rope in a sheave may cause undersize grooves to wear in the sheave. These undersized grooves will cause severe or immediate damage to the proper size rope when it is reeved into the block. Rope that is run through sheaves larger in diameter than the rope will become distorted and damaged when load is applied to the system. Conversely, rope that is run through sheaves with a diameter too small for the rope will cause damage to the rope when a load is applied, damage to the cheeks of the block as it rubs the sides, and increase the friction load on the system. Sheave size is determined by the manufacturer of the block as the smallest angle the rope can be bent around a smooth object without inflicting damage to the rope. Using undersize or oversize sheaves will damage the rope, the sheave, and the frame. It can also cause the *safe working load* (SWL) of the system to decrease due to the increased friction load (Table 4–1).

A quick rule of thumb is to multiply the rope diameter by four to get the approximate sheave size.

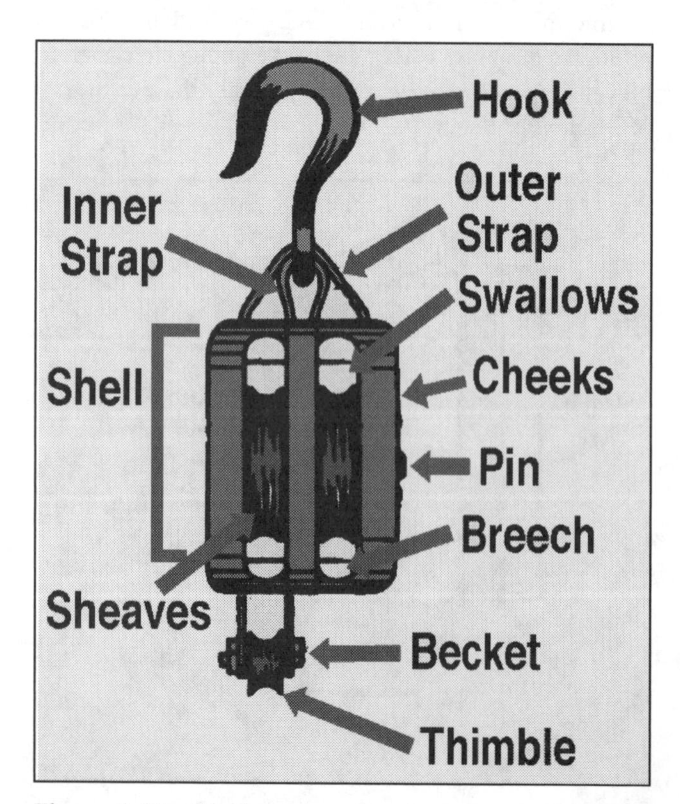

Figure 4–15 Block.

Table 4–1
SWL and friction load

Block Size in Inches	*Rope Size Diameter in Inches*
4	½
6	¾
8	⅞
10	1
12	1¼
14	1½

Care of Block and Tackle

As with all rescue tools, blocks should be inspected after each use. Inspection should also occur on a regular schedule based on the frequency and period of usage and of the environment in which the block has been operated and/or stored. During block inspections look for:

- The wear on pins or axles, rope grooves, side plates, bushings or bearings, and fittings.
- Misalignment or wobble in sheaves.
- Securement of bolts, nuts, and other locking methods such as stacked nuts.

In caring for blocks, follow the manufacturer's specific recommendations. Some manufacturers recommend the use of a lithium-based grease of medium consistency for the bearings.

Blocks that are infrequently used should be inspected and lubricated as needed at 90-day intervals, contingent upon the storage and exposure to various environments.

If the cheeks of the blocks are made of metal, first check them for burrs that could easily cut the rope as it passes through the block. Wooden blocks can cause wooden splinters to enter the rope and, in turn, enter the rescuer's hands as the rope is handled.

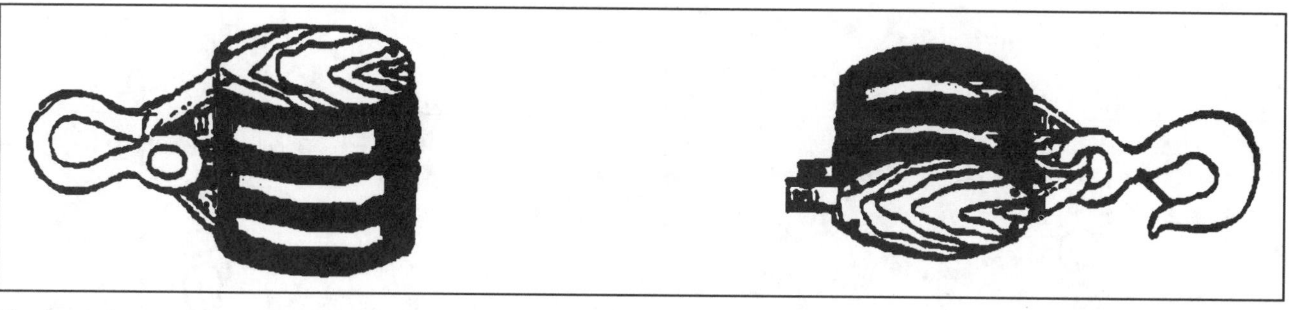

Figure 4–16 Standing (left) and running (right) block.

Safety Points

Ten safety points to remember are:

1. All lines should be clear of kinks and twists including the fall line.
2. All hooks must be moused.
3. Block and tackle should always be carried and never dragged across any surface.
4. Suspended loadings should be eased off uniformly and in a steady manner. Extreme jerks and shock loading should be avoided.
5. Teamwork is essential in using block-and-tackle systems.
6. Blocks should be reeved in a manner that prevents twisting.
7. After the blocks are reeved, the rope should be pulled back and forth through the block several times to allow the rope to adjust to the blocks.
8. The antitwisting device for the block-and-tackle system includes lashing rod or pipe to the outer shell or insertion of a stick between the returning ropes.
9. Blocks should be inspected after each use and properly maintained.
10. Snatch blocks with locking devices moused should be utilized to change the direction of pull. It is easier to pull at ground level than from other positions.

REEVING BLOCK AND TACKLE

The left-hand block in Figure 4–16 is the *standing* block in a normal system. It will also receive the running end of the rope when reeving the tackle. The right-hand block is the *running* block, or the one normally attached to the load. Note that the left-hand block is lying with the sheaves parallel to the surface, while the right-hand block is lying with the sheaves perpendicular to the surface. The hooks on both blocks are pointing away from each other. The left-hand block should also be the block with the most sheaves if both blocks do not have the same number of sheaves (e.g., a two-sheave to a one-sheave block or three-sheave to a two-sheave block). Consistently placing the blocks in this fashion eliminates errors in reeving.

The becket that accepts the running end of the rope will always be on the left-block when reeving even-sheaved blocks in a lifting system (1 to 1, 2 to 2, or 3 to 3). Therefore, if a block has a damaged or missing becket, make sure that it is the right-hand block.

Two blocks drawn together as close as possible (Figure 4–17) are termed *chock-a-block*. The quantity of

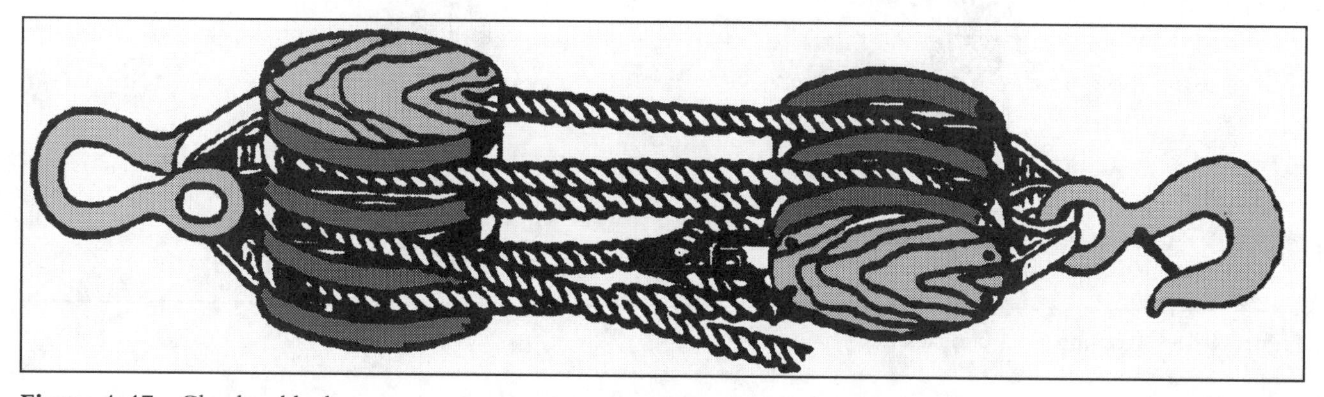

Figure 4–17 Chock-a-block.

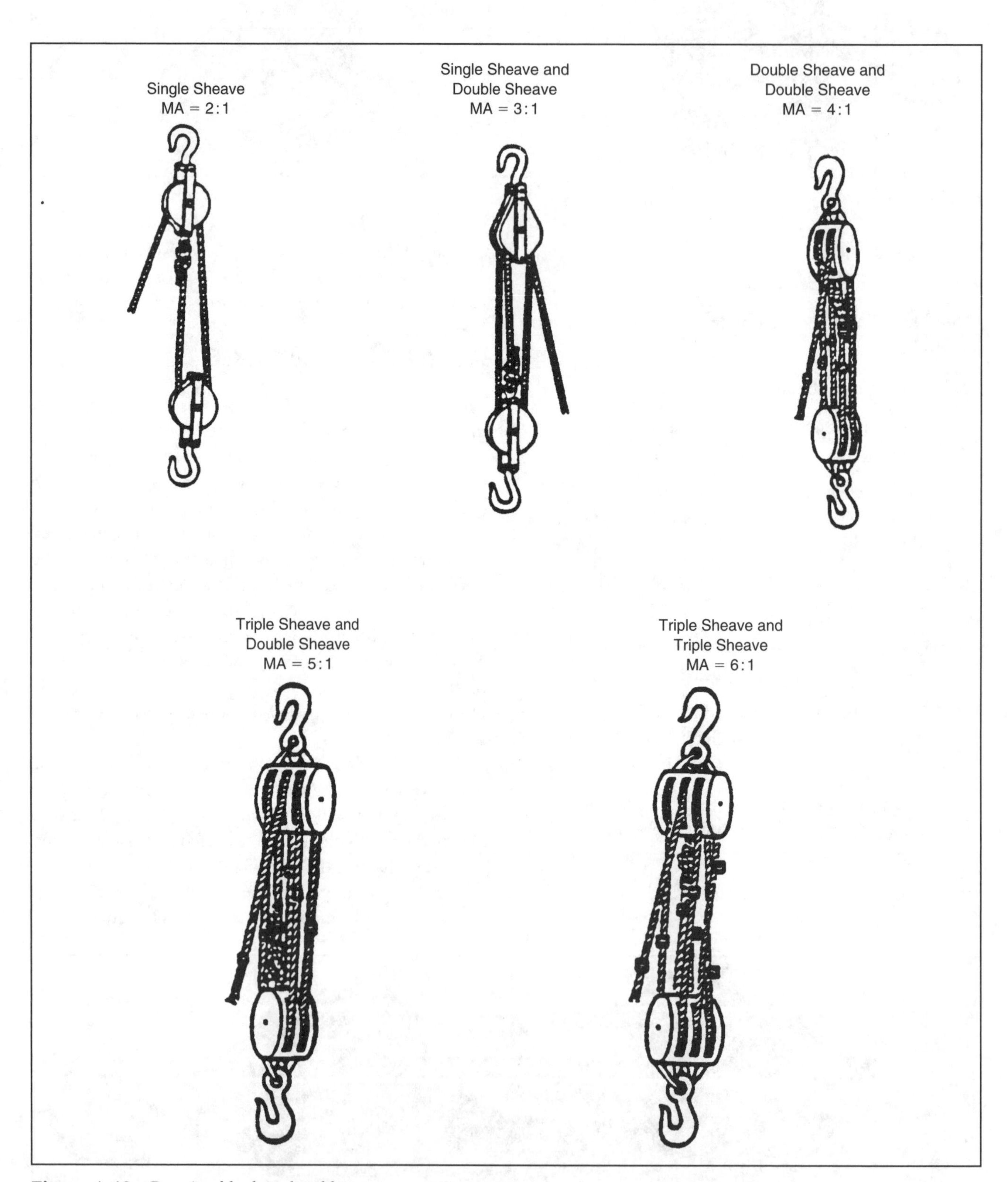

Figure 4–18 Reeving block and tackle.

rope involved in chock-a-block is computed as 4 ft. per pair of sheaves.

Figure 4–18 illustrates the proper method of reeving the various combination of blocks to be used during this section of training.

COMPUTING ROPE LENGTH AND MECHANICAL ADVANTAGES

Lifting and Hoisting

When computing the maximum load of a lifting tackle, only the returns between the blocks are used in computing the strength of the system. The weight is attached to the running end or lower block. The fall line is pulled off the standing block (upper block). The fall line is moving in the opposite direction of the weight being lifted; therefore it does not assist in the lifting process (MA 4:1; Figure 4–19).

Factors to be considered in calculating the maximum load of a lifting block and tackle include using an SWL of rope, the number of returns at the moving block (including the standing part if it is attached to the moving part), the SWL of the block, and the friction loss which reduces the efficiency of the block and tackle 10% to 15% throughout the entire system.

Hauling Systems

In a hauling system, the running end of the fall line comes off the moving block where the weight is attached. The standing block is secured to a holdfast. Factors to be considered in calculating the strength of a hauling block and tackle apply in the lifting as well as the hauling. These factors include:

1. When computing the strength of a hauling block and tackle, the fall line is pulled in the same direction as the weight and therefore assists the returns in moving the weight (gains additional line for MA).
2. Because of the assist, it must be considered as a return (MA 5:1; Figure 4–19).
3. Computations for figuring the strength of the hauling tackle remain the same except for the adjustment in the returns.
4. Example: Using a two-over-two block and tackle reeved with nylon rope:

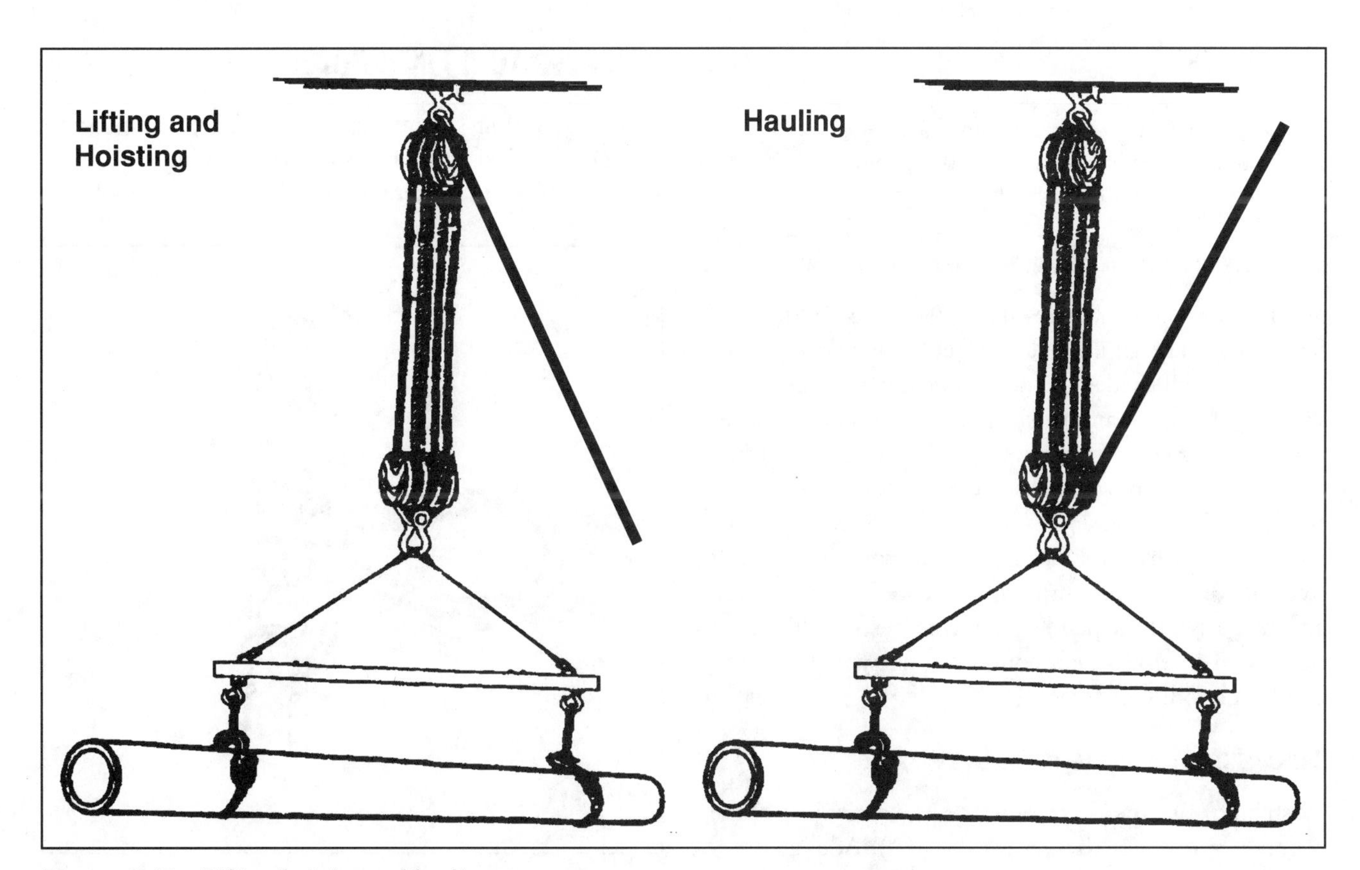

Figure 4–19 Lifting/hoisting and hauling systems.

(SWL) × (returns plus the fall line) − 10% FL

SWL × # of returns − 10% FL or
500 × 5 × .90 = 2500 − 250 = 2250

SWL × # of returns − strength = 90%

Note: Consideration must be given to a safety line whenever lifting/hoisting loads. A true safety is a second line firmly attached to the load through an appropriate belay to an adequate anchor.

Computing Length of Rope

When computing the amount of rope needed or required to lift or lower a victim, object, or weight a given distance, these following factors should be considered:

1. Number of sheaves plus the fall line.
2. Distance the object, victim, or weight has to be moved.
3. Overall length of a tackle when chock-a-block standard established is 4 ft. (4 ft. of length is added for *each* pair of sheaves).

To compute:

utilize the number of returns
+ 1 × the distance + chock-a-block
= footage of rope needed for the task.

For example:

Given two-over-two block and tackle,
with a required movement of 20 ft (4 plus 1) × 20
= 100 ft. + 8 ft. = 108 ft.

Determining Mechanical Advantages—Block and Tackle

Machines are utilized by rescue personnel to multiply the force exerted by an individual using levers, screws, jacks, and blocks and tackles. To determine the mechanical advantage of a block and tackle, add up the number of returns in the tackle. This gives the theoretical mechanical advantage of the block and tackle not accounting for friction loss of ropes passing over sheaves. For example, using a three-over-two block and tackle, there is a total of five sheaves or five returns. The theoretical mechanical advantage is 5:1, depending on whether it is lifting or hauling. Therefore, each pound of pull would result in exertion of 5 lbs. of force.

Compounding Block-and-Tackle Systems

With block-and-tackle systems, the MA varies (count the number of ropes or sheaves for the MA). Adding a second block and tackle attached to a lead line becomes a multiplier of the MA. If the original MA is 4:1; the compounded MA raises it to 16:1. That being insufficient, an additional block and tackle with an MA 6:1 can be added to reduce the effort still further. Multiplying the 16:1 by the additional MA of 6:1 equals a final MA of 96:1, less friction loss in each set of blocks being used.

Several major obstacles prevent the full use of compounding systems:

1. Insufficient room to rig out the reeved systems
2. Inadequate lengths of rope available
3. System weight

HAULING SYSTEMS

When using mechanical rope grabs, prusiks, and carabiners to construct hoisting devices, it is possible to build both simple and compound systems with minimum effort. Use single triple-wrapped prusik knots for hauling and lifting systems (Figure 4–20). The use of mechanical rope grabs is not recommended for lifting and hauling systems.

Figure 4–21 depicts a "Z" hauling system (simple) while Figure 4–22 depicts a "piggyback" hauling system (compound).

SECURING TO A FIXED OBJECT

Once the lifting system has been designed, it must be properly secured or anchored to the standing end of the system. Most times there are natural or in-place objects

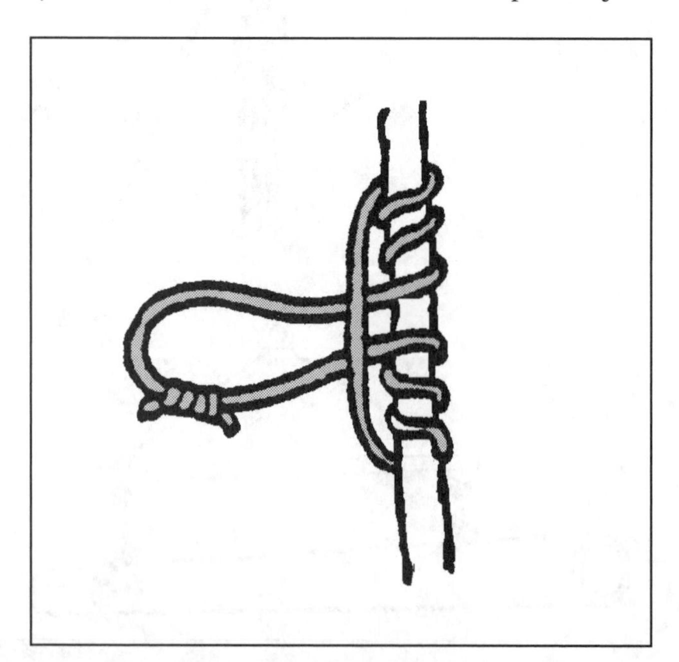

Figure 4–20 Triple-wrapped prusik knot.

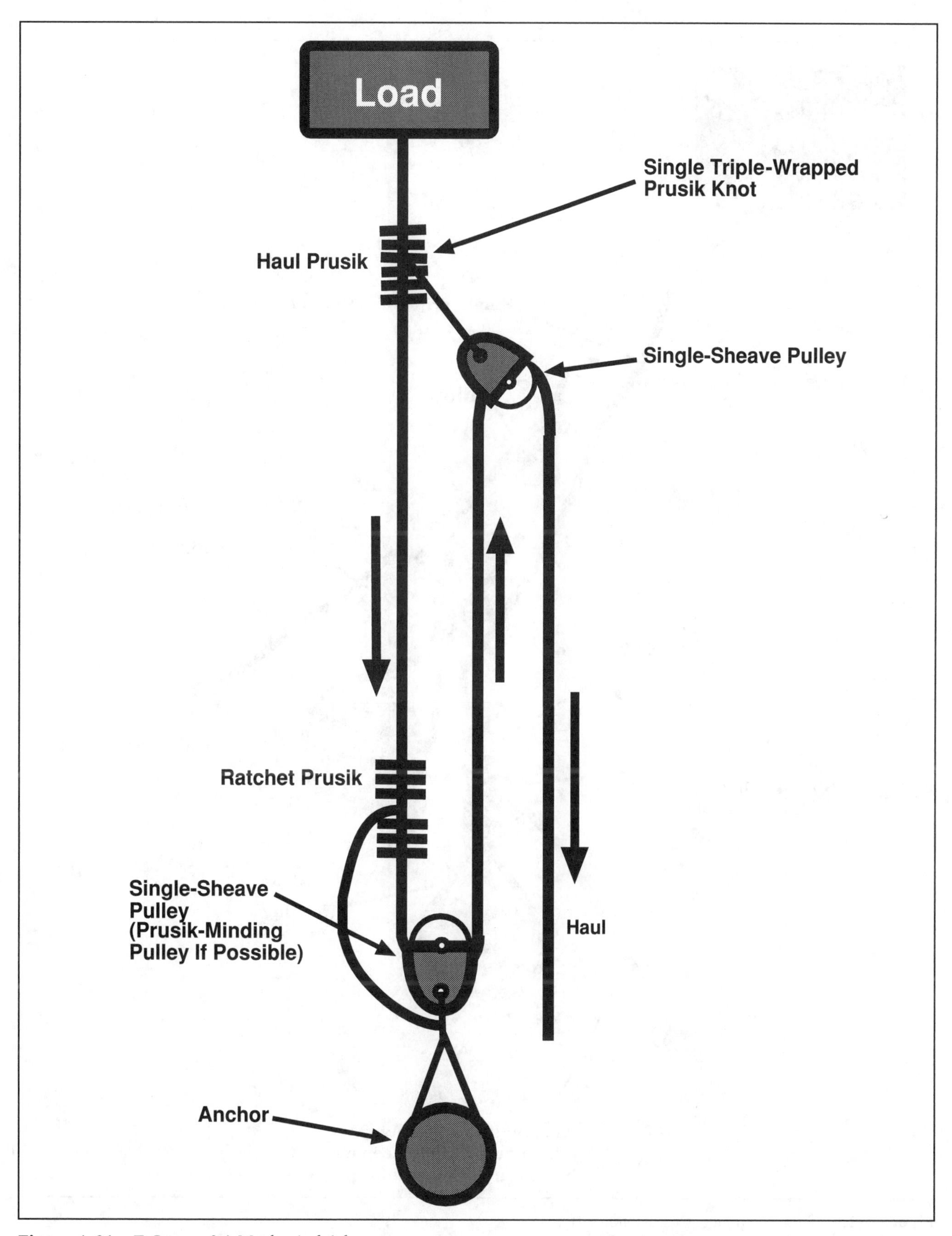

Figure 4–21 Z-System 3:1 Mechanical Advantage.

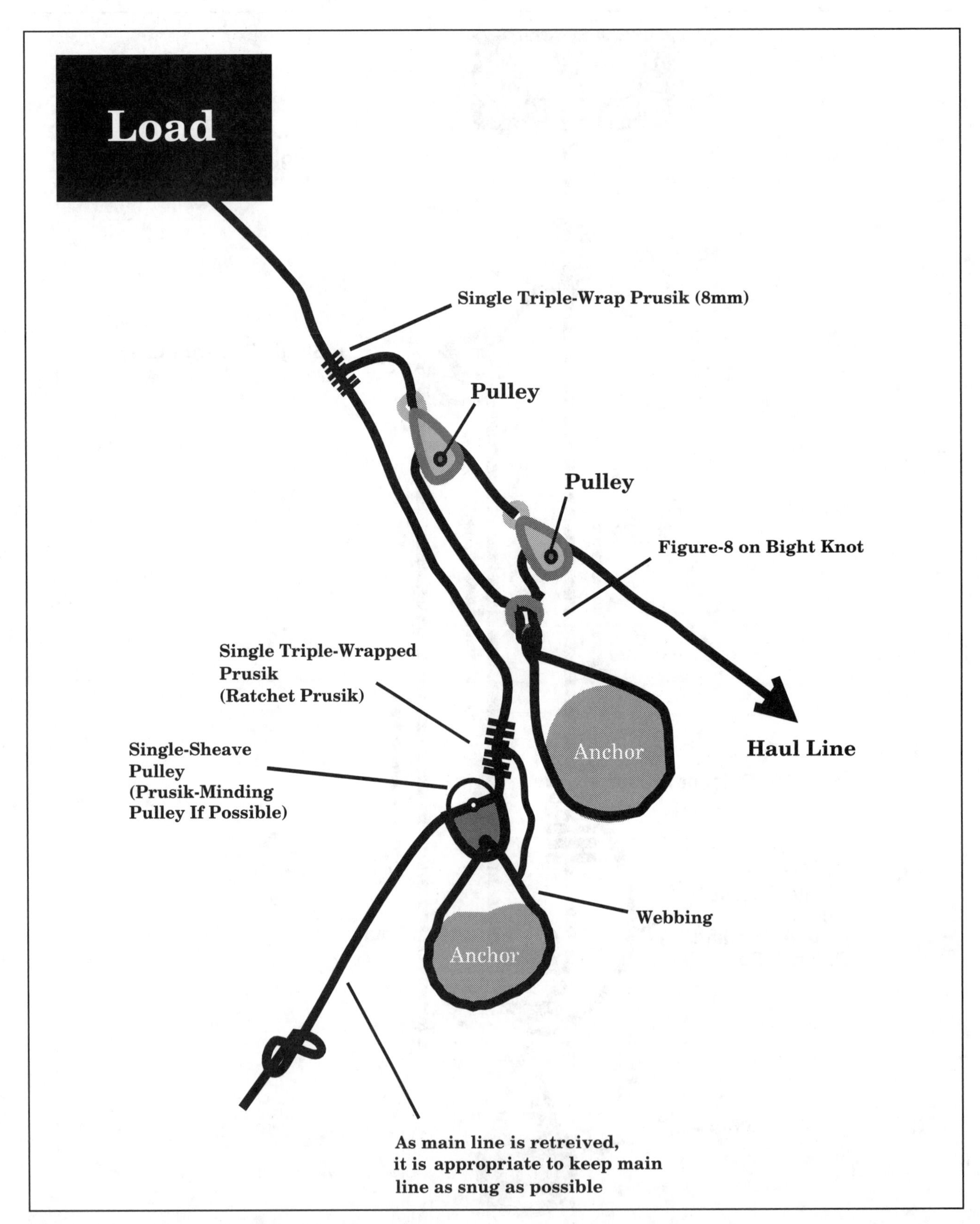

Figure 4–22 Compound piggyback hauling system.

that can be safely used as anchor points. When working in or off of buildings, there are usually a myriad of stationary objects available. However, double-check the selected object to make sure it will support the total load that will be applied to it and not collapse at the point the load is tied. Large trees are natural anchor points. While large stationary boulders or rocks will also work, be sure to protect the rope or sling that is placed around these objects from abrasion or cutting.

Where anchor points are not available or their ability to hold the expected load is questionable, it will be necessary to construct them. There are various methods of constructing anchor points. The type of soil will dictate the type of anchor needed. When selecting an anchor, remember it must be of sufficient size and strength to hold the total weight of the system and its load, both static and dynamic.

HOLDFASTS AND PICKETS

The picket holdfast can be used in most any material that will accept stakes or rods driven into it. Wooden pickets should be made from ash or oak. They should be at least 5 ft. long and a minimum of 4 ins. thick. If they are to be made with softer wood, then a minimum thickness of 5 ins. is required.

The use of steel pipe or rods vastly increases the shear strength of the device, thus reducing the thickness requirement (at least 1 in. in diameter). The increase of shear strength between wood on the transverse angle and structural steel of the same size could be as much as 16:1. The soil mechanics is more limiting than the ability of the picket to hold the applied weight. The recommended 5 ft. length is not unreasonable, particularly in sand or in soft or wet soil. The pickets should be driven into the ground at a minimum distance of 3 ft. apart to a maximum of 6 ft. apart. A 5 ft. long picket should stick out of the ground a maximum of 2 ft. (Figure 4–23). They should penetrate the ground to approximately two thirds of their length.

Table 4–2
Shear stress

Holdfast	*Pounds*
Single Picket	700
1–1 Picket Holdfast	1,400
1–1–1 Picket Holdfast	1,800
2–1 Picket Holdfast	2,000
3–2–1 Picket Holdfast	4,000

Steel reinforcing rods ½ in. diameter or larger are easily obtainable and work well as a picket in most applications. The shear strength of a ½ in. rod is in excess of 30,000 lbs.—high enough for normal rescue applications. When the applied weight is suspect, or it is necessary to reduce the possibility of bending the rods, add one or more pickets at each point.

Soil conditions will also dictate the holding power of a picket holdfast. Different setups of picket holdfasts will allow for greater pounds in holding power.

Notice that shear strength is discussed as being so many pounds (Table 4–2). This shear stress is not to be confused with bending stress or the point where the material will begin to distort. To shear a piece of steel, one would place the bar on the shear table and clamp the bar in place. A knife blade would drop down and cut or shear the bar in half. A wire or fiber rope presents a very small area of pressure to the picket, not unlike a shear blade. To reduce this tendency to shear and bend, the bar increases the area of exposure presented by the rope. As the rope's exposure area is increased, the pressure exerted on a spe-

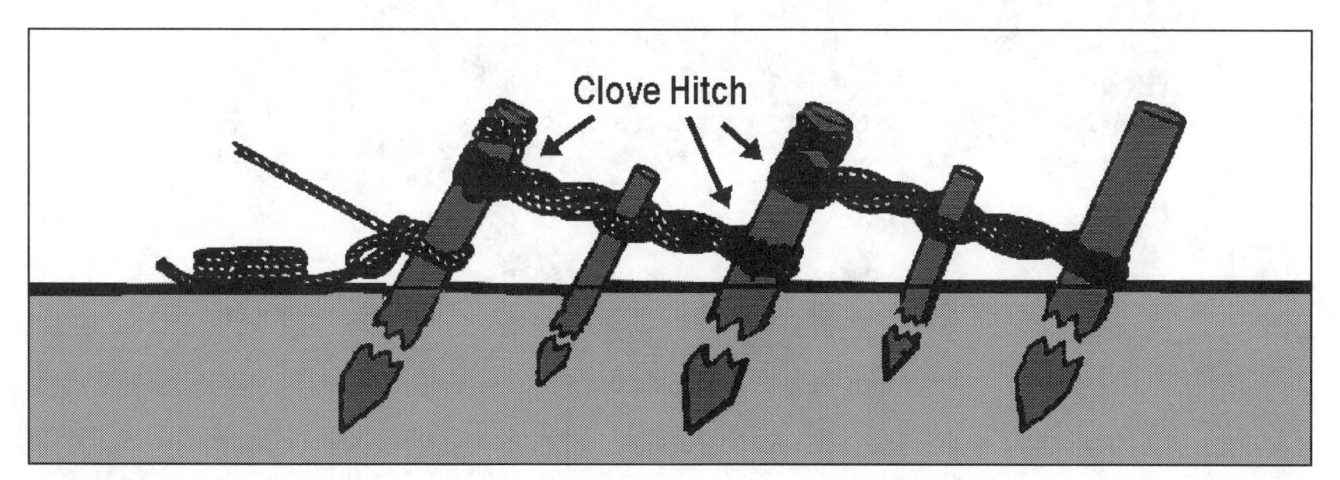

Figure 4–23 Picket holdfast.

cific area of the picket is reduced. To increase the pressure area, use straps or other devices to spread the load over a wider area, employing the same theory as using wide boards under jacks in vehicle stabilization.

In the figures presented here, the pickets were driven into the ground at a 90° angle to the load being applied. Reducing this angle could substantially reduce the holding power of the picket and further reduce the shear strength, particularly in wood. The reduced pressure angle presented to the picket increases the shear to the longitudinal axis or along the grain where wood is at its weakest.

Remember, sheaves are designed to allow the rope to bend at a radius that would not damage it. After the picket holdfast is built, a method is needed to safely attach the load line to the picket without damaging the rope. A thimble would be the ultimate device. Since thimbles are not readily available on the rescue scene, place a folded blanket around the picket. This will present a wide, more graceful radius to the load-bearing line.

If a block is attached to the picket, use either a fabric, chain, or cable sling, or tie a base lashing to the picket with a utility rope.

When the hook of the block is attached to either the load or the anchor point, it is necessary to ensure that the hook cannot jump out of or off of the device. This jumping occurs when a shock load has been applied to the block. To eliminate this possibility, depend on the factory-installed safety latch. If it is missing or not working properly, "mouse" the hook.

Constructing Combination Pickets

1. Drive three pickets into the ground in the same line as the guyline being supported.
2. Pickets should be spaced at least 3 ft. apart
3. Lashing commences with 50 ft. section of ½ in. rope.
4. A clove hitch is tied to the top of the first picket.
5. The rope is then passed around the second picket at least six times leading from the top of the first picket to the bottom of the second picket.
6. The rope is then fastened to the second picket with a clove hitch and safety just above the turns.
7. Repeat the same steps, starting with the second picket and going to the third picket as outlined above. Proper tensioning results in an integrated, load sharing anchor.
8. Place a short picket spinner through the turns of the lashing rope between each set of pickets. Tensioning results in transfer of loading from one picket to another.

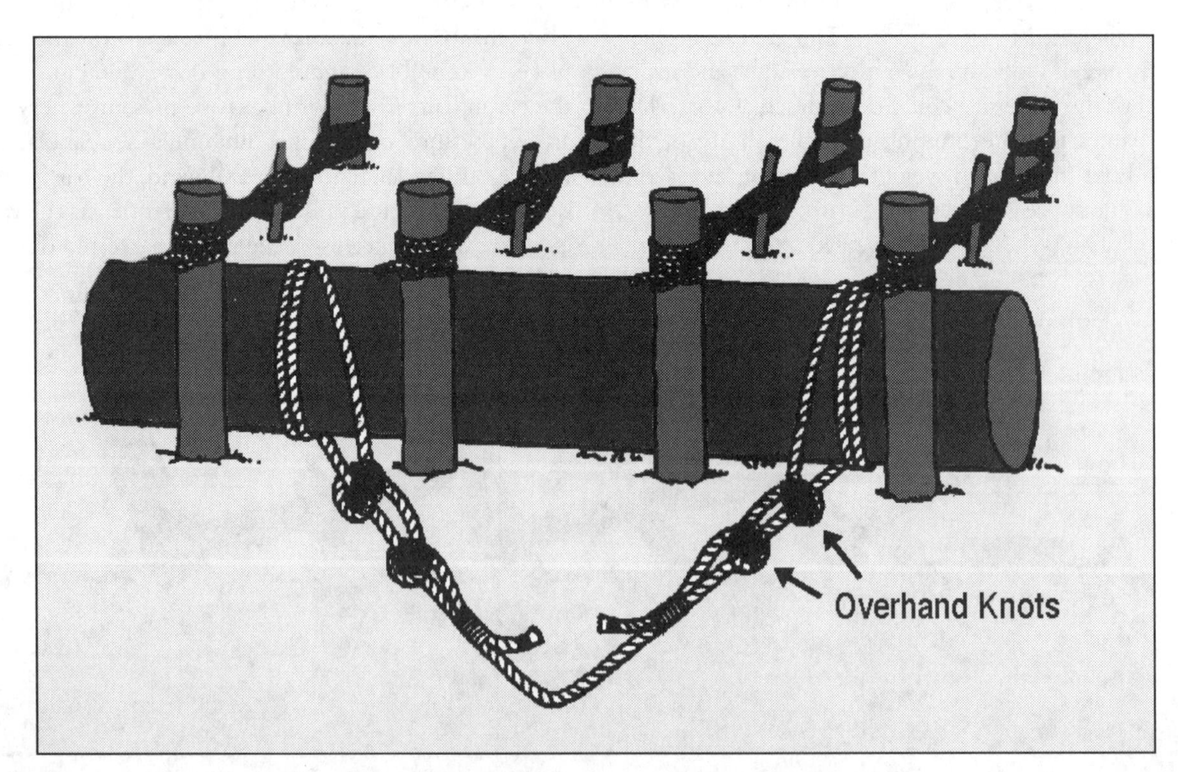

Figure 4–24 Combination log-and-picket holdfast.

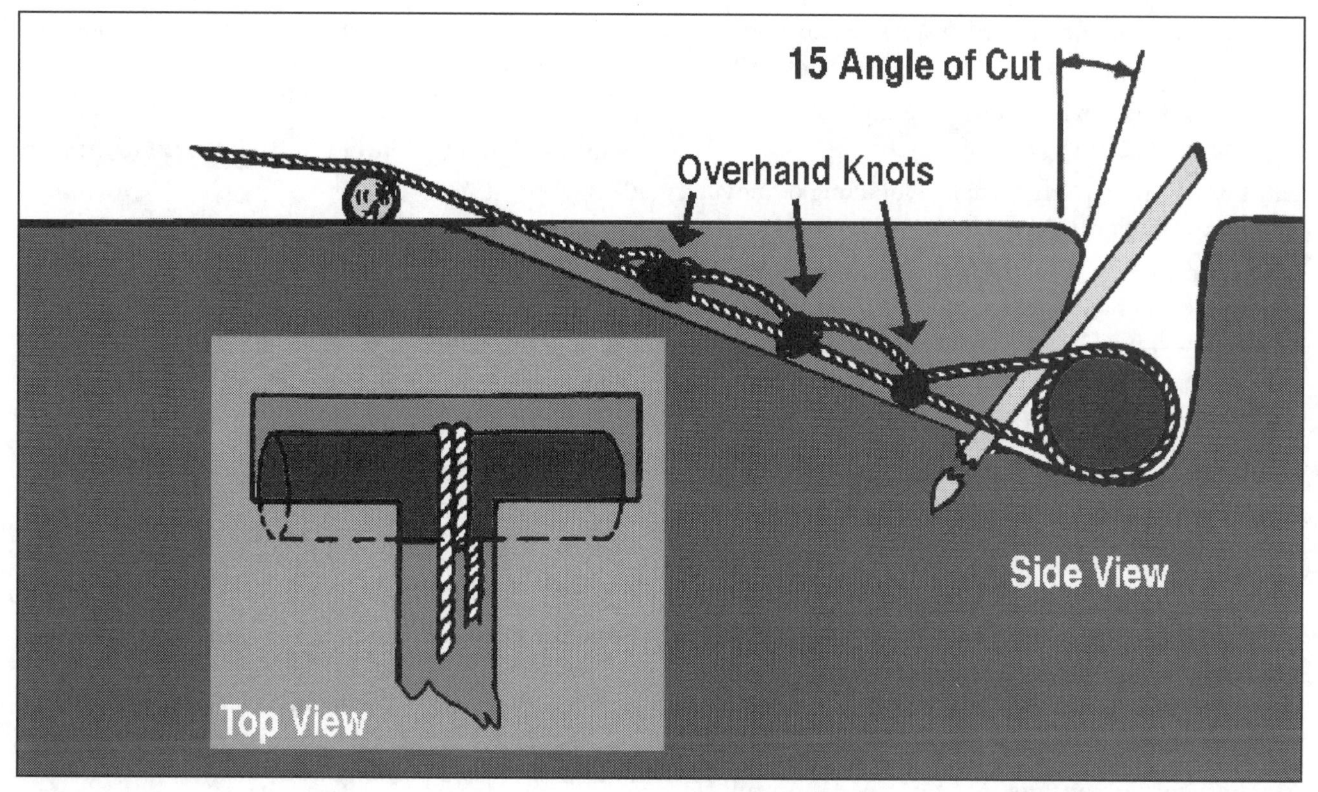

Figure 4–25 Deadman holdfast.

9. Twist the spinner until the lashing is taut, and then drive the short pickets into the ground

Combination Log-and-Picket Holdfast

A good holding device is provided when there is major concern about the shear strength of the pickets versus the load being applied or the method of application. This device is named *combination log-and-picket holdfast.* Naturally, if there is another object that would have greater strength than available logs, then use it. Note that the bridle attaching the holdfast is constructed with wire rope. This could also be accomplished utilizing the appropriate size "lifeline quality" rope (Figure 4–24).

Deadman Holdfast

A deadman holdfast is one method of providing an anchor point and is one of the few that will work well in sand or very loose material. The log or item used in its place must be in good condition or it will collapse or break apart under load.

The holding device may be of any substantial material. It is preferable that it be solid or of heavy wall construction. The lifter or guide at the top of the cut keeps the line from digging into the material. Note the 15° angle of the undercut. This is done to prevent the holding device from rolling up the side of the trench (Figure 4–25).

Safety with Holdfasts

When utilizing holdfasts to secure lifting devices via guylines, it is imperative that a safety person monitor each and every holdfast for indications of excessive strains. Normally the weakest point in a lifting device formulated for rescue purposes is the holdfast system.

DEFINITIONS

Anchor: An immovable object to which a standing block is attached.

Block: A grooved pulley or sheave set in a frame or shell connected with a hook or strap by which it may be attached to another object: (a) Three sheave; (b) Two sheave; (c) Single sheave; (d) Snatch block.

Block and tackle: Blocks with associated rope or cable for hoisting or lowering.

Carabiner: An oblong steel ring with a gated opening.

Chock-a-block: Position of blocks when the two blocks have been run in as far as they can possibly move.

The distance when measured from hook to hook on blocks is 4 ft. per pair of sheaves.

Compound hauling system: Consists of more than one rope and/or block and tackle.

Fall line: The rope that is pulled for lifting or moving an object with block and tackle.

Gibbs ascender: A mechanical device used by mountain climbers and spelunkers to assist them in climbing up rope. It is also used by rescue personnel in rigging.

Gun tackle: A block and tackle attached to a load with the running block reeved with the haul line.

Haul line: The running end of a line.

Hauling: Rescuers exerting a pulling force on the rope (Fall line).

Lashing: Places lifting/lowering device in position over object.

Leading block: Usually a snatch block utilized to change the direction of pull in a block-and-tackle system without affecting the MA of the system.

Mechanical advantage (MA): (MA) Advantage gained by use of mechanism in transmitting force. Rate of force that performs useful work of a machine to the force that is applied to the machine.

Mousing: Safety cord or line tied across the throat of a hook to prevent a sling or anchor from jumping out of the hook.

Overhauling blocks: Process of separating the two blocks to a distance at least equal to the length of move desired. (Accomplished prior to attaching running block to the load.)

Paying out: Easing off or slackening a rope.

Pulleys: Develops the MA and allows rope to change directions.

Reeve: To pass a rope through a hole or opening; to pass a rope through a block.

Reeving: The process of passing correct size rope over sheaves in the proper direction and order.

Returns: Moving sections of rope between blocks.

Rigging: The use of rope in a variety of applications wherein objects are secured against movement, or they are moved under controlled conditions with reduced effort.

Running block: The block that is nearest to the load. Also known as the fall block.

Running end: The active part of a rope.

Sheave or pulley: The grooved well in which a rope passes over and changes direction.

Shell: Portion of the block that supports or holds the sheave, and to which the strap, hook, or ring is attached.

Simple hauling system: Uses a single line throughout the entire hauling system.

Sling: A looped line, strap, cable, or chain used to hoist, lower, or carry.

Snatch block: A single-sheave block with an opening gate on one side of the shell, through which the rope can be engaged or snatched without having to thread the end of the rope through the block. (Opening is closed by a hinged or pivoted portion of the strap.)

Standing block: The block attached to an anchor point or the fixed block. Normally the haul line comes from this block.

Standing end: The inactive part of a rope.

Strap: Portion of the block to which the hook is attached.

Tackle: A group of ropes and pulleys arranged for lifting, lowering, or hauling.

REFERENCES

Frank, J.A., and J.B. Smith. 1992. *Rope rescue manual.* 2d ed. Santa Barbara, CA: CMC Rescue, Inc.

Maryland Fire and Rescue Institute. 1989. *Rescue technician course.* Berwin Heights, MD: MFRI.

National Fire Academy. 1993. *Rescue systems I.* Washington, DC: United States Fire Administration and California State Fire Marshal's Office, Fire Service Training and Education System.

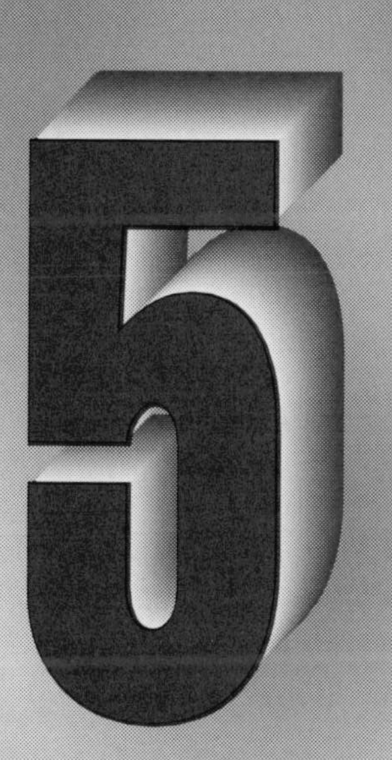

Principles of Rigging, Anchoring, and Mechanical Advantage Systems

OBJECTIVE

Working as a member of a team, the student will be able to reeve blocks, construct anchoring systems, and reeve a simple and compound hauling system, from memory, without assistance, to an accuracy of 70% and the satisfaction of the instructor.

OVERVIEW

Principles of Rigging, Anchoring, and Mechanical Advantage Systems

- Reeving Blocks
- Anchoring
- Hauling Systems

ENABLING OBJECTIVES

5-1-1 Demonstrate reeving blocks to obtain mechanical advantage (e.g., 3:3, 3:2, 2:2, 2:1, 1:1).

5-1-2 Given a simulated rescue, be able to:

- Select an anchor
- Prepare anchor for use
- Rig an appropriate anchor or sling on the anchor(s):
  - —simple anchor sling
  - —tensionless anchor
  - —backed-up tensionless anchor
- Construct a two-point self-equalizing system
- Construct a picket holdfast

5-1-3 Demonstrate both a simple and a compound hauling system.

I. Practical Work Station I
Reeving blocks to achieve mechanical advantage (50 minutes)

Reeving	*Yields*
A. 3:3	6:1 MA
B. 3:2	5:1 MA
C. 2:2	4:1 MA
D. 2:1	3:1 MA
E. 1:1	2:1 MA

II. Practical Work Station II
Anchoring/anchor preparation and attachment (50 minutes)
   A. Select an anchor/point
   B. Prepare an anchor for use
   C. Rig an anchor
      1. Simple anchor sling <120°
      2. Tensionless anchor
      3. Backed-up tensionless anchor
   D. Construct a two-point self-equalizing anchor
   E. Construct a picket holdfast

III. Practical Work Station III
Hauling Systems (50 minutes)
   A. Construct a Z-rig system (yields 3:1 MA)
   B. Construct a compound (piggyback or "Pig Rig") system (yields 4:1 MA)

Note: Each practical work station should have an instructor assigned. Students should be divided into 3 groups (e.g., 30 students = 3 groups of 10 students). Safe practices must be observed.

REFERENCES

Frank, J.A., and J.B. Smith. 1992. *Rope rescue manual.* 2d ed. Santa Barbara, CA: CMC Rescue, Inc.

Maryland Fire and Rescue Institute. 1989. *Rescue technician course.* Berwin Heights, MD: MFRI

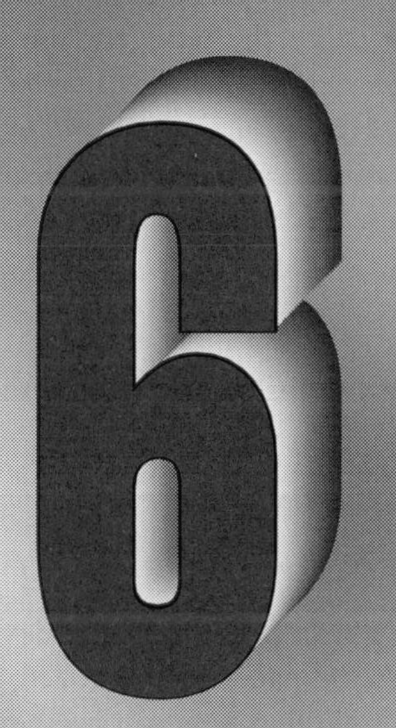

Incident Scene Approach to Patient Packaging and Transfer

OBJECTIVE

The student will be able to identify and demonstrate the proper methods of using various patient transfer devices in patient removal and transfer, functioning as a team member, from memory, without assistance, to an accuracy of 70% and the satisfaction of the instructor.

OVERVIEW

Incident Scene Approach to Patient Packaging and Transfer

- Lifting and Moving Patients
- Safety Inspection of Patient Transfer Devices
- Five Goals for Patient Packaging
- Patient Packaging on Transfer Devices
- Triage

ENABLING OBJECTIVES

6-1-1 Demonstrate the proper methods of lifting or loading a patient onto various patient transfer devices using the following devices or techniques:
- Log roll
- Straddle lift
- Orthopedic (Scoop) stretcher

6-1-2 Identify the critical points of each patient transfer device that require a safety inspection.

6-1-3 Identify the five goals for selecting a patient transfer device prior to patient packaging.

6-1-4 Demonstrate the proper methods for packaging a patient on each of the following (as available):
- LSP halfback extrication/rescue vest
- Miller full-body splint/litter
- Plastic basket litter with and without long backboard
- Wire basket litter (Stokes) with and without long backboard

- SKED stretcher with and without long backboard

6-1-5 Describe the objective of triage and the four priorities for classifying patients.

LIFTING AND MOVING PATIENTS

Once a patient has been located, access gained to him/her, and injuries properly stabilized by EMS providers, he/she must then be placed on an appropriate transfer device for evacuation. It is extremely rare that a patient must be moved without any emergency care being provided. When patient injuries are vague or uncertain, rescuers should treat injuries suggested by the mechanism of injury, choosing to err on the side of good patient care rather than ease of transport. Where injuries have occurred, and the route of egress prohibits the use of backboards and other standard immobilizing devices, a flexible or narrow profile device (e.g., a SKED stretcher, Miller board, or LSP Halfback) should be considered. If available devices prove to be unacceptable, a consultation between the EMS rescue provider and a doctor, if obtainable, should be held to determine the safest method of preparing the patient for movement under existing conditions and protols.

Patient care should be supervised by the senior patient care provider on scene from the phase of victim access until the rescue is terminated and patient care is transferred to the next level of medical care.

A patient should never be transferred without first being properly secured to the patient transfer device. There are too many documented cases where the patient has fallen from the stretcher resulting in the patient suffering more profound injuries. Exceptions to this guideline include removal under conditions that are immediately dangerous to life and health (e.g., fire, explosion, other hazardous conditions posing imminent threat to life) and movement over water when there is no spinal trauma or head trauma.

Manual techniques for lifting or the use of an orthopedic (scoop) stretcher should be used to place patients on transfer devices with appropriate precautions for spinal trauma and proper lifting technique.

When conditions prohibit full stabilization prior to transfer (such as those described above) the patient should, wherever possible and practical, have an extrication collar placed around his/her neck and have manual stabilization applied to the head. This will reduce the possibility of further injury to the patient.

The national standard of care for patients with potential or suspected cervical spine (c-spine) injuries requires that cervical/spinal stabilization be applied prior to transfer.

The log roll tends to be the most commonly used technique for placing backboards under patients, but it is not necessarily the best technique.

Whatever technique is chosen, patient care should be the first consideration in making the selection.

Log Roll (Figure 6–1)

Follow these steps when using the log roll technique:

1. Rescuer #1 kneels at the patient's head and holds manual stabilization on patient's head.

Note: Do not pull!

2. Rescuers #2–4 position themselves side-by-side along one side of the patient to be rolled, leaving enough room to roll the patient toward them, with the rescuers' arms parallel and extended as indicated in the steps that follow.
3. Rescuer #2 kneels at the patient's shoulder, with one hand positioned on the patient's far shoulder and the other hand positioned at the patient's far hip.
4. Rescuer #3 kneels at the patient's hip, with one hand positioned on the patient's lower torso at approximately the base of the far scapula and the other hand positioned on the patient's far buttock.
5. Rescuer #4 kneels at the patient's knees, with one hand positioned on the patient's far thigh and the other hand positioned on the patient's far calf.
6. On command from Rescuer #1, the patient is rolled evenly, as a single unit, to a point that is approximately 135° toward Rescuers #2–4.

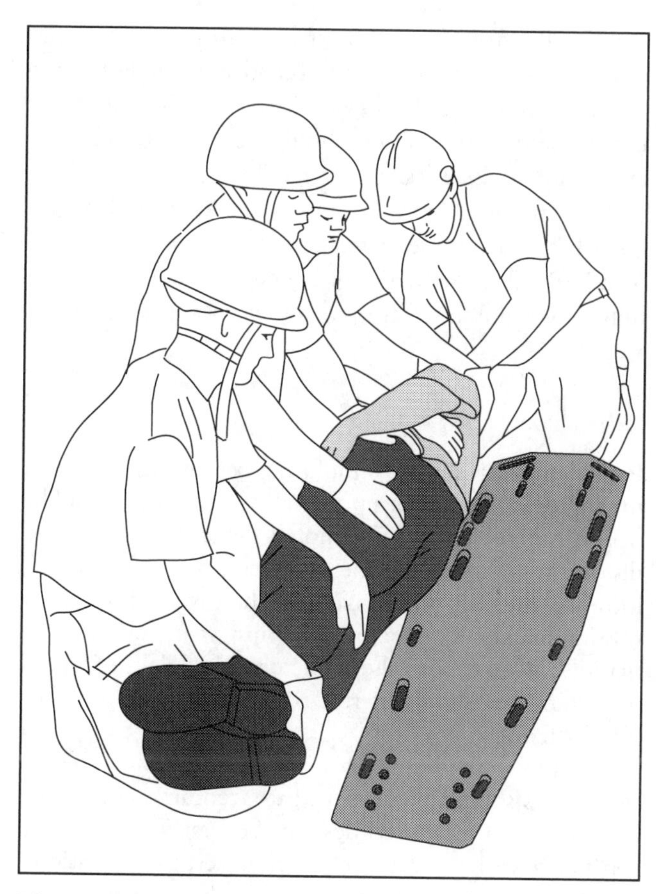

Figure 6–1 Log roll.

7. While the patient is supported against the thighs of Rescuers #2–4, Rescuer #5 examines the patient's backside for injuries and places a full backboard on the ground, directly behind the patient with the top edge of the board aligned with the top of the patient's head.
8. A trauma pad should be placed on the board in the area of the lumbar spine and another should be placed in the area behind the back of the patient's head. Trauma pads placed at anatomical void spaces and behind the head enhance the stabilization of the long backboard and maintain the c-spine in more neutral alignment. The trauma pads also decrease patient discomfort and possible soft tissue injuries that result from prolonged immobilization on hard, unyielding surfaces.
9. On command from Rescuer #1, the patient is rolled evenly, as a unit, back onto the backboard. Unless the patient is obese, the patient will not be centered on the backboard at this time.
10. In order to center the patient on the board, rescuers straddle the patient and slide him/her evenly, as a unit, first toward the foot of the board and then back toward the head at a slight angle toward the center of the board each way. This so-called "straddle slide" technique is an old standard in patient care. The technique may, however, aggravate spinal injuries due to the extension and compression of the spine.

Straddle Lift

The straddle lift technique is equally effective and holds far less potential to injure the patient.

Follow these steps when using the straddle lift technique:

1. Rescuer #1 kneels at the patient's head and holds manual stabilization on patient's head.

Note: Do not pull!

2. Rescuer #2 straddles the patient, facing the patient's head, and grasps the patient's upper torso under the armpits.
3. Rescuer #3 straddles the patient, facing the patient's head, and grasps the patient under the hips.
4. Rescuer #4 straddles the patient, facing the patient's head, and grasps the patient's legs just below the knees.
5. On command from Rescuer #1, the patient is lifted evenly, as a single unit, 2 to 3 ins. above the ground. During all lifting operations, proper lifting technique must be exercised. Rescuers should squat as low as they can, look straight ahead at the back for the rescuer in front of them and arch their backs. This posture will place the majority of all lifting effort on the rescuer's legs, rather than their backs. Rescuers with recent history of back, c-spine or shoulder injuries should refrain from participation in this part of the evolution.
6. Rescuer #5 centers a backboard on the ground, under the patient. On command from Rescuer #1 the patient is lowered onto the backboard, centered and with the top of his/her head aligned with the top edge of the backboard.

Orthopedic (Scoop) Stretcher

Follow these steps when using an orthopedic stretcher:

1. First rescuer kneels at the patient's head and holds manual stabilization on patient's head.

Note: Do not pull!

2. Rescuers #2 and #3 release the locking mechanism on the lower part of the stretcher, extend the

stretcher to a length that is 4 in. past the patient's head and 4 ins. past the patient's feet and reengage the locking pins.

3. Rescuer #2 depresses the latch at the head cushion from the stretcher if so equipped.
4. Rescuer #2 depresses the latch at the head end of the stretcher while Rescuer #3 depresses the latch at the foot end of the stretcher. With latches depressed, both rescuers pull the two halves of the stretcher apart, breaking it into two pieces which are then placed with one half on either side of the patient.
5. Rescuers #2 and #3 work together to slide the two halves under the patient being careful not to pinch the patient between the two rescuers maintaining c-spine stabilization.
6. Rescuers #2 and #3 lock the two stretcher halves together, head latch first.

SAFETY INSPECTION OF PATIENT TRANSFER DEVICES

Devices

There are many types of patient transfer devices used by the rescue services. The most common is the ambulance wheeled-type stretcher. This is a very good unit and fulfills its intended job well. However, it is not practical to use when moving patients over rough terrain or from open elevation to another where steps or ramps are not available.

The basket litter has proven to be one of the best devices for this type of transportation. Basket litters are shell-like in design and are made of either a tubular metal frame with wire-mesh lining or of semi-rigid plastic and shaped like the outline of a human body.

Plastic basket litters and SKED stretchers are well suited for rescues over snow and ice. Their closed structure allows for sliding the basket along the surface, making them ideal for snow and ice rescue applications. Plastic basket litters may be at risk of developing fractures during patient transfers. The two-piece models are a less desirable design due to questions about their structural integrity during vertical hoisting and lowering evolutions. In general, plastic devices are undesirable for transfer over moving water or when being hosted or used in fixed-line helicopter flyouts without special preplanning and training. In moving water, plastic basket litters create drag and act like boats when afloat. When filled with water, they become too heavy to manage. When using plastic baskets under helicopters, tag lines and trained crews are mandatory for control during hoisting. During fixed-line flyouts, plastic baskets act as airfoils and spin wildly making them a poor choice for those operations. Therefore, the use of plastic basket litters should be restricted to slope evacuation and ice rescues over still water.

The one-piece wire Stokes basket long used by the navy has proven adequate for most rescue evolutions. The LSP halfback extrication/rescue vest and the Miller full-body splint/litter are two other patient transfer devices.

Inspection

Patient transfer devices should be visually inspected for the following conditions prior to each use and should be placed out of service until noted defects are corrected: distortions of any components; cracks; rust; weld failure; loose or missing bolts, rivets, or hardware; broken or missing buckles, connectors, or strips; or any other irregularities. Wire baskets should be tipped while the inspector listens for sounds of rust particles sliding inside the tubular frame.

The metal dividers in Stokes baskets to isolate the patient's legs should be removed to accommodate a long backboard (of a tapered design). Several failures of the top rail have been reported during vertical operations. You are encouraged to modify all Stokes baskets as recommended by the National Aeronautics and Space Administration (Figure 6–2), including

1. Grinding and cleaning the existing weld.
2. Fabricating a 16-gauge sleeve that is long enough to span the space between the two ribs at the end of the litter. The inside diameter of the sleeve should correspond to the outside diameter of the tubular rail stock.
3. Installing a sleeve.
4. Welding, cleaning, and painting.

FIVE GOALS FOR PATIENT PACKAGING

When preparing to package a patient for transfer, there are five goals that rescuers need to consider.

1. Packing Should Protect the Patient from Further Injury

Helmets that do not cause hyperflexion of the patient's neck and safety glasses to protect the patient's eyes from falling debris and the ends of lashing materials should be provided at a minimum. Removable litter shields provide an even greater degree of protection for the patient's head

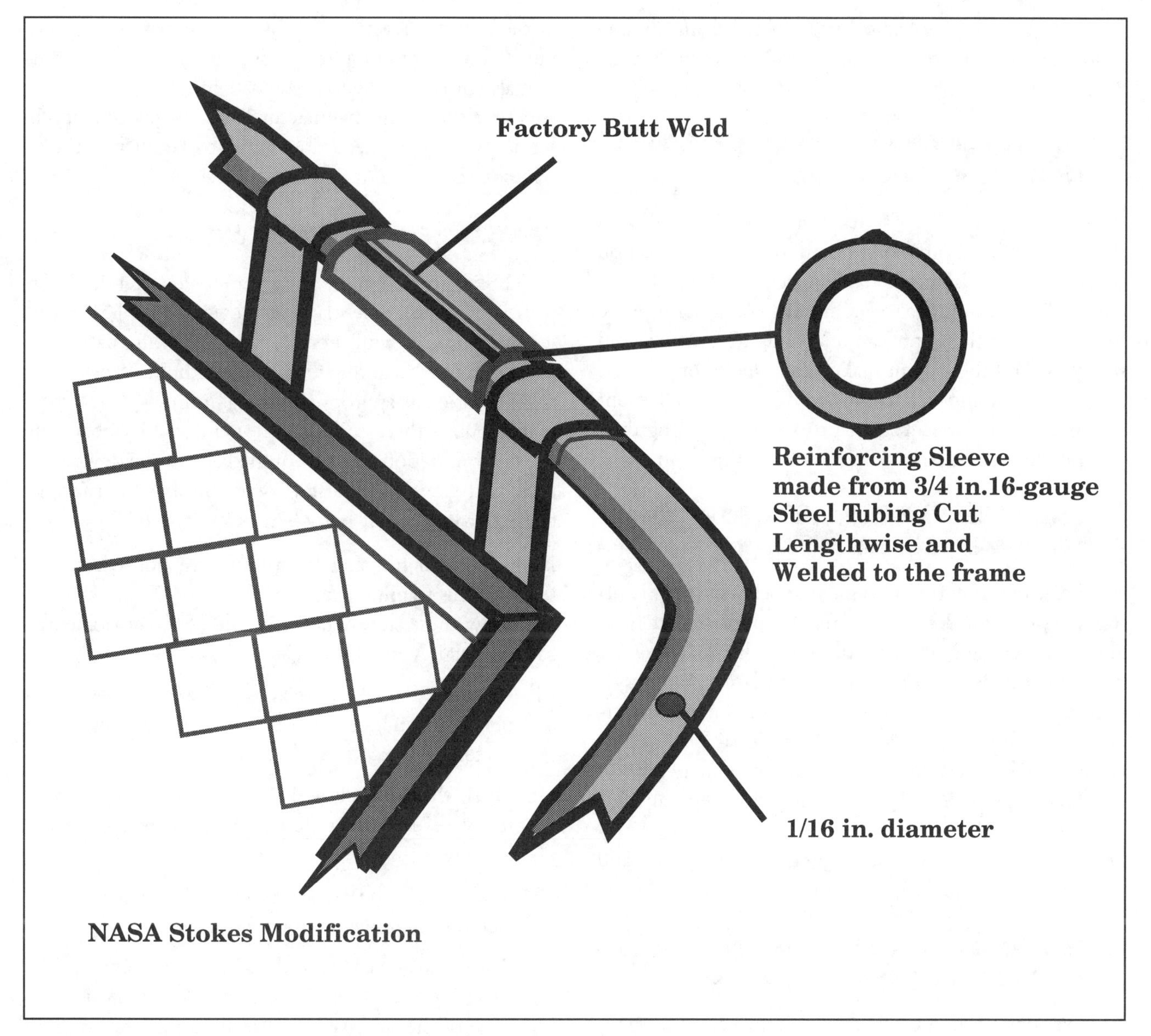

Figure 6–2 NASA Stokes modification.

and face. Lashing should protect the patient from falling out or from being ejected during a spin. Rescuers should always prepare for the worst possible conditions. The litter may be dropped, inverted, or turned upside down. Make certain that the patient is secured in the basket and stays there until you are ready to remove him/her.

2. Packaging Should Include Provisions for Patient Comfort

Patients who are immobilized for extended periods of time on rigid backboards or on wire mesh may develop soft tissue injuries at the points of contact with the underlying surface. Knees that are tied down into hyperextended positions can cause extreme joint pain. Padding placed at anatomical void spaces and behind the head enhance the stabilization and maintain the c-spine in more neutral alignment. Padding also decreases patient discomfort and reduces the possibility of soft tissue injuries that result from prolonged immobilization on hard, unyielding surfaces. Remember, this is probably the patient's first rescue, don't leave a lasting impression that your organization or rescue group is callous or unfeeling. Remember the charge to prehospital care providers everywhere: "Do no harm." Patient comfort includes making provision for the efficiency of the patient's shelter. Patients must be insulated against heat loss where appropriate and must be protected from overheating during warmer weather. Patients must also be protected from cooling caused by exposure to inclement weather or windy conditions.

3. Packaging Should Provide Adequate Stabilization of Fractures and Adjacent Joints

Patients with suspected spinal trauma or head injuries must be stabilized on a long board or other stabilization device prior to placing the patient in the transfer device. Cervical collars must also be applied using appropriate techniques for their application. Filling all existing void spaces around the patient makes them feel more secure, aids in insulating from the cold during inclement weather, and prevents patient or extremity shifting during movement which may aggravate existing injuries.

4. Packaging Should Include Provisions for Rescuers to Carry or Move the Patient Transfer Device

Examples of such provisions include belay systems, hauling systems, and detachable litter support wheel. Rescuers must consider the terrain, time of day, and weather conditions to be encountered during transfer. Rope systems may be useless over clear, flat terrain but are the vital link in high-angle or vertical terrain. Rescuers performing a flat carry over long distances may tire of carrying their share of the litter with one hand. The addition of a shoulder strap to help redistribute the load may reduce rescuer fatigue. Remember, rescuer fatigue and discomfort has a direct impact on patient care.

5. Packaging Should be Compatible with the Mode of Transport and Specific Rescue Environment

For example, if the patient is to be transported by helicopter, no plastic basket litters for exterior hoisting and no ambulance stretchers for confined space rescue should be used. As mentioned in the "Safety Inspection of Patient Transfer Devices" section, there is no ideal device for all rescue situations. Companies who are responsible for rescue in their area should acquire an assortment of devices to handle the types of calls they may respond to.

PATIENT PACKAGING ON TRANSFER DEVICES

It would be unrealistic to attempt to list packaging techniques for every device that is currently available from retailers or is being carried on the inventory of every fire/rescue agency in Maryland. Instead, this program has addressed equipment that is used in many EMT-B training classes across the state. This does not constitute an endorsement or recommendation for purchase of any device that is mentioned here. It is incumbent on the individuals who are likely to participate in rescues, to acquire data sheets from the manufacturers of any device that is in service with their department and to familiarize themselves with the use of that device.

LSP Halfback Extrication/Rescue Vest

The LSP is applied in the same manner as a Kendrick Extrication Device. The major advantage of the LSP is that it can be used as a full-body harness for lifting patients as in a confined space rescue with or without suspected c-spine injuries. If appropriate, the aluminum "back stay" that stabilizes the c-spine can be removed by detaching the hook and loop straps from the back of the device and then withdrawing the "stay" with the head harness attached, from the full-body harness (Figure 6–3).

Note: Vertical hoisting techniques are not within the scope of this training program.

Follow these steps who using the LSP halfback extrication/rescue vest:

1. Remove patient's eyeglasses and any articles in patient's shirt pockets after treating any obvious or suspected injuries.
2. Open the halfback and make certain that the back stay is secured with the velcro straps on the back of the device.
3. Remove the head harness from the device by detaching the hook and loop fasteners.
4. Place the device behind the patient such that the back stay is centered behind the patient and the top edge of the side flaps sit directly under the patient's armpits.
5. Release all straps from the strap pockets. Connect each color-coded buckle to the corresponding colored snap hook.
6. Adjust the length for the shoulder straps so that the top edge of the side flaps sit directly under the patient's armpits.
7. Adjust the two torso straps so that the device is snug against the patient's torso.
8. Adjust the leg straps so that they are not crossed, the foam pad is located in a position of comfort for the patient, and the length provides a snug fit.
9. Disconnect the chin and head straps from the head harness.

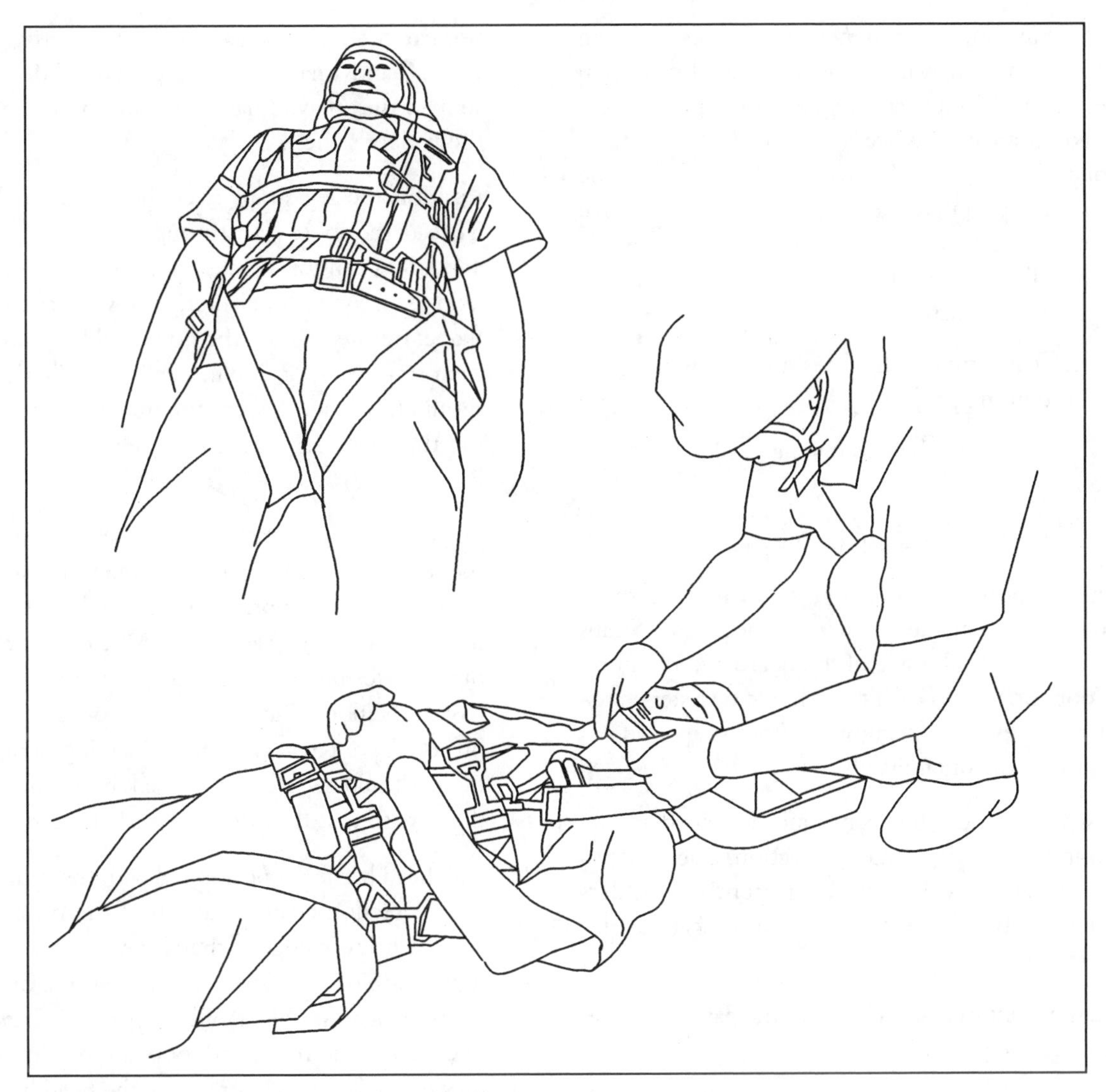

Figure 6–3 LSP halfback extrication/rescue vest.

10. Position the patient's head in the foam "V" of the back stay.

Note: It may be necessary to move the "stay" forward to contact the patient's head.

11. Position the head harness so that it is centered and resting against the top of the patient's head. Secure the harness in place by fastening the hook and loop fasteners to the corresponding surface on the back of the stay.
12. Secure the patient's head to the device by positioning the forehead strap across the patient's forehead above the eyebrows and securing both ends to the hook and loop surface on the head harness.
13. Connect the chin strap to both sides of the head harness by connecting the hook and loop fasteners to both sides in a manner such that the patient's mouth can be opened for airway maintenance.

Warning: Under no circumstances should the chin strap be so tight that a rescuer would be unable to perform adequate airway maintenance. Failure to comply with this warning could result in the death of the patient from aspiration of vomitus or other foreign bodies and body fluids that may be in the patient's oropharynx.

Miller Full-Body Splint/Litter

The Miller full-body splint/litter is a radioparent, chemical-resistant spinal immobilization board used for patients ranging in size from small children to large adults. Fabricated from a yellow plastic resin exterior and closed-cell foam interior, the board can be used in conjunction with Stokes type baskets with leg dividers to stabilize the potential c-spine injured patient. In addition to being chemical resistant and waterproof, the closed cell-foam core gives the board approximately 200 lbs. of buoyancy, which makes it an appropriate device for in-water stabilization of c-spine injuries. The narrow dimensions of the board make it appropriate for all types of confined-space evacuation. When used with the LSP halfback and optional vertical lift strap assembly, the Miller board can be used for vertical evacuations.

Note: Vertical hoisting techniques are not within the scope of this training program.

Follow these steps when using the Miller full-body splint/litter:

1. Position the board next to the patient.
2. Open the hook and loop straps and remove them from the pins on the left side of the board. Straps should be laid to the side of the board and the hook and loop surfaces on each strap should be fastened together to prevent tangling with other straps and accumulation of contaminants.
3. Using the straddle lift technique described in the "Lifting and Moving Patients" section, place the patient on the board with the patient's shoulders aligned evenly with the shoulder pins so that the pins are just visible.
4. Place the chest strap loosely across the patient's chest, excluding the patient's arms.
5. Slide the shoulder straps into position, aligned with the shoulder pins on their free end and positioned slightly to the outside of the patient's sternum on the fixed end.
6. Adjust the tension on the chest strap first while fastening the hook and loop surfaces together. Tension should be sufficient to hold the patient in position, but not so tight that it obstructs normal chest expansion.
7. Adjust the tension on the shoulder straps while fastening the hook and loop surfaces together. Tension should be sufficient to hold the patient in position, but not so tight that it obstructs normal chest expansion.
8. Place the torso strap across the patient's abdomen. Thread the strap through the corresponding pin on the board at the patient's left side, and adjust the tension on the strap while fastening the hook and loop surfaces together. Be careful not to overtighten. Patient's hands may either be placed inside the torso strap or they may remain unsecured and be placed on the patient's chest.
9. Position the leg straps over the corresponding leg. Thread the loose end through the appropriate pin and adjust tension on the strap so that the patient is held securely without interfering with circulation in that extremity. Fasten the hook and loop surfaces for each strap back on itself. Small or pediatric patients should have their lower extremities secured by passing the right leg strap completely across both their legs.
10. For full-sized patients, position the ankle straps over the corresponding ankle. Thread the loose end through the appropriate pin and adjust tension on the strap such that the patient is held securely without interfering with circulation in that extremity. Fasten the hook and loop surfaces of each strap back on itself. Rescuers who are packaging pediatric patients should secure the unused ankle straps out of the way so that they do not snag during transfer.
11. The head harness is positioned with the center foam-rubber section against the top of the patient's head and the bottom edge of the center section against the top surface of the board. Gently press the outer foam sections against the stabilized patient's head while connecting the hook and loop fasteners on the harness to the board. Placement of the head harness can also be accomplished with a cervical collar in place.
12. Connect the forehead strap to both sides of the head harness by connecting the hook and loop fasteners to both sides so that the strap is positioned squarely and securely across the patient's forehead above the eyebrows.
13. Connect the chin strap to both sides of the head harness by connecting the hook and loop fasteners to both sides so that the patient's mouth can be opened for airway maintenance.

Warning: Under no circumstances should the chin strap be so tight that it prevents the patient from opening his/her mouth or that a rescuer would be unable to perform adequate airway maintenance. Failure to comply with this warning could result in the death of the patient from aspiration of vomitus or other foreign bodies and body fluids that may be in the patient's oropharynx.

Plastic Basket Litter

Follow these steps when using a plastic basket litter:

1. Litter preparation.
   a. During periods of inclement weather, periods of extremely cold temperatures, or during windy conditions, line the litter with a tarpaulin or salvage cover that is large enough to completely surround the patient without being unmanageable.
   b. Place padding in litter at locations that correspond to knees, lumbar spine, neck, and back of patient's head (thin, closed-cell foam pads used as mattresses for campers can also be used).
   c. When weather conditions suggest a need to insulate the patient, place blanket #1 in the litter with the long axis lengthwise and centered in the litter, extending from the anticipated area of the patient's rib cage to 1 ft. more past the foot end of the litter.
   d. Blanket #2 is laid with the long axis across the litter and centered from side to side. The blanket edge that corresponds to the head of the litter should extend approximately 1 ft. past the end of the litter.
   e. Blanket #3 (hypothermia blanket) is laid on top of the second, with its long axis rotated 45° from that of the second blanket.

2. Position the patient in the litter either with or without c-spine stabilization devices in place as patient injuries dictate.

3. Apply wrap [hypothermia wrap (blanket #3) in cot].
   a. The diagonally placed blanket head end is folded down approximately 6 ins.
   b. The head end is folded down onto the forehead. (This will resemble the fold of a nun's habit.)
   c. The blanket point at the foot end should be folded up, toward the patient's head, and brought up between the patient's legs in the manner of a diaper, covering as much of the chest and neck area as possible.
   d. The blanket points on either side of the patient should be folded in across the chest area, leaving the arms exposed.

4. Apply "interior lashing." Tie leg loops on each of the patient's legs to prevent sliding toward the foot end of the litter.
   a. Pass a 15-ft. section of 1-in. tubular webbing under the patient's buttocks at the level of the groin area.
   b. Locate the center of the webbing length and form a bight at the center and pull this bight up between the patient's legs.
   c. Form two leg loops, one around each of the patient's thighs. Using the free end of the webbing, form an overhand knot around the side of the webbing bight and on top for the patient's thigh and on the leg that corresponds to the side that the free end is coming from.
   d. Pass each free end of webbing between the blanket and the litter to a point where it can be passed around the interior section of perimeter rope that is as close to the position of the patient's armpit as possible without crossing the patient.
   e. Remove all slack from the webbing and secure each free end of webbing to the perimeter rope with two round turns and two half hitches. A trauma dressing or surgipad placed between each of the webbing "leg loops" and the patient's groin area may help in minimizing patient discomfort and reduce the potential to restrict circulation through the femoral arteries.

5. Apply head blanket.
   a. Fold corners of blanket #2, at head end, in at a 45° angle toward foot end, approximately 18 ins. × 18 ins.
   b. Fold the edge of the blanket that extends past the head of the litter down over the patient's head, staying just above the eyebrows.
   c. Fold each side of that blanket completely across the patient's arms and chest in sequence.

6. Apply foot blanket.
   a. Fold the bottom end of blanket #1 up across the patient's feet.
   b. Fold each side of that blanket completely across the patient's legs and lower torso in sequence.

7. Apply foot lashing to prevent the patient from sliding toward the head of the basket.
   a. Using a 10 ft. to 12 ft. section of 1 in. tubular webbing, form a round turn around the patient's ankles by first passing the webbing across the top of the patient's foot, behind the ankles, and then crossing on top a second time. A trauma dressing or surgipad can be placed between the patient's ankles to minimize discomfort from snug ankle hitches.
   b. Form a stirrup in the webbing by passing one of the two sides of the round turn under the other, and then looping over that same section.

c. Position the stirrup under the patient's instep and adjust the tension on both ends of the webbing ankle hitch to make it snug around the ankles without causing any patient discomfort.

d. Secure each end of the ankle hitch to the perimeter rope with two round turns and two half hitches, making certain that there is no slack in the webbing.

8. Fill all void spaces around the patient to prevent shifting, provide additional padding and insulation, and to further stabilize any fractures.

9. Apply "exterior lashing" to prevent patient from falling out of the basket.
   a. Using one piece of 1 in. tubular webbing, rope, or a combination of shorter pieces that is approximately 25 ft. to 30 ft. in length, girth hitch the center of the length to the perimeter rail at the foot of the basket.
   b. Lash the patient in an X configuration, from foot to shoulder level by passing the girth-hitched webbing across the patient and through the space between the perimeter rail and the basket.

Note: Make certain that the lashing does not cross the patient's neck.

   c. Remove all slack from the lashing and secure the ends by forming two round turns around the perimeter rail at the level of the patient's shoulder and finishing with two half hitches.

Wire Basket Litter

Follow these steps when using a wire basket litter:

1. Litter preparation.
   a. During periods of inclement weather, periods of extremely cold temperatures, or during windy conditions, line the litter with a tarpaulin or salvage cover that is large enough to completely surround the patient is without being unmanageable.
   b. Place padding in litter at locations that correspond to knees, lumbar spine, neck, and back of patient's head (thin, closed-cell foam pads used as mattresses for campers can also be used).
   c. When weather conditions suggest a need to insulate the patient, place blanket #1 in the litter with the long axis lengthwise and centered in the litter, extending from the anticipated area of the patient's rib cage to 1 ft. or more past the foot end of the litter.
   d. Blanket #2 is laid with the long axis across the litter and centered from side to side. The blanket edge that corresponds to the head of the litter should extend approximately 1 ft. past the end of the litter (Figure 6–4).
   e. Blanket #3 (hypothermia blanket) is laid on top of the second, with its long axis rotated 45° from that of the second blanket (Figures 6–5 and 6–6).

2. Position the patient in the litter either with or without c-spine stabilization devices in place as patient injuries dictate.

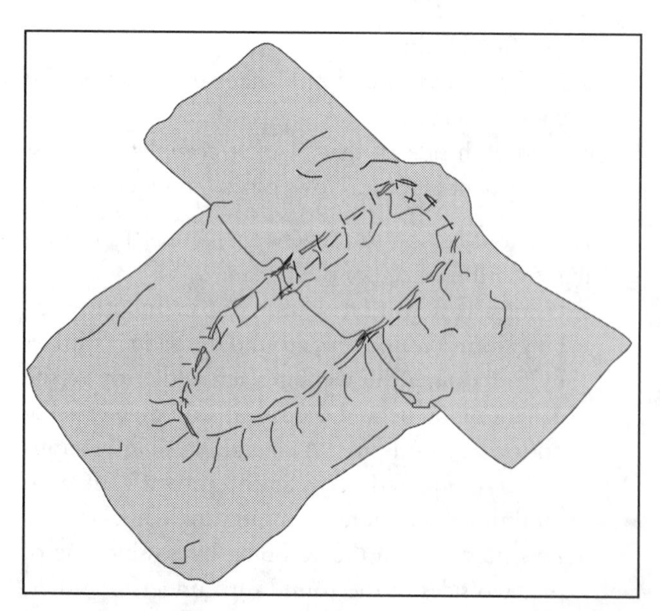

Figure 6–4 Blanket #2.

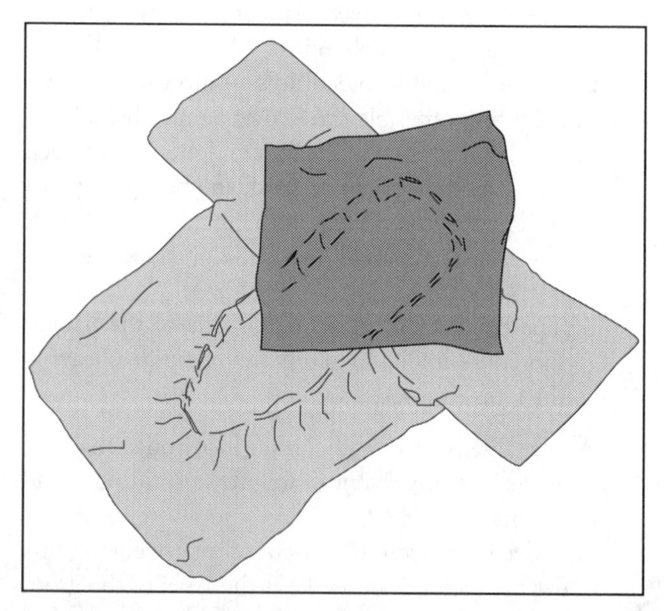

Figure 6–5 Blanket #3.

3. Apply wrap [hypothermia wrap (blanket #3) in cot].
   a. The diagonally placed blanket head end is folded down approximately 6 ins.
   b. The head end is folded down a second time, over the patient's forehead. (It will resemble the fold of a nun's habit.)
   c. The blanket point at the foot end should be folded up, toward the patient's head, and brought up between the patient's legs in the manner of a diaper, covering as much of the chest and neck area as possible.
   d. The blanket points on either side of the patient should be folded in across the chest area, leaving the arms exposed.
4. Apply "interior lashing." Tie leg loops on each of the patient's legs to prevent sliding toward the foot end of the litter.
   a. Pass a 15-ft. section of 1 in. tubular webbing under the patient's buttocks at the level of the groin area.
   b. Locate the center of the webbing length, form a bight at the center and pull this bight up between the patient's legs.

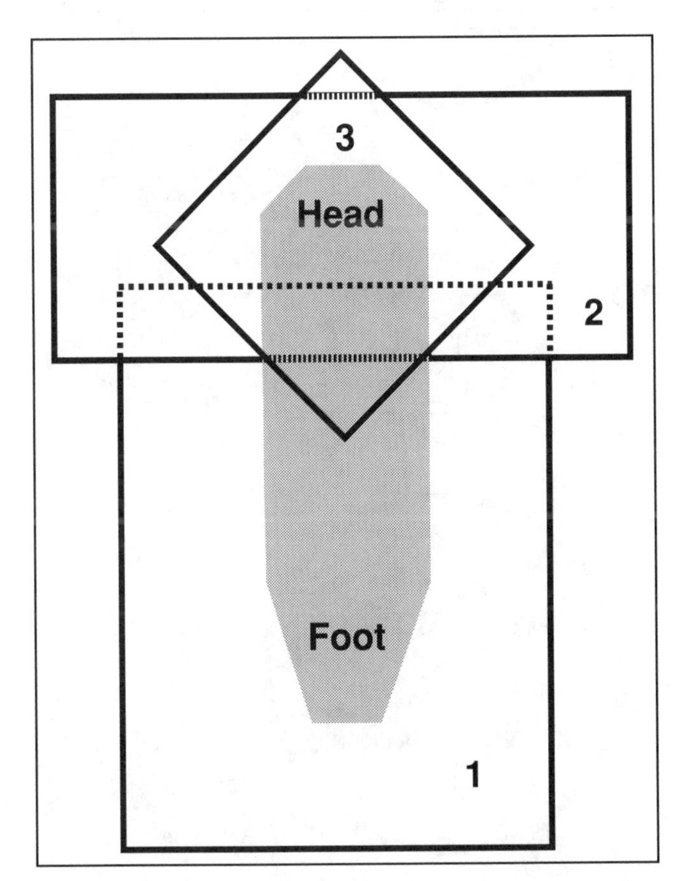

Figure 6–6 Blanket #3.

   c. Form two leg loops, one around each of the patient's thighs. Using the free end of the webbing, form an overhand knot around the side of the webbing bight, on top of the patient's thigh, on the leg that corresponds to the side that the free end is coming from. A trauma dressing or surgipad placed between each of the webbing "leg loops" and the patient's groin area may help in minimizing patient discomfort and reduce the potential to restrict circulation through the femoral arteries.
   d. Pass each free end of webbing between the blanket and the litter to a point where it can be passed around the basket rib that is as close to the position of the patient's armpit as possible without crossing the patient.
   e. Remove all slack from the webbing and secure each free end of webbing to the basket rib with two round turns and two half hitches (Figure 6–7).
5. Apply head blanket
   a. Fold corners of blanket #2, at head end, in at a 45° angle toward foot end, approximately 18 ins. × 18 ins.
   b. Fold the edge of the blanket that extends past the head of the litter down over the patient's head, staying just above the eyebrows.
   c. Fold each side of that blanket completely across the patient's arms and chest in sequence.

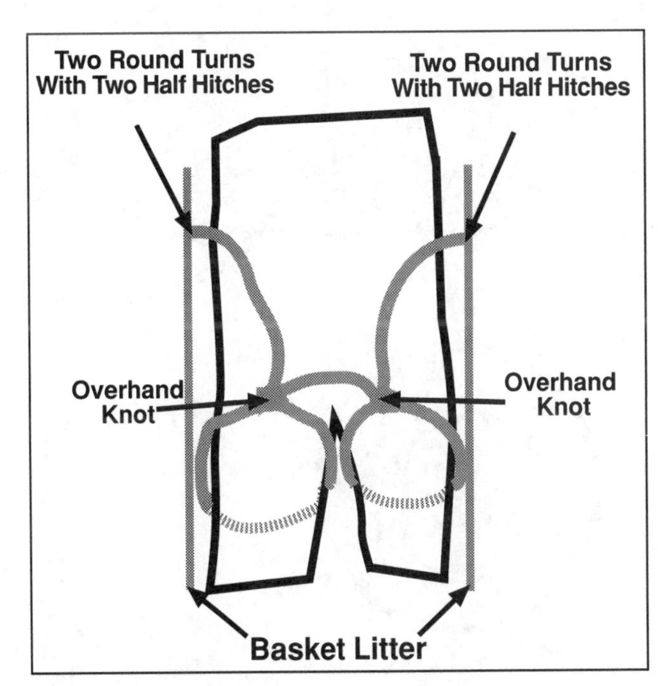

Figure 6–7 Secure each free end of webbing to the basket rib.

6. Apply foot blanket.
   a. Fold the bottom end of blanket #1 up across the patient's feet.
   b. Fold each side of that blanket completely across the patient's legs and lower torso in sequence.
7. Apply foot lashing to prevent the patient from sliding toward the head of the basket (Figures 6–8, 6–9, 6–10).
   a. Using a 10 ft. to 12 ft. section of 1 in. tubular webbing, form a round turn around the patient's ankles by first passing the webbing across the top of the patient's foot, behind the ankles, and then crossing on top a second time. A trauma dressing or surgipad can be placed between the patient's ankles to minimize discomfort from snug ankle hitches.
   b. Form a stirrup in the webbing by passing one of the two sides of the round turn under the other, and then looping over that same section.
   c. Position the stirrup under the patient's instep and adjust the tension on both ends of the webbing ankle hitch to make it snug around the ankles without causing any patient discomfort.
   d. Secure each end of the ankle hitch to the basket rib with two round turns and two half hitches, making certain that there is no slack in the webbing.
8. Fill all void spaces around the patient to prevent shifting, provide additional padding and insulation, and to further stabilize any fractures.
9. Apply "exterior lashing" to prevent patient from falling out of the basket (Figures 6–11 and 6–12).
   a. Using one piece of 1 in. tubular webbing, rope, or a combination of shorter pieces that is approximately 25 ft. to 30 ft. in length, girth hitch the center of the length to the top rail at the foot of the basket.
   b. Lash the patient in an X configuration, from foot to shoulder level by passing the girth-hitched webbing across the patient and around each rib encountered on the basket.

Note: Make certain that the lashing does not cross the patient's neck.

   c. Remove all slack from the lashing and secure the ends by forming two round turns around the basket rib at the level for the patient's shoulder and finishing with two half hitches.

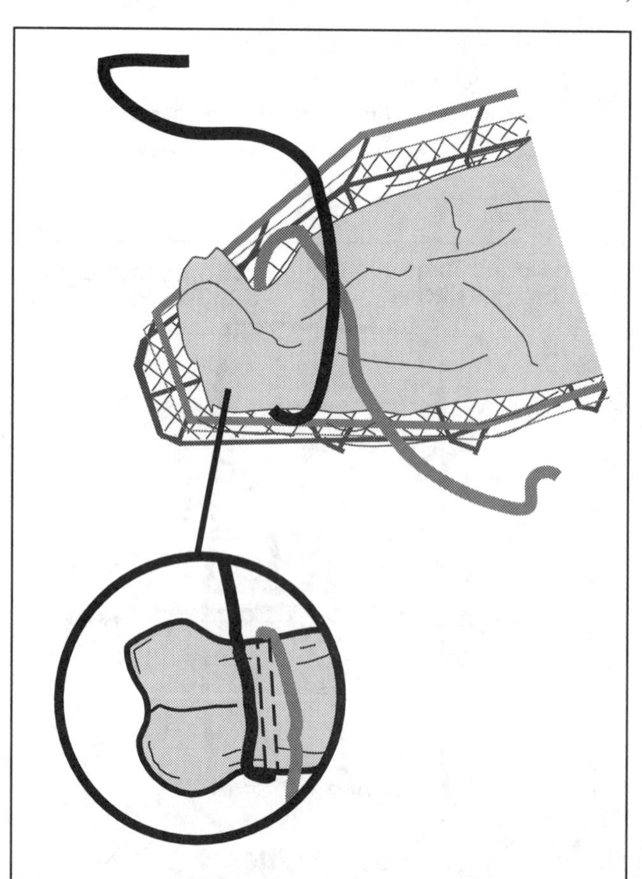

Figure 6–8 Foot lashing.

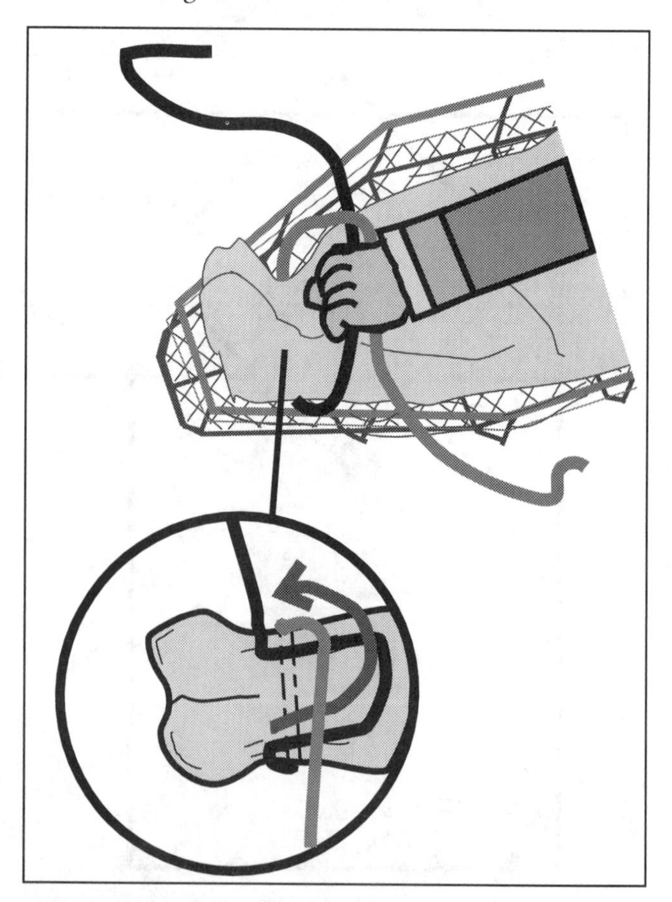

Figure 6–9 Foot lashing.

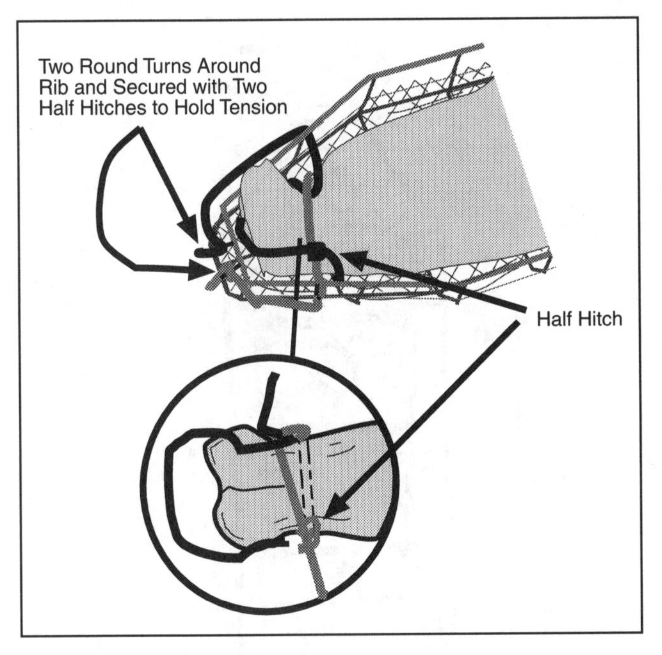

Figure 6–10 Foot lashing.

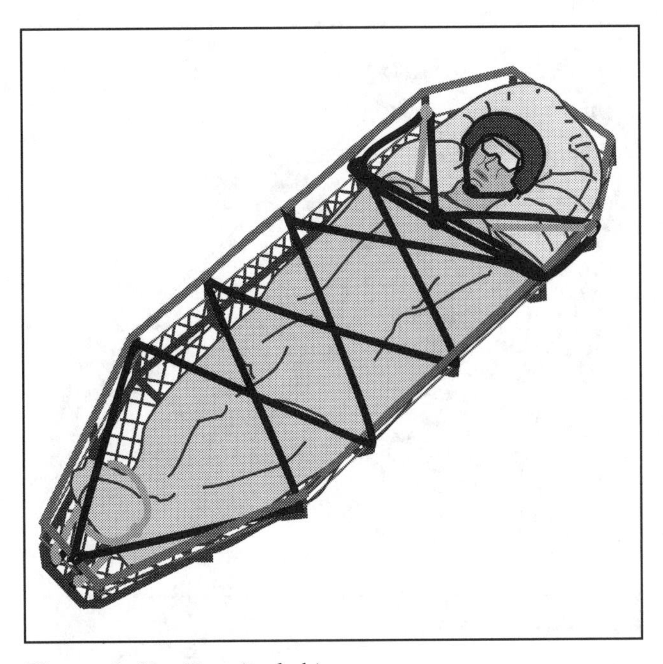

Figure 6–12 Exterior lashing.

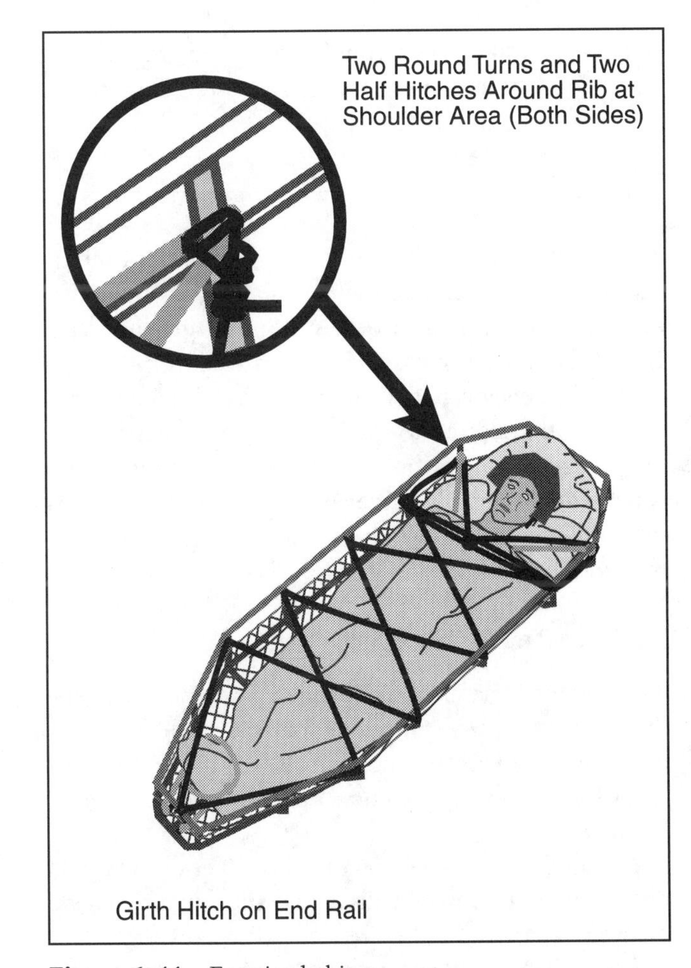

Figure 6–11 Exterior lashing.

SKED Stretcher

SKEDco Incorporated has developed a "complete rescue system" (Figures 6–13, 6–14, and 6–15) that has the ability to be rolled up for compact storage and ease of handling. It can be easily backpacked into remote areas or handled through small openings. There is a documented responses where a victim was inside a 6 ft. diameter tank that was 10 ft. long. He was packaged in the SKED then passed out through the tank hatch which was 11 in. × 15 in.

Another incident found the responders lashing two SKEDs together and packaging a 807-lb. victim then lowering him via a ladder slide from the second floor to the ground. Lowering the 807-lb. victim required eight rescuers. Experience has shown the SKED to be ideal for both vertical- and low-angle litter evacuation. The stretcher is radioparent and is easily applied and removed, reducing possible further injury to victims with spinal injuries.

The SKED stretcher provides a means for patient transfer, however, it is not a spinal immobilization device and should not be used for patients with suspected spinal injuries without separate, full-spinal immobilization. Also, when lifting one end of the SKED as in vertical-hoisting techniques, the patient's head can be hyperflexed due to the lack of rigidity of the device, therefore appropriate caution must be exercised to avoid this undesirable effect on the patient.

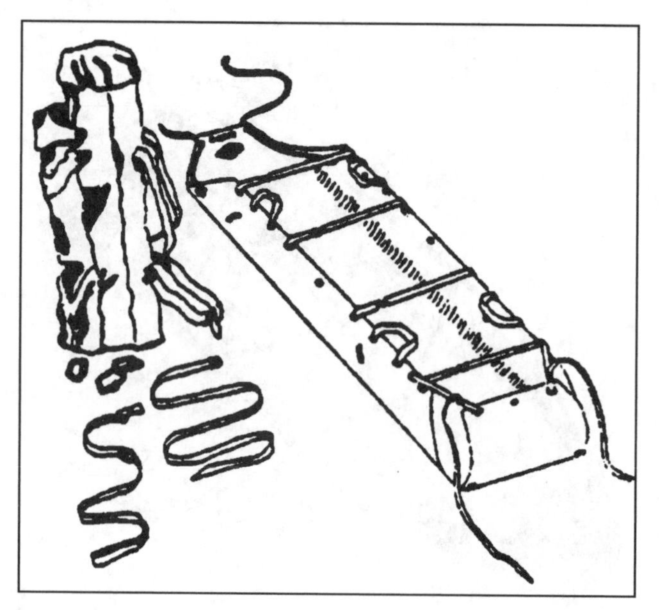

Figure 6–13 SKED device.

Note: Vertical hoisting techniques are not within the scope of this training program.

Follow these steps when using the SKED stretcher:

1. Unroll the SKED.
   a. Remove the SKED from pack.
   b. Unfasten strap, step on end of SKED, and unroll the device completely.
   c. Bend the SKED in half and roll each end toward the center, in the reverse direction from the direction used during storage.
   d. The device should lay flat after these preparations.
2. Position patient on the SKED using one of the techniques already described.
3. Secure the patient in the SKED.
   a. Lift both sides of the SKED and fasten the four cross straps to the buckles that are positioned directly across from them on the opposite side of the stretcher.

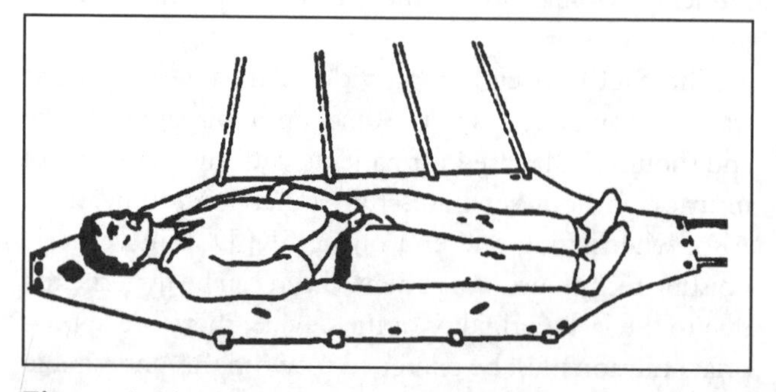

Figure 6–14 Securing patient to SKED lashing.

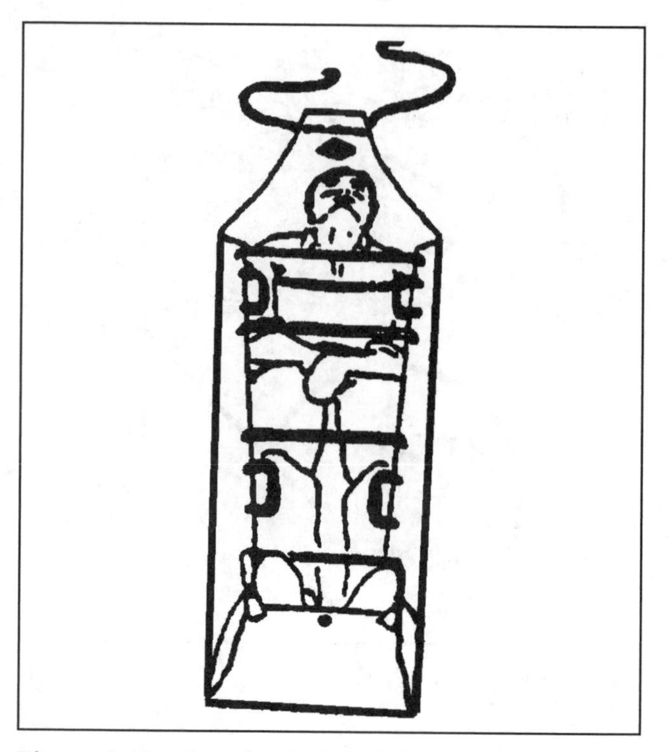

Figure 6–15 Completed SKED lashing.

   b. Feed foot straps through the unused grommets at the foot end of the SKED and fasten them to the corresponding buckles.

TRIAGE

Triage is the sorting of patients at mass casualty or multicasualty incidents and allocating resources for their care based on a system of priorities. During such incidents EMS personnel would decide which victims should receive emergency care first and in what order the injured are to be transported to medical facilities. Triage is defined as the sorting of, and the allocation of, treatment to patients and especially battle and disaster victims according to a system of priorities designed to maximize the number of survivors.

Four Priorities for Classifying Patients

The state of Maryland has designed a program whereby the victims are placed in one of four categories. The priorities are based on the assessment of the illnesses and injuries suffered by each victim. Patients are prioritized as follows:

Priority One Critically ill or injured person who will die or suffer permanent disability without immediate medical attention.

Priority Two Patients with less serious conditions that

require medical care who are not in immediate danger of dying or disability.

Priority Three Patients who require some degree of medical care but not on an emergency basis.

Priority Four Persons who do not require medical care or transport (e.g., obviously dead).

First responders must follow a logical sequence during these casualty incidents to maximize the use of available resources and afford the greatest potential for recovery of all the patients. The decisions are difficult at best and only through conformity to the standardized plan can the first responders on the scene make the proper decisions. Such decisions are perhaps the most difficult tasks to perform for anyone regardless of their training or experience. Unfortunately, it is a task that must be performed and followed in order for the available equipment and personnel to be used to the best advantage for all concerned.

The hardest decision confronting a first responder will probably be when the attending patient care provider advises that their patient is a Priority One but that major efforts are required to free them from entanglement while there are Priority Two or Three patients also in need of extrication who can be freed in a much shorter time. Who comes first? Some of the questions that need to be addressed are:

1. Will any of the victims with lower priority deteriorate before the first victim can be extricated?
2. Might the first victim die before extrication?
3. Who has the best chance of recovery?

The Maryland State Protocol for response to mass casualty or multicasualty incidents defines the responsibilities of the first arriving unit on a mass casualty incident as:

1. Conduct a quick "survival survey" while employing only basic life support skills for establishing airways or controlling profuse bleeding.
2. Direct "walking wounded" and those individuals being assisted by others to an area of relative safety to await assistance.
3. Attach colored flagging to patients to identify their priority for treatment:
   Red: Priority One
   Yellow: Priority Two
   Green: Priority Three
   Black: Priority Four
4. Once prioritized and immediately accessible patients are collected in an area of relative safety. First responders should administer emergency medical care (within the limits of their training) to the patients with the highest priority, until relieved by senior patient care providers.

First responders and rescue personnel must never lose their focus on the patient. Far too often the focus of the rescue incident is on transportation (getting to and from the rescue site) or on entanglement and entrapment issues (displacing metal, disassembly of machinery, etc.). While these are all vital issues for the Rescue Sector Officer, the focus must remain on the patient, without whom there would be no reason for any evolutions.

The intent for participants in this period of instruction is to focus on the skills necessary to ensure the welfare of the patients. As a collateral benefit of good patient care skills, rescuer safety is also enhanced.

REFERENCES

American Academy of Orthopaedic Surgeons. 1990. *Basic rescue and emergency care.* Park Ridge, IL: The Academy.

Grant, H.D., R.H. Murray, and D.J. Bergeron. 1990. *Emergency care.* 5th ed. Englewood Cliffs, NJ: Prentice Hall.

Maryland Institute for Emergency Medical Services Systems (MIEMSS). 1986. *The Maryland way.* 3rd. ed. Baltimore, MD: MIEMSS.

Segerstrom, J., and B. Edwards. 1994. *Low to high angle rescue technician.* Elk Grove, CA: Rescue 3, International.

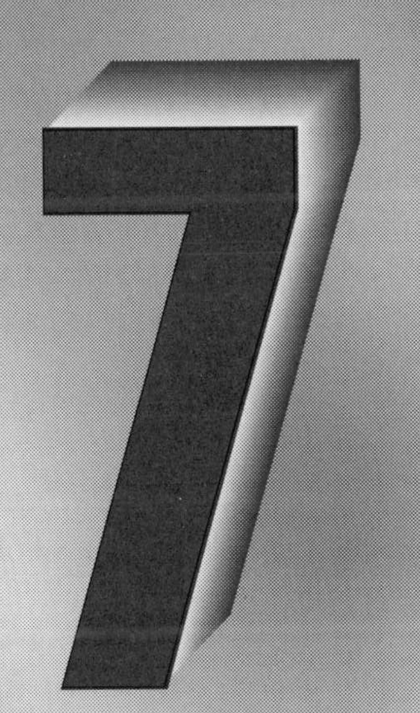

Slope Evacuation

OBJECTIVE

The student will be able to identify and demonstrate the practical skills and knowledge required to rig a rope system to assist rescuers who are transporting patients either up or down sloping terrain, while functioning as a team member, from memory, to an accuracy of 70% and the satisfaction of the instructor.

OVERVIEW

Slope Evacuation

- Definitions
- Terrain Evaluation
- Litter Rigging and Litter Bearer Tie-ins
- Vehicle Anchors
- Roadside Rigging
- Methods of Transporting the Litter
- Commands Used During Litter Slope Evacuations

ENABLING OBJECTIVES

7-1-1 Define the terms used in slope evacuations.

7-1-2 Identify the characteristics of flat, low-angle, steep-angle, and high-angle terrain and describe the role and necessity for rope systems and specially skilled rescuers in each different type of sloping terrain.

7-1-3 Demonstrate the proper method of attaching belay lines and hauling and lowering lines to the head of various patient transfer devices including litter bearer tie-ins using the following:
- Direct tie-in
- Webbing/rope "bridle"
- Prefabricated low-angle litter harnesses

7-1-4 Demonstrate anchoring to a vehicle for an "over-the-embankment" type of rescue including precautions to prevent vehicle movement. Distinguish between acceptable and unacceptable vehicle anchor points.

7-1-5 Demonstrate the applicable systems and proper procedures for roadside rigging down a slope from a vehicle anchor.
- Rescuer lowered
- Second rescuer lowered utilizing two-wrap prusik self-belay
- Litter bearers lowered
- Rappel utilizing figure-8 DCD
- Prusik belay system
- Lower litter utilizing figure-8 DCD with a prusik belay on second line

7-1-6 Demonstrate litter passing and hauling uphill:
- Using a caterpillar pass with a prusik belay
- Using a 1:1 system with ample staffing
- Using a 1:1 counter-balance system
- Using a 3:1 Z-rig anchored to a second vehicle

7-1-7 Define the commands used during slope evacuations.

INTRODUCTION

According to the National Safety Council, accidents (which are defined as violence that is not associated with suicides, homicides, acts of war, or for those incidents where the cause of the violence is uncertain) are the leading cause of deaths and injuries in the 1- to 44-year-old age group of the population. The leading cause of accidental deaths and injuries is motor vehicle accidents, followed in descending order of occurrence by drowning, falls, and fires.

Census surveys have shown that more and more Americans are relocating from high-density population centers to suburban and rural communities. As a result, increasing numbers of citizens have ventured out on roads and highways at younger ages and with lower experience and judgement levels to reach schools, shopping, employment, and recreation. America's increased mobility is reflected in increases in high-speed road construction and increases in motor vehicle ownership.

Advancements in highway and automobile designs coupled with America's traditional love affair with driving and owning automobiles, have made it possible for record numbers of inexperienced drivers to travel farther at higher speeds than ever before in U.S. history.

This increased mobility, coupled with newly developed action and adventure sports and opportunities, have opened new avenues to adventure for the adventurers among us. Those who wish to "go for the gusto" by leaping from heights, scaling mountains, braving savage rivers, or by swimming with sharks (with little or no requirements for skill or training) need only produce the required cash and sign the release forms. Some get themselves into trouble in locations and ways never even heard of before, knowing full well that the heroes of "911" will come to their aid when they are in trouble.

Couple all this high-speed, long-distance travel and the desire for the "ultimate rush," with alcohol or drugs and the results are a recipe for disaster.

What is the impact of these trends on rescuers? At minimum, first responders and patient care providers must be prepared to respond to emergencies at off-road, remote, previously uninhabited, or inaccessible locations where conventional patient transfer devices being wheeled along paved city streets and sidewalks are inappropriate. The objective of this session is to prepare students for that eventuality.

DEFINITIONS

Prior to developing technical skills in any field of rescue, students must first "learn the language" of the rescue discipline they are studying in order to avoid misunderstanding or misconception when rescuer's and their patient's lives are hanging in the balance between the hazards they are confronted by and the tools and the techniques being used in the rescue. The following definitions will aid the student in gaining an understanding of slope evacuation technical rescue.

Brakeperson: Person operating the descent control device that regulates the rate of descent of a litter during a slope evacuation.

Counter-balance haul system: A 1:1 hauling system in which a hauling team employs gravity to assist with the haul by descending a slope while hauling the litter and litter bearers up a slope.

Descent control device (DCD): A piece of rope rescue hardware that slows the rate at which rope slides through it by creating friction at the points of contact where the rope is reeved through the device. May be used in a "standing" or stationary configuration where the device is attached to a stationary anchor point and a rescue load is lowered on a rope that passes through the device. More commonly used as a "traveling brake" or rappel device which is attached to a descending rescuer or rescue load and travels on a fixed-descent line. Figure-8 plates and rappel racks are two examples of DCDs.

Girth hitch (ring hitch, larksfoot): A means of attaching a line or rope to an object where both the running end and the standing end of the line or rope are passed around the point of attachment and through the loop formed in the standing part of the rope.

Note: Similar to a prusik knot with a single wrap around the point of attachment.

Haul Team: The group of rescuers who provide the manual effort in a hauling system.

Prusik-minding pulley: A pulley designed to prevent a prusik knot from passing through it during hauling operations.

Rappelling: Descent on a fixed line by attaching a DCD to the rescue load so that friction is under the control of a descending rescuer.

Slope evacuation: The movement of a rescue subject over terrain that is so rugged or angled that it requires the litter to be safely tied with a rope and its descent controlled by a braking device or its ascent assisted with a hauling system.

Three-bight anchor: An anchor using webbing or rope tied into a fixed loop. That loop is passed around the anchor in a bight configuration. Easily recognized by the bight at either end of the loop as well as the third bight formed around the anchor.

TERRAIN EVALUATION

Within the state of Maryland most rescues occur in areas where patients can be transferred to the transport vehicle on a rolling, wheeled stretcher over pavement or at worst by performing a flat carry of a patient for a short distance on a backboard or in a basket litter.

Sometimes, however, rescuers are so conditioned to using these transfer mediums that they attempt to use them in inappropriate circumstances, with less-than-desirable results. Attempting to roll a wheeled stretcher through a heavily wooded area or attempting to use a conventional basket litter to remove a worker from the inside of a tank through a small opening are two such examples. In each case, the environment of the rescue dictates the type of transfer device to be used. A basket litter would be perfectly acceptable in the wooded environment rescue but is too large for passage through most tank scuttles.

The slope of terrain and the condition of the walking surface have a similar impact on the need for rope systems to support patient transfer operations and the degree of technical expertise required to construct and manage such a system.

Slope is only part of the formula. Rescuers may carry a basket litter up a small rise with little or no difficulty under dry weather conditions but find the same slope almost impossible to climb after periods of rain or snow. Therefore, a knowledge of how to read and anticipate the impact of the angle of terrain under varied weather conditions is essential to a successful patient transfer operation.

For the purpose of this discussion, the angle of terrain is divided into four categories:

- Flat terrain
- Low-angle terrain
- Steep-angle terrain
- High-angle terrain

Flat Terrain

Flat terrain is 0° to 15° off a horizontal plane.

The following are characteristic of flat-terrain evacuations:

1. Carries require five to six litter bearers walking upright with one foot in front of the other and scouts ahead of the litter bearers to select a route of travel, warn of obstacles and hazards in the path, and assist with passing over any obstacles encountered.
2. No external rope systems required. Footing is adequate for balance such that litter bearers can focus on carrying the litter without fear of dropping it, instead of using their hands to reach for handholds and struggling to maintain balance and footing.
3. No tie-ins required for bearers. Since the litter bearers are able to walk upright with one foot in front of the other, bearers have no need to be tied to a system to help them walk or to maintain balance and footing.
4. No technical gear or expertise required. Without a need for rope systems, there is no need for expertise to rig such a system.

5. Litter bearers carry 100% of the rescue load instead of having the load partially or completely supported by a rope.
6. Risk of falling injury is minimal. Aside from normal risks of tripping and falling, there is no significant threat of a fall at this inclination.

Low-angle Terrain

Low angle terrain is 15° to 40° off a horizontal plane.

The following are characteristic of low-angle terrain evacuations:

1. Carries require five to six litter bearers walking upright with some degree of difficulty due to the incline. Litter bearers may have a need to side step or walk in a slightly forward leaning direction to aid in balance and footing.
2. Belay line with a prusik knot to litter required for added safety. As the difficulty of walking increases, the need to use hands and careful foot placement also increases. In these circumstances, a safety line or belay may be desirable in the event that the litter is dropped.
3. No tie-ins required for bearers. Since litter bearers are, for the most part, able to walk without reaching for handholds, they do not have a need for a rope system to protect them from falling or to assist with moving the litter uphill.
4. Anchor system with single belay line as required. The use of simple anchor systems without being reinforced by supplemental tie-backs or multiple points of attachment are adequate for this minimal loading application.
5. Litter bearers carry 100% of the rescue load as they did on flat terrain.
6. With an increase in the angle of inclination, there is some risk of minor injury as a result of falls.

Steep-angle Terrain

Steep angle terrain is 40° to 65° off a horizontal plane.

The following are characteristic of steep-angle terrain evacuations:

1. Carries require three to four litter bearers sharing the weight of the litter with a supporting rope due to the steeper angle.
2. Rope lowering/hauling system required with belay. As the terrain becomes steeper, the litter bearers support the litter as it is moved forward by a rope and attached hauling system. Any attempt to climb a slope of this angle while carrying 100% of the weight of the litter would likely be unsuccessful if not disastrous.
3. Since the litter bearers hands are used to support the litter, the litter bearers must be tied into the rope system to protect them from falling and to move them up the slope.
4. Any failure in the rope system, from anchor failure caused by poor selection of anchor points, breakage of substandard hardware or software, or human error on the part of the haul team, could have catastrophic results. This application, therefore, requires a double-line system, prusik belay, and problem-solving capability.
5. As mentioned previously, on this angle of terrain, the rescue load is shared between the bearers and rope system with the rope system acting both as fall protection and means of moving uphill.
6. Without their hands to assist with climbing, litter bearers would almost certainly fall and be injured without rope systems.

High-angle (Vertical) Terrain

High-angle terrain is 65° to 90° off of a horizontal plane.

The following are characteristic of high-angle terrain evacuations:

1. Carries require one to two litter *attendants*. (Note that the terminology for the litter bearers changes as they cease to carry the weight of the litter and focus exclusively on providing patient care and assistance.)
2. Sophisticated rope-lowering and rope-raising systems with prusik belays are mandatory. In these extreme rescue challenges, the ability to build and operate mechanical advantage (MA) systems and belays for rescue loads is critical.
3. Litter attendants are suspended on a line separate from the litter bridle. This tie-in could be the running end of the main line tied into a long tail bowline or a short piece of life line attached to the main line via an end of the line loop such as a figure-8 on a bight or an appropriately tied bowline and a locking carabiner.

4. Any system failure in this environment will most likely result in the death of those suspended on the line. Thus, high-angle rescue specialists with a vast array of technical equipment and expertise are mandatory for building "bomb proof" anchors and complex raising and lowering systems.
5. Litter attendant(s) guide the litter over irregularities and administer patient care as required. In this type of evacuation, 100% of the rescue load is on the rope.
6. Unquestionably, any fall will result in serious injury or death.

LITTER RIGGING AND LITTER BEARER TIE-INS

When the terrain over which the patient will be transferred dictates the need for rope systems, the exact procedure for connecting the patient transfer device to the rope often poses a different set of problems. Many fire/rescue departments have basket litters but lack any clear procedure for attaching lines to the litter. Other departments may have invested in prestitched bridles that are designed for high-angle or vertical applications that do not easily convert to the linear movement configuration used in low/steep-angle rescue applications. Rescuers should be familiar with a variety of techniques for litter rigging, especially if they anticipate patient transfers on devices that belong to neighboring companies.

Direct Tie-in to Basket Litters, Full Backboards, and the Miller Board

1. Form a figure-8 knot approximately 4 ft. to 5 ft. from the running end of the main haul/lower line.
2. Pass the running end:
   a. Around the top rail of the wire basket litter, at the head end, in a spiral fashion, beginning outside one of the basket ribs that runs the length of the basket.
   b. Continue spiraling from outside to inside and then back to the outside of the corresponding basket rib on the other side of the basket litter.
   c. For plastic basket litters, the Miller full-body splint/litter, or for full backboards, proceed in a similar fashion to the description above, but instead of spiraling (since there are only two handholds for openings) form a girth hitch on the top rail passing through both hand-holds.
3. Retrace the figure-8 knot with the running end and finish with an overhand safety, allowing an extending tail of 10 ins. to 12 ins. (Figure 7–1).

Bridle Attachment Using Webbing/Rope

Basket Litters, Miller Boards, and Full Backboards

1. Tie a piece of 10 tubular webbing that is 10 ft. to 12 ft. in length into a fixed loop with a water knot leaving a tail of 3 ins. to 6 ins. protruding past both sides of the knot.
2. Form a bight in the fixed loop being careful not to include the water knot in the bight.
3. Pass the bight around the top rail of the wire basket, at the head end, in a spiral fashion, beginning outside one of the basket ribs that runs the length of the basket.
4. Continue spiraling from outside to inside and then back to the outside of the corresponding basket rib on the other side of the basket litter.
5. For plastic basket litters, the Miller full-body splint/litter, or for full backboards, proceed in a similar fashion to the description above, but instead of spiraling (since there are only two handholds for openings) form a girth hitch on the top rail passing through both handholds.
6. Join the two ends of the fixed loop together with a locking carabiner. The carabiner that attaches the bridle to the haul/lowering line is to be oriented with the open end toward the transfer device and the pivot pin toward the haul/lowering line. The gate should be on top to prevent it from being dragged over obstructions and the locking sleeve should be screwed closed tight over the gate opening and then unscrewed one-quarter turn.
7. Form a figure-8 on a bight knot at the end of the haul/lowering line so that the loop is no greater than 6 ins. to 8 ins. in length, there is sufficient length to the running end to tie an overhand safety knot directly behind the figure-8 on a bight knot, and there is a tail of 10 ins. to 12 ins. left protruding from the knot.
8. Attach the bridle for the patient transfer device to the impact end of the haul/lowering line using a carabiner.

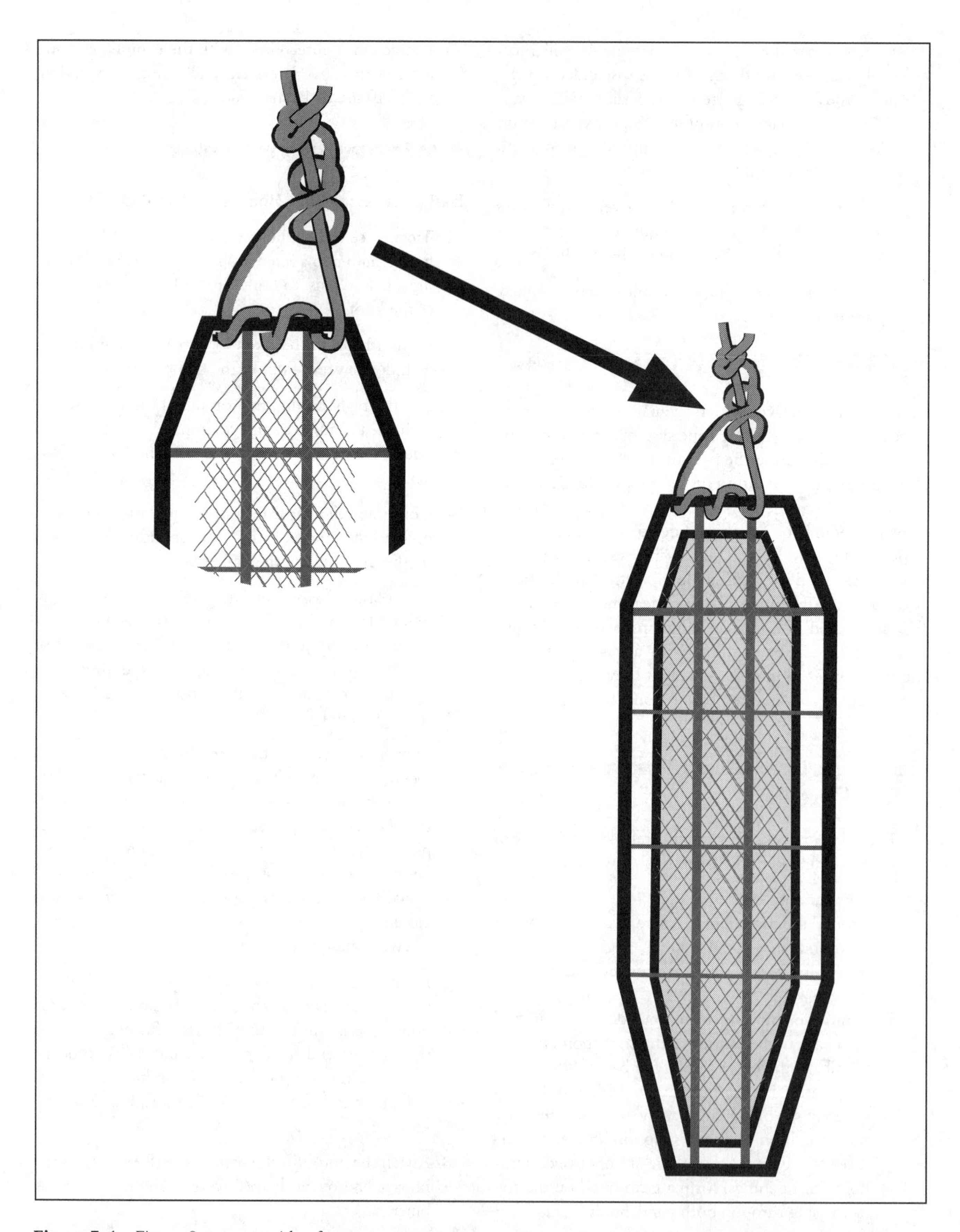

Figure 7–1 Figure-8 reweave with safety.

SKED Stretcher

This system for attaching a SKED stretcher to a haul/lowering line works equally well for all applications where linear movement of the SKED is desired, whether it is for steep-angle evacuations or for linear movement in a high-angle evacuation (Figure 7–2).

Note: Vertical hoisting techniques are not within the scope of this training program.

1. Pass each end of the 30 ft. × ⅜ in. static kernmantle line provided, through the grommets on each side of the head end of the SKED.
2. Feed the bridle line through all unused grommets and through all handles between the head and the foot of the SKED, making certain to keep both ends even and leaving a bight of rope at the head that is approximately 3 ft. to 4 ft. long.
3. Pass the ends of the bridle line through the grommets at the foot end of the SKED and tie them together on the outside of that end with a square knot.
4. Take all remaining excess back toward the head of the SKED, pass the ends through the carrying handles that are closest to the foot, and tie them together with a second square knot that is backed-up with overhand safety knots.
5. Tie the bight at the head end of the SKED into a loop with a figure-8 on a bight.

Prefabricated Low-angle Litter Harness

1. Attach the bridle to the haul/lowering line.
2. Form a figure-8 on a bight knot at the end of the haul/lowering line such that: the loop is no greater than 6 ins. to 8 ins. in length, there is sufficient length to the running end to tie an overhand safety knot directly behind the figure-8 on a bight knot, and there is a tail of 10 ins. to 12 ins. left protruding from the knot.
3. Attach the bridle for the patient transfer device to the loop at the end of the haul/lowering line using a carabiner. The carabiner that attaches the bridle to the haul/lowering line is to be oriented with the open end toward the transfer device and the pivot pin toward the haul/lowering line. The gate should be on top to prevent it from being dragged over obstructions and the locking sleeve should be screwed closed tight over the gate opening and then unscrewed one-quarter turn.

VEHICLE ANCHORS

Likely scenarios for slope evacuations include autos over embankments, sledding accidents, and obese patient transports from dwellings with narrow outside stairways. Many of these incidents will be in locations that are immediately adjacent to roadways where fire service vehicles will be parked. Rescuers should familiarize themselves with acceptable anchor points on fire service vehicles that could be used in the event of such a need. Beware of anchoring to ornamental "brite work," mirrors, etc.

Vehicle Startup and Movement

Vehicle startup and movement must be prevented by:

1. Removing keys or otherwise disabling the vehicle to prevent movement.
2. Tagging with a high-visibility sign or tag in the driver's position to advise that the vehicle is not to be moved.
3. Make certain that manual transmission vehicles are in gear and that automatic transmission vehicles are left in park.

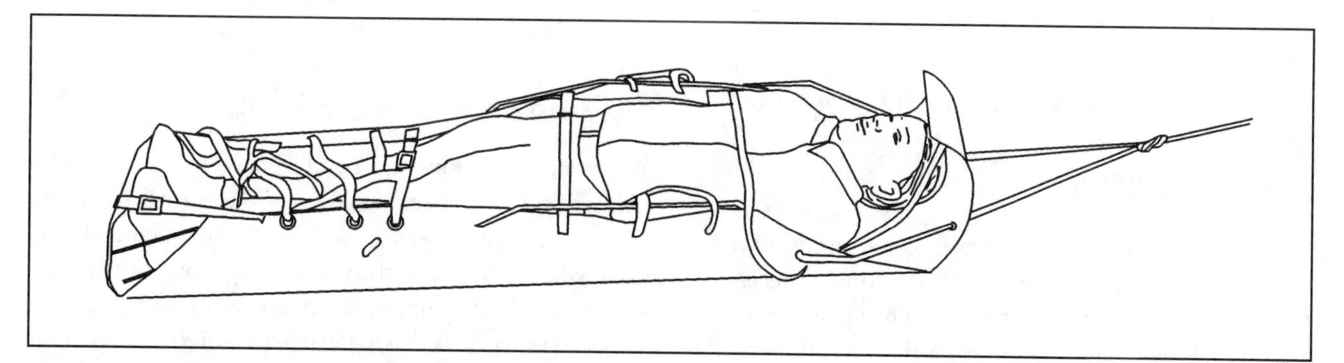

Figure 7–2 Use of SKED in linear movement.

4. Engage the parking brake.
5. Place wheel chocks in conspicuous locations at wheels to prevent movement.

Three-bight Wheel Anchors

Three-bight wheel anchors are the most secure and have the lowest probability of failure.

1. Anchors through holes in the rim and around the tire may expose anchor material to brake dust, however, there is some potential for contamination from bearing grease or for brake lines to be damaged. This is the most secure wheel anchor.
2. Three-bight anchors can be placed around tires at the road surface, however, there is some potential to pull the anchor material out from under some vehicle tires especially when sitting on gravel, mud, snow, etc.
3. Three-bight anchors can be placed through *moused* towhooks (hooks with the opening closed off with tape, twine, or wire to prevent anchor materials from coming unhooked).
4. Three-bight anchor through tow "eye" brackets.
5. Three-bight anchor around leaf springs, axles, frame components. (Watch out for brake lines.)
6. Three-bight anchor around "B" posts and roll bars with padding to prevent damage to painted surfaces.

Constructing a Three-bight Anchor

To construction three-bight anchors:

1. Select a length of 1 in. tubular webbing or ½ in. diameter static kernmantle rope that is at least six times the diameter of the anchor object.
2. Tie a fixed loop using either a water knot for webbing or a figure-8 retrace for rope.
3. Pass the loop around the back side of the anchor object.
4. Join the two free ends together with a carabiner.

ROADSIDE RIGGING

For a search-and-rescue operation to be successful, rescuers must reach the victim with the resources necessary to stabilize him/her prior to transfer. The victim becomes a patient of the rescuers once they arrive with their packaging and stabilization resources.

Once rescuers have reached the victim, provided initial patient care, and have packaged the patient for transfer, rescuers who are supporting the litter bearers/patient care providers contribute to the means of transfer. They either control the rate of descent down the slope or haul the rescue team and patient back up the slope. Routes of access to awaiting-patient transport vehicles determine which way to go on the slope. Given any choice in the matter, rescuers should choose to lower the rescue team wherever conditions permit. Remember the keep it simple stupid (KISS) principle, the more complex the rescue the greater the potential for problems. By far, lowering usually offers the least technical problems so long as the anchors and equipment are adequate for the rescue loads (including rope that is long enough to reach the bottom).

This step-by-step explanation will guide the student/rescuer through an assortment of practical evolutions for descending slopes via rescue lines with "standing brakes," "traveling brakes," and by utilizing prusik knots in short loops of accessory cord attached to the rescuer's harness as a "self-belay" to prevent him/her from falling down the slope while descending to the victim.

Rigging for a Rescuer to be Lowered Down a Slope

1. Using a carabiner, attach a figure-8 DCD to a vehicle anchor after threading a rescue rope of adequate length through the DCD.
2. Attach a loop of 7 mm or 8 mm accessory cord to the rope with a two-wrap prusik and attach the loop to the same carabiner as the DCD.
3. Tie a figure-8 on a bight knot in one end of the rescue rope and use a carabiner to attach the rope to the attachment point on a harness being worn by a rescuer.
4. After a safety check, and with a safety line tender wearing gloves, lower the rescuer until the patient is reached and tie off the figure-8 DCD.

Descending a Slope Using a Prusik "Self-Belay"

After safety checking a second rescuer for gloves and a helmet, and after checking all straps and harness hardware for correct assembly, the second rescuer descends the slope while attached to the first rescuer's lowering line by a short length of 7 mm or 8 mm accessory cord tied with a two-wrap prusik "self-belay" to assist with patient packaging.

Rigging for a Team of Litter Bearers to be Lowered Down a Slope from a Vehicle Anchor

1. Construct a second anchor using the same size webbing as close to the first anchor as possible.
2. Reeve a second line of adequate length through a figure-8 DCD and attach it to the new anchor with a carabiner.
3. Construct a field-fabricated bridle on the head end of the litter to be lowered/raised.
4. Attach the lowering line to the litter bridle with an in-line figure-8 knot and a carabiner.
5. Make sure there is patient packaging material and any needed medical supplies in the litter prior to sending it down the slope.
6. After safety-checking the two litter bearers as described above, use a carabiner to attach their harnesses to loops of 7mm or 8mm accessory cord that are girth hitched around the top rail of the litter at three o'clock and nine o'clock positions.
7. Safety-check the system and lower the litter and the two bearers.
8. Once in position to load the patient, tie off the figure-8 DCD.
9. The four rescuers work together to load the patient into the litter and attach both interior and exterior lashings.
10. First two rescuers disconnect from the first lowering line and each one attaches to the litter rail by a girth hitched, 2 ft. loop of 7mm or 8mm accessory cord, one at the four o'clock position and one at the eight o'clock position. The first two litter bearers adjust their position as necessary.

Descending a Slope by Rappelling

1. Disconnect the unattached line and the DCD from its anchor point.
2. Reattach the disconnected line to the three-bight anchor with a carabiner after tying a figure-8 on a bight knot in the rope.
3. After safety-checking a fifth rescuer for gloves, helmet, and harness, the fifth rescuer descends the slack rope by rappelling with a figure-8 DCD to assist with litter transport.
4. The fifth rescuer uses a carabiner to connect to a 2 ft. loop of 7mm or 8mm accessory cord which is girth hitched at the six o'clock position on the top litter rail. This litter bearer is designated as the "litter captain" who directs all hauling and lowering activities.
5. The fifth rescuer disconnects the DCD from the rappel line.

Construction of a Prusik Belay System

1. Rescuers at the top of the slope disconnect the rappel line from the three-bight anchor that it was attached to.
2. Those same rescuers attach a loop of 7mm or 8mm accessory cord using a three-wrap prusik to the disconnected line and attach the other end of the loop to the carabiner that the line had previously been attached to. A tandem prusik belay system can also be used.
3. The litter bearers on the slope add the figure-8 on a bight loop that is tied in the free end of the rappel line to the carabiner that already attaches the lowering line to the litter bridle.

Lowering the Litter and Litter Bearers with a DCD and a Prusik Belay

1. One rescuer is designated as the brakeperson to control the rate of descent for the litter bearers using the figure-8 DCD.
2. One rescuer is designated as the belayperson who prevents the prusik from setting on the belay line during desired movement by manually holding on to the prusik during lowering operations.
3. On command, the litter bearers lift the litter and the brakeperson, as directed by the litter captain, lowers it down the slope. Litter bearers must assume a position that is at a right angle to the surface of the slope for best footing. On steep slopes this position is effectively the same as the position one assumes when on rappel with the weight of the rescuers fully supported by the loops that are attached to the basket litter.

METHODS OF TRANSPORTING THE LITTER

There are locations where lowering the litter and the litter bearers down the slope is an inappropriate evacuation route. In those situations, a variety of hauling options are available that employ varying numbers of personnel for haul teams.

Litter Ascent of a Slope Using a "Caterpillar Pass"

This technique for moving a litter up a slope takes on the appearance of a caterpillar (a small wormlike larva having many pairs of legs) by having one column of rescuers standing abreast of the other rescuers in their column, facing a second column of similarly positioned rescuers while the litter is passed from hand to hand up the slope between the two columns.

1. Unwrap the figure-8 DCD and allow enough line out for the prusik on the belay line to set on the belay line and take the load.
2. When the load has been transferred to the belay line, disconnect the lowering line from the bridle and remove the rope from the DCD.
3. Remove the DCD and the carabiner from the three-bight vehicle anchor.
4. Remove the three-bight anchor from the vehicle.
5. Position the rescuers in two rows facing each other along the anticipated path of travel of the litter.
6. Pass the litter up the slope through the rescuers' hands as the belayperson pulls the resulting slack in the belay line uphill and through the prusik knot.
7. As the litter leaves the hands of the rescuers that are positioned the farthest down the slope, they climb to a position at the head of the line, closest to the top of the slope, to receive the litter and pass it on from that position.

Litter Ascent of a Slope Using Ample Personnel as a Hauling Team

When the skill or understanding of the rescuers is inadequate to perform the caterpillar pass or when safety considerations deem that technique inappropriate, alternate litter ascent options must be considered. On occasions where personnel is in bountiful supply, a simple change of direction pulley on a separate haul line from the belay line, along with multiple rescuers acting as a haul team to pull the litter team up the slope, may be employed.

1. Establish the belay line as detailed above.
2. Attach a separate three-bight vehicle anchor as close to the anchor for the belay as possible.
3. Tie a figure-8 on a bight in the end of a second rope and attach it to the carabiner at the litter bridle.
4. Attach a short loop of 7 mm or 8 mm accessory cord to the second rope using a three-wrap prusik.
5. Attach a prusik-minding pulley (PMP) to the second line at a point on the opposite side of the prusik from the litter.
6. Use one carabiner to attach the loop and the PMP to the new three-bight anchor.
7. On command from the litter captain, while the designated belayperson pulls slack in the belay line through the belay prusik, all necessary/available personnel act as a hauling team and haul the litter and team of litter bearers up the slope by pulling the rope as they walk away from the vehicle anchor. The number rescuers in the hauling team is determined by the difficulty of moving the litter and litter bearers up the slope.
8. Hauling team pulls the second line at a 90° angle to the slope.

Litter Ascent of a Slope Using a 1:1 Counter Balance System

When less personnel are available or when patient condition or conditions at the rescue site dictate that the evacuation be expedited without waiting for the arrival of additional personnel, smaller hauling teams can employ gravity to assist with the hauling operation.

1. Establish the belay line as detailed above.
2. Attach a separate three-bight vehicle anchor as close to the anchor for the belay as possible.
3. Tie a figure-8 on a bight in the end of a second rope and attach it to the carabiner at the litter bridle.
4. Attach a short loop of 7 mm or 8 mm accessory cord to the second rope using a three-wrap prusik.
5. Attach a PMP to the second line at a point on the opposite side of the prusik from the litter.
6. Use one carabiner to attach the prusik loop and the PMP to the new three-bight anchor.
7. On command from the litter captain, while the designated belayperson pulls slack in the belay line through the belay prusik, personnel act as a hauling team and descend the slope while attached to the hauling line using prusiks to aid in gripping the rope.

Litter Ascent of a Slope Using a 3:1 Z Rig

When the angle of the slope is steep or when the footing is treacherous such as snow covered, muddy, wet grass or loose flowing rock or gravel, the amount of support required by the litter bearers may exceed the capabilities of a hauling team with a 1:1 system. Treacherous footing also rules out the option of a caterpillar pass and a counter-balance system. During these circumstances, or any others when skilled rope rescuers and hardware are available, large numbers of rescuers are not required for the haul team if MA haul systems are employed.

While there are several MA options available, only one will be addressed in this program due to the simplicity in constructing it and to economize on the amount of time spent on this area of expertise.

1. Establish the belay line as detailed above.
2. Attach a separate three-bight vehicle anchor as close to the anchor for the belay as possible.
3. Tie a figure-8 on a bight in the end of a second rope and attach it to the carabiner at the litter bridle.
4. Attach a short loop of 7 mm or 8 mm accessory cord to the second rope using a three-wrap prusik.
5. Attach a PMP to the second line at a point on the opposite side of the prusik from the litter.
6. Use one carabiner to attach the prusik loop and the PMP to the new three-bight anchor.
7. Position a second vehicle on the shoulder of the road, in line with and approximately 30 ft. away from the end of the vehicle to which the PMP is attached.
8. Attach a three-bight anchor to the second vehicle, preferably on the same side of the vehicle as the anchors are attached on the first vehicle, and on the end of the second vehicle that is closest to the first.
9. Attach a single sheave rescue pulley to the new anchor.
10. Use a carabiner and a 7 mm or 8 mm accessory cord loop with a three-wrap prusik knot to attach a single-sheave rescue pulley to the haul line at a point between the PMP on the first vehicle and the single-sheave pulley on the second vehicle.
11. Pass the standing end of the haul line through the pulley on the second vehicle.
12. Double the standing end of the haul line back toward the first vehicle and pass the standing end through the pulley that was last attached to the haul line with the loop of accessory cord.
13. On command from the litter captain, while the designated belayperson pulls slack in the belay line through the belay prusik, all necessary/available personnel act as a hauling team and haul the litter and team of litter bearers up the slope by pulling the rope as they walk away from the first anchor vehicle toward the second.

COMMANDS USED DURING LITTER SLOPE EVACUATIONS

While each rescue presents different conditions and circumstances, certain aspects of all rescues remain fairly constant. Rescues usually occur at the worst possible times and in the worst locations. Whether the rescue is in the middle of a busy interstate or at the side of a rain-swollen creek, the lives and safety of both the rescuers as well as the patients rely on coordination of efforts within the rescue team. Effective communications between team members and sectors within the incident are critical to that coordination.

The following list of commands represents only the bare essential messages that may need to be communicated. Augmentation with hand and arm signals, whistle blasts, etc., ensures that your rescue team is always getting the correct message.

"On belay" (litter captain to belayperson) The litter bearers are attached to the system and are ready to ascend or descend the slope.

"Belay on" (belayperson to litter captain) The belay device is in place and the belayperson is ready to catch the rescue load.

"Down slow" or "Down fast" (litter captain to brakeperson) Describes the desired rate of descent for the litter bearers.

"Stop" (may be given by anyone who sees danger of a potential problem developing) All activities stop and the brakeperson and litter captain communicate what problem has been identified.

"Off belay" (litter captain to belayperson) The litter has reached the desired location and has been set down in a secure spot.

"Belay off" (belayperson to litter captain) The belay is no longer being tended.

Note: With the terms "Off belay" and "Belay off," remember that a belay should always be attended until your patient reaches safety. These terms are considered interactive communications between the litter captain(s) and the belayperson(s).

"Prepare to haul" (haul team captain to haul team and litter team) The haul team is to grasp the end of the haul line and prepare to haul the load up the slope.

"Set" (means "set the safety"; given by the haul team captain to belayperson) Hauling has stopped and the rescue load is to be secured to prevent slippage.

"Safety is set" (belayperson to haul team captain) The safety device has been affixed to the haul line to prevent slippage.

"Slack" (means overhaul/reset the system; given by the haul team captain to the haul team) The safety is holding the rescue load, extend the hauling system out to its full range of travel.

"Haul" (litter captain to haul team captain) The litter bearers have raised the litter and are prepared to continue their ascent of the slope. Can also be given by the haul team captain to the haul team when they begin/resume pulling the load up the slope by pulling on the haul line.

Every year hundreds of rescuers and public safety personnel sustain back and joint injuries as a result of improper lifting of patients. Transporting patients over sloping terrain poses an exceptional hazard of personal injury to rescuers and patients alike. By practicing slope evacuation techniques, rescuers develop proficiency in skills which may prevent injuries as well as increase operational effectiveness on calls in sloping environments.

REFERENCES

American Academy of Orthopaedic Surgeons. 1990. *Basic rescue and emergency care*. Park Ridge, IL: The Academy.

National Fire Academy. 1993. *Rescue systems I.* Washington, DC: United States Fire Adminstration and California State Fire Marshal's Office, Fire Service Training and Education System.

Thorne Group, Inc. 1989. *Introduction to rope rescue, #1A*. Lake Elizabeth, CT: Thorne Group.

Vines, T., and S. Hudson. 1989. *High angle rescue techniques*. Dubuque, IO: Kendall/Hunt Publishing Co.

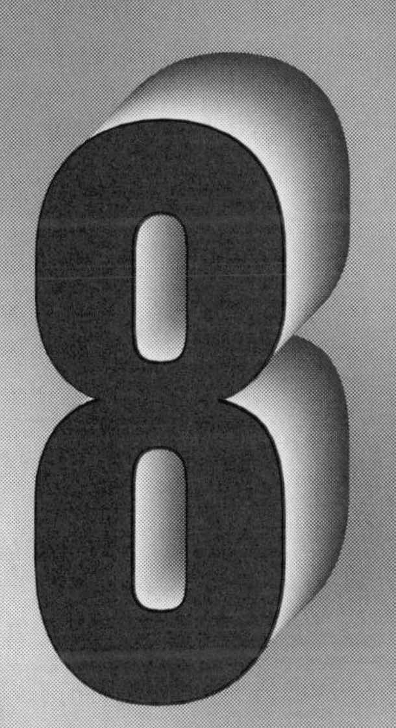

Skills Proficiency Evaluation: Rope Rescue Systems and Exam #1

OBJECTIVE

The student will be able to demonstrate knowledge and understanding of the skills learned in sessions 1 through 7, on a written exam and skills proficiency evaluation, from memory, without assistance, to an accuracy of 70% and to the satisfaction of the instructor. **This is a pass/fail point in the program.** Satisfactory completion permits the student to continue in the program.

OVERVIEW

Rope Rescue Systems

- Rescue Knots and Harnesses
- Mechanical Advantage and Anchor Systems
- Patient Transfer Devices

ENABLING OBJECTIVES

8-1-1 Demonstrate the correct tying of all knots, proper donning and doffing of a harness as selected by the instructor, and correctly prepare for slope rappel.

8-1-2 Demonstrate the reeving of block-and-tackle systems as selected by the instructor, rig both a simple and a compound hauling system, and correctly anchor the system using an anchor selected by the instructor.

8-1-3 Demonstrate the securing of a patient in a transfer device as selected by the instructor and correctly prepare the transfer device for horizontal movement.

I. Skill Station 1
Rescue Knots and Harnesses (Individual Skill Evaluation)
Correctly tie the following family of figure-8s:

1. Figure-8
2. Figure-8 reweave
3. Figure-8 bend
4. Figure-8 bight

Correctly tie the following clove hitch knots:

5. Clove hitch *around* an object
6. Clove hitch *over* an object
7. Split clove hitch
8. Correctly *don and doff* harness specified by the evaluator
9. Using the donned harness, correctly prepare for slope rappel

II. Skill Station 2
Mechanical Advantage and Anchor Systems (Team Evaluation)
Correctly demonstrate the following:

10. Reeve a mechanical advantage block-and-tackle system specified by the evaluator
11. Reeve a Z-system
12. Reeve a piggyback system
13. Anchor the system using a natural anchor point
14. Anchor the system using an anchor point on vehicle
15. Anchor the system using a picket holdfast

III. Skill Station 3
Patient Transfer Devices (Team Evaluation)
Correctly demonstrate the following:

16. Secure a patient in a Stokes basket
17. Secure a patient in a SKED stretcher or LSP
18. Prepare the transfer device for horizontal movement

REFERENCES

See Reference Section, Sessions 1–1 through 7–1

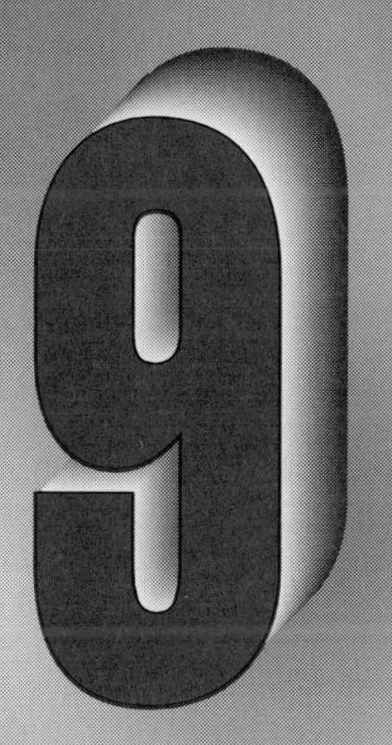

Principles of Vehicular Construction and Associated Technology

OBJECTIVE

The student will be able to describe the components of vehicular construction as they relate to passenger vehicles using models and diagrams, from memory, without assistance, to an accuracy of 70% and the satisfaction of the instructor.

OVERVIEW

Principles of Vehicular Construction and Associated Technology

- Types of Vehicular Construction
- Construction Components
- Component Reactions in Collisions
- Developing an Extrication Plan
- Vehicular Fuel Systems

ENABLING OBJECTIVES

9-1-1 Describe types of vehicular construction.

9-1-2 Describe vehicular construction components.

9-1-3 Describe vehicular component reactions during collisions.

9-1-4 Describe the parts to keep in mind when developing an extrication plan.

9-1-5 Describe the various types of vehicular fuel systems.

TYPES OF VEHICULAR CONSTRUCTION

By far the most common rescue operations performed today involve the passenger vehicle. For the extrication to be effective and efficient, the rescuer must be familiar with the construction of these vehicles. Passenger vehicles come in too many styles and makes to develop a procedure for each. Common elements of all vehicles is the way in which they are constructed. This section introduces the rescuer to the common elements of modern vehicle construction.

Prior to the oil crisis of the 1970s, vehicles were very large and heavy. Materials and welding techniques applied to a frame, produced vehicles which could withstand large impacts. With the sudden shortage of fuel, manufacturers were forced to develop vehicles that would be able to use fuel more efficiently, producing more miles to the gallon.

There are three ways to achieve efficient fuel use: decrease the weight of the vehicle, improve the power plant's use of the fuel, and improve the fuel. Manufacturers developed better methods of construction which produced lighter and stronger vehicles. The development of these vehicles continues today.

Full-frame Construction

Full-frame construction was the most common method prior to the 1970s. This method uses a steel frame to support the floor, suspension, drivetrain, and body. Molded steel was used in the frame and rolled sheet metal in the body. Due to the strength of the these materials, the hydraulic rescue tool was developed. Using lighter and stronger materials, full-frame construction is currently found in pickup trucks, station wagons, and some mini vans.

Unit Body Construction (Uni-body)

Unit body construction was developed to decrease the weight of various vehicles and to improve gas mileage. This was a radical change in vehicle construction methods. With unit body construction there is no frame, and

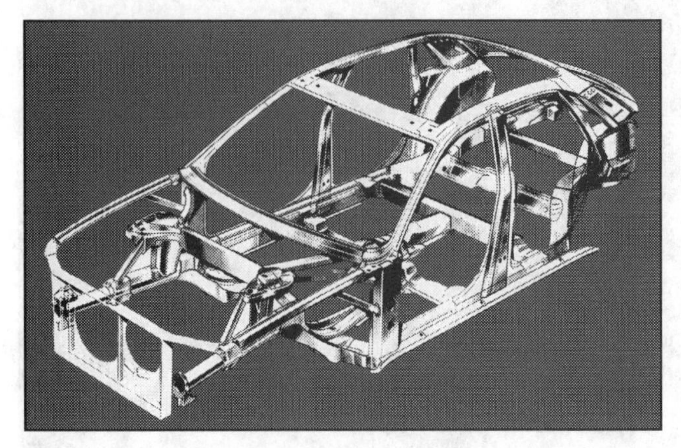

Figure 9–1 Space frame construction.

materials are lighter in weight and gauge. Rails, posts, floor, doors, and roof are welded together to support the drivetrain and suspension systems. The effect is much like the truss system used in building construction. All parts support the others to increase the overall strength. Remove any one component and the structural stability of the vehicle will be weakened.

Space Frame Construction

Vehicles of the future will be constructed using the space frame method. This is a new technology being developed currently by the Saab Motor Company. This method uses aluminum materials in its frame design. This construction is based on two parts. The weight of the vehicle demands 70% of fuel consumption and the rigid side impact standards that are mandated in the United States for the 1997 model year. The aluminum space frame has 50% the weight with twice the strength when compared to steel unit body construction. The weight and strength of aluminum make it the material of the future in vehicle construction and design (Figure 9–1).

CONSTRUCTION COMPONENTS

Figure 9–2 depicts the vehicle terminology used in vehicle construction.

The most prevalent material used in the construction of unit body is sheet metal. Rolled sheet metal has enhanced strength. Consider a soda can. While made of aluminum, it has similar properties of sheet metal. Roll the sheet out like paper, the sheet is very weak. To strengthen its ability to support any weight, the sheet must also be supported. If you roll the sheet and stand it on end, the same sheet will support many times its own weight.

Check Your Knowledge

_____ **A Pillar**	_____ **Roof Rail**
_____ **B Pillar**	_____ **Rear Quarter Panel**
_____ **C Pillar**	_____ **Rocker Channel**
_____ **Hinge Side**	_____ **Kick Panel**
_____ **Latch Side**	_____ **Corner / V Space**

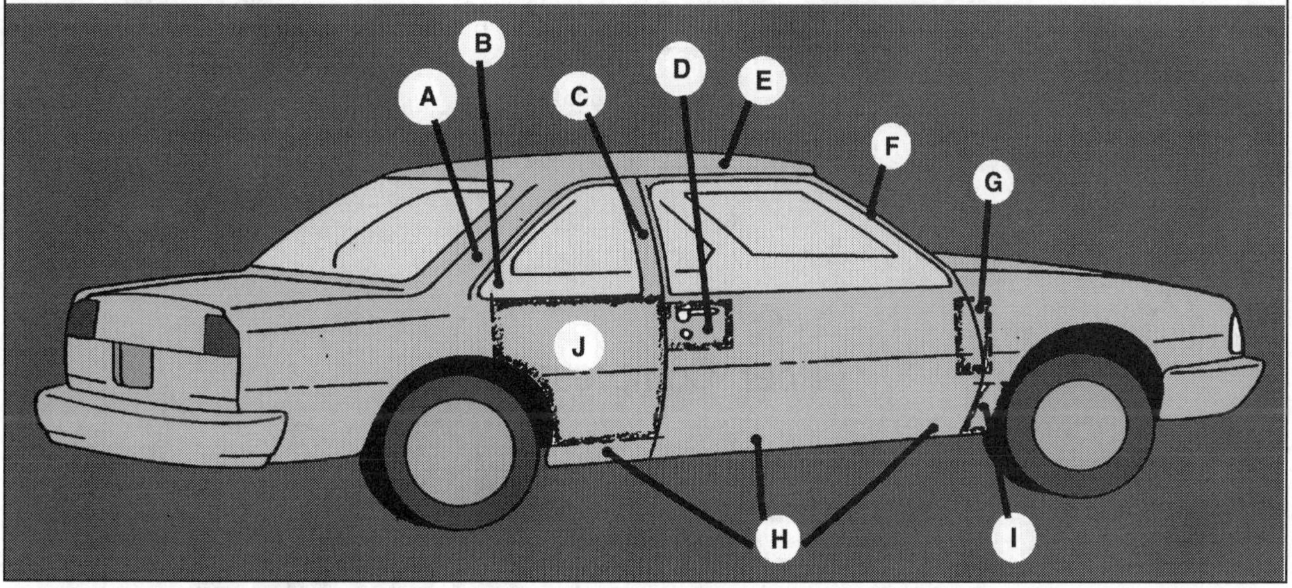

Figure 9–2 Vehicle terminology.

Plastics are the material of choice inside the vehicle. The dash and all moldings are constructed of plastic—lightweight and strong. During extrication, most of this material can be pried away manually. In vehicle fires, this material will give off toxic fumes.

Increasingly, polycarbonite *composites* are used as the outer skin of doors in today's vehicle. The Saturn and Lumina van are two examples. Composites were developed by the aerospace industry to absorb energy on impact and then return to its original shape. While this results in a decrease in the cost of repairing dents and dings, it causes problems during vehicle extrication due to its ability to absorb applied energy from various rescue tools.

Exterior Components

The exterior components of the vehicle include the bumpers, engine compartment, post and rails, window glass, doors, roof, and trunk areas. These areas are the most visible during the extrication process, and will influence gaining entry/access to the occupants.

Bumper: The evolution of the bumper began with the 1973 "5-miles-per-hour" standard. This standard required that front bumpers be able to absorb the energy generated in an impact of 5-miles-per-hour. In 1974 the standard was amended to include the rear bumper. This standard produced four different bumper mechanisms found throughout the automotive industry.

The earliest energy-absorbing bumper allowed the bumper support to travel back along a channel. This is commonly referred to as the *leaf-spring assembly*.

The next evolution produced the *rubber-cushion assembly*. This assembly consists of a steel tube and steel pipe. At the rear of the tube is a thick piece of rubber which absorbs the energy as the pipe is compressed. The rubber cushion allows the pipe to return back to its original position.

The *hydraulic piston assembly* was the next and most prevalent assembly. *Energy-absorbing bumpers* (Figure 9–3) are designed to absorb low-speed impact (2.5 mph to 5.0 mph) energy and return the bumper to its original position without major damage. The unit consists of two subassemblies: the *piston tube* and *cylinder tube*.

The piston tube assembly is filled with a pressured gas and consists of a bumper bracket, piston tube, orifice, seal, piston, and stop ring. The cylinder tube assembly is

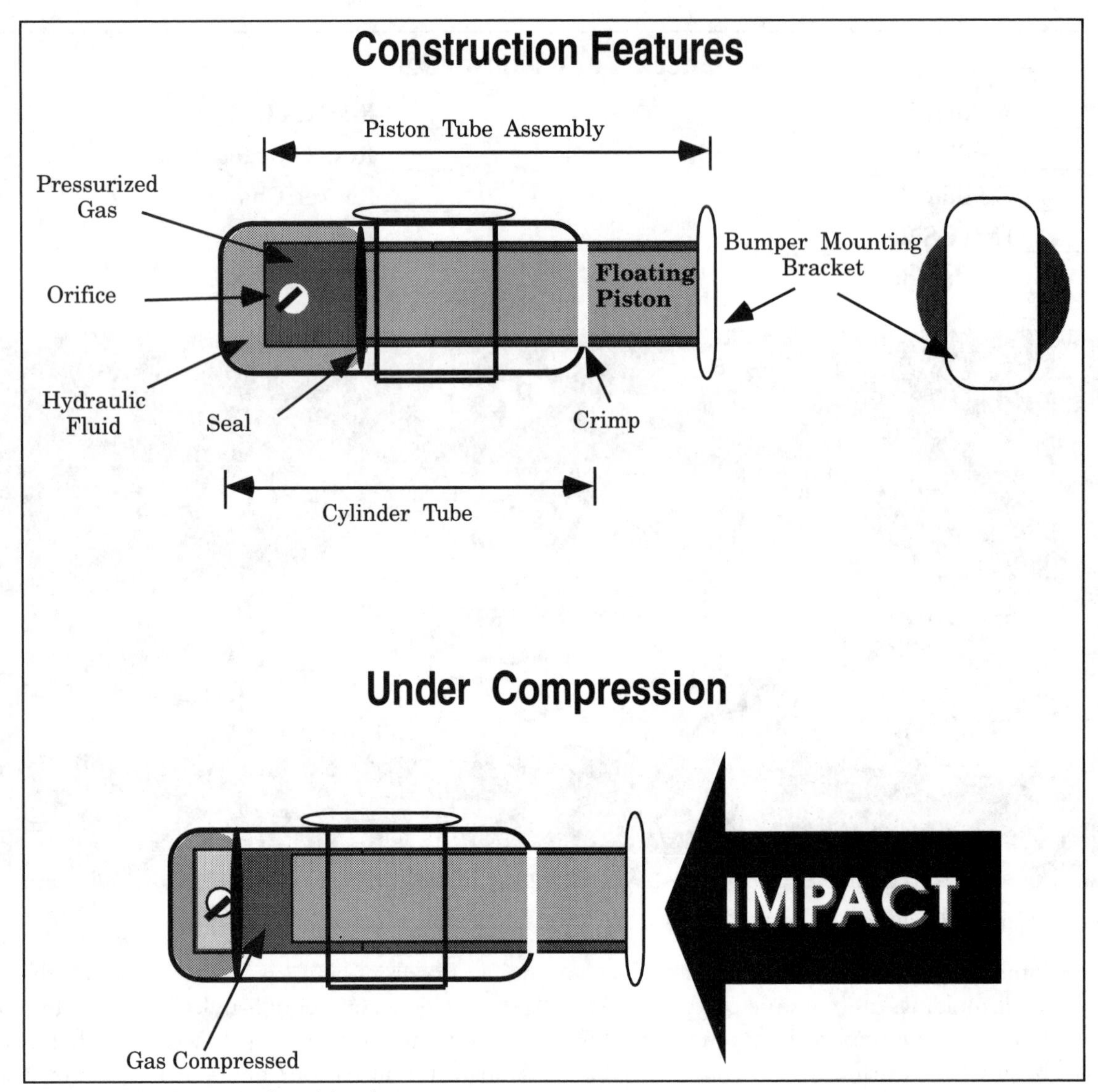

Figure 9–3 Energy-absorbing bumper.

filled with a hydraulic fluid and consists of a frame bracket, cylinder tube, mounting stud, and metering pin.

The piston tube assembly is inserted into the cylinder tube assembly and the cylinder tube is crimped. The crimp mates with the stop ring to hold the unit together. The recess in the stop ring area is filled with grease to keep out foreign material. When attached to the vehicle, the piston tube attaches the bumper to the vehicle, and the cylinder tube to the frame.

The gas pressure in the piston tube assembly maintains the unit in the extended position. Extension is limited by the top ring on the outside of the piston tube engaging the matching contour of the crimp on the cylinder tube. The engagement is also intended to provide strength to withstand jacking and towing stresses.

As the energy absorber is collapsed upon impact, the hydraulic fluid in the cylinder tube is forced into the piston tube through the orifice. The metering pin controls the rate at which the fluid passes through the orifice. This controlled passage of fluid provides the absorbing action. The hydraulic fluid that is forced into the piston tube displaces the floating piston compressing the gas behind the floating piston. After impact, the pressure of the compressed gas behind the piston forces the hydraulic fluid back into the cylinder tube extending the unit to its original position.

This assembly has some inherent dangers for rescue personnel. Should the bumper be restricted from returning to its normal position by bent metal, it may spring forward very rapidly during extrication injuring rescuers standing in front of it. In a fire situation the compressed gas may expand and violently *BLEVE,* propelling the bumper forward to distances of 50 ft. to 100 ft.

Note: Always assess the bumper prior to working in the front of any vehicles that are subjected to fire conditions. This is an area that should be avoided.

During the 1990s, the bumper standard was reduced to a 2.5-mile-per-hour impact. Technology changes also affect plastics, composites, and styrofoam. The *honeycomb assembly* is now the industry standard on unit body construction. This assembly uses an outer shell of plastic or composite and a thick inner layer of styrofoam to absorb impact energy. These components are then mounted on metal reinforcement brackets.

Engine Compartment: The engine compartment in today's vehicle is designed to house the drivetrain and to absorb the impact energy of frontal collisions. Commonly referred to as collapse zones, the hood, and engine supports will direct the engine away from the occupants during a rapid deceleration collision.

Hood: The hood is constructed of sheet metal and is supported by formed sheet metal beams. Beware—some models use hydraulic pistons to control the hood and trunk hatches when open. These may be under pressure after impact or explode during fire conditions. The hood and truck areas have two latching assemblies to prevent premature opening.

Battery: Attempt to locate the battery on all extrications. If it can't be located, don't worry, it's there. The battery may be under the window washer reservoir or may not be in the engine compartment at all. Batteries are often destroyed or fail on impact.

Posts and Rails: Posts are constructed of formed sheet metal to support the roof and floor, giving strength laterally and from top to bottom. The post connecting the front door and windshields is referred to as the "A" post by the fire service. Continuing to the rear of the vehicle, the lettering B, C, D, etc., is used. Rails and posts are constructed similarly and support floors and roofs and give strength front and back. Posts and rails are joined by a weld and supported by metal coves to give additional strength. Remember, posts and rails are hollow and are used as chases for wires. Supports for rails may conceal fuel lines (Figure 9–4).

Glass: When gaining entry/access to occupants, the window glass may be a consideration. The windshield is of a different construction than the other windows. The front window is designed to keep occupants in the vehicle and required not to shatter on impact. The common design is two layers of safety glass with a layer of plastic laminate between them. This design reduces the amount of broken glass inside the vehicle.

The windshield was, at one time, mounted in a rubber gasket that could be cut to remove the glass. Modern construction has eliminated the gasket in favor of mastic glue. The mastic is very strong and difficult to remove in extrications. In most cases the windshield glass should be removed in concert with the A posts and the roof unit.

Another windshield design, Securi-flex, uses a single layer of glass with a stronger layer of plastic on the inside. The thickness of the glass may be thinner than in the laminated windshield.

The side and rear glass is tempered construction. Tempered glass is heated to its melting point and then poured into a mold to form the pane. This high heat treatment gives the pane high surface tension. To break this glass, strike it with a sharp object. The spring-loaded center punch works well.

Doors: The next obstacle to occupant access is the doors. Doors are constructed of a rolled sheet metal frame with inner and outer panels. The outer panel is made of either sheet metal, plastic, or composite material. The inner panel is made of sheet metal, and serves as the foundation for mounting accessories, such as motors for electrical windows and locks. Remember the characteristics of sheet metal and composite material when attempting to force a door. Sheet metal has little or no strength at its edges when flat. Composite material, however, absorbs energy and returns to its original shape.

In the 1960s Ralph Nader lobbied Congress to increase the safety standards for passenger vehicles. His strong lobbying effort lead to the 1973 mandate which changed vehicle construction, seat belts, and the construction components of doors. This mandate requires that doors must be able to sustain a side impact of 2.5 mph to 7.5 mph depending on the model year. The door must also remain closed in frontal and rear impacts. To meet this mandate, a crash bar was placed inside the door and the latching assemblies reengineered.

There are two configurations of the crash bar. The "guard-rail" configuration consists of three layers of rolled steel corrugated into guard-rail fashion. The rail is 7 ins. high and 2 ins. thick. The ends are welded to the inner frame of the door and are situated about lap level in the door and run from front to rear. In a T-bone collision at normal speeds (greater than the collision bar is designed to withstand), the victim can be injured by the door moving into the passenger compartment.

Many of these collision bars have a new design; they are made of tubular steel with spot-welded plates in the

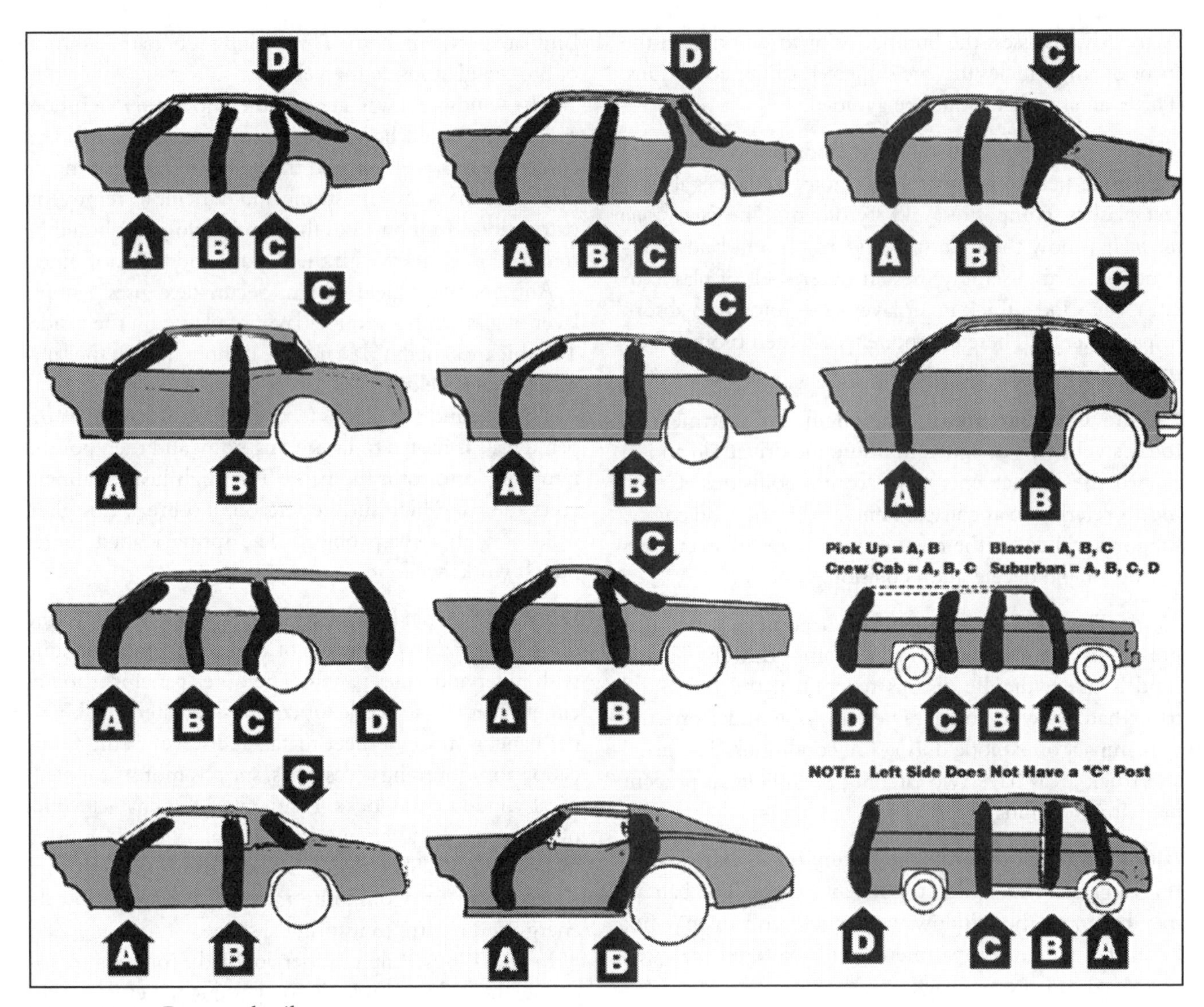

Figure 9–4 Posts and rails.

area between the hinges and the area of the striker bolt. As a result of its placement, the collision bar contributes to the overall integrity of the vehicle.

In the closed position the door is secured to the vehicle by the latching assembly and its hinges. In the past, hinges that were accessible after impact presented a viable option for dealing with jammed doors. An impact wrench or a socket set used on the four or six hinge bolts, along with a pair of wire cutters to deal with the wiring, was generally a fast technique with low impact on the victim. Hinges are constructed of solid cast, stamped, or pressed metal. They are then bolted to the post using ½ in. to 9/16 in. or 10 mm to 15 mm bolts. Some bolts may be welded to a post. While some doors may have bolts that appear to be inside out and difficult to unbolt, remember that *all* hinges are bolted to the door. Striker bolts on the door frame are, by design, one of the strongest components of the vehicle. They are typically backed by ¼-in. steel and normally the bolt itself does not fail during impact or through rescuer's efforts. One of the concerns that rescuers tend to forget is: Don't tear metal when you are popping a door. It is important to remember that if you tear metal around the striker bolt, you will have difficulty freeing the door.

The latching assembly of the passenger vehicle door is very similar to that of an entry door to a building. The two parts are the striker and the keeper. The *keeper* is located on the door. It is attached to the door frame at the level of the crash bar. The crash bar serves as reinforcement for the keeper. The keeper grasps the striker to keep the door shut.

The *strikers* are located on the B and C posts. There are various types of strikers. The striker bolt, commonly referred to as the "Nader bolt" in the fire service, is the strongest part of this assembly. The striker bolt is reinforced at the post, and is rated to withstand 2,500 psi to 4,000 psi.

Foreign models may have a *U* bolt as a striker. This bolt is formed from tempered steel and is also reinforced at the post. The latest version of the striker is the *mini wedge*. This striker is constructed of two tempered steel posts connected to a wedge. This design allows the keeper to grasp two posts and increases strength to withstand side impacts.

There are two techniques for forcing these assemblies. Using a hydraulic jaw, place one jaw on the post just above the striker and the other jaw at the keeper using the crash bar as support. Using the post as a support, force the door open. A reciprocating saw can also be used to cut the striker if it is visible.

When using a hydraulic rescue tool on unibody construction, remember: Don't force the door until the tips of the tool are on the inner surface of the door. Watch the metal as you work the inner surface. Look for metal stressing and stop before it tears.

Take small bites, each a little deeper than the previous, until you reach the inner surface of the door, then force the door with the hydraulic rescue tool. This will force the striker bolt off the latch mechanism, and the door will usually come free.

Remember, once the door is free of the latch, it may still be jammed by the impact. This typically occurs in the hinge area. A ram placed against the B post and the forward portion of the door (such as the window handle area) will move the door out of the way with minimal impact on the victim.

The striker bolt, or mini wedge, will have a similar impact on rescue operations. Forcing a door with a hydraulic rescue tool or cutting with a reciprocating saw used to be a simple, standard operation. Like the hinge operation when the hinge is visible, when the striker bolt is visible, a fast, simple, low-impact cutting operation can be used.

The mini wedge is difficult to cut. Using a reciprocating saw with a 6-in. Lenox Hackmaster 18-tooth-per-in. blade and a one part soap to six parts water spray solution generally results in a quick operation. The Nader bolt could be cut in 15 to 30 seconds, the U-bolt in 30 to 45 seconds, and the mini wedge in 90 to 120 seconds.

Roof: The roof is simple in construction but very important to the strength of a vehicle. It is constructed of sheet metal (sometimes two layers thick) and supported by formed sheet metal beams resulting in the roof being lightweight. Remember the roof is the structure that ties and holds the sides together. Remove the entire roof and the vehicle becomes very weak along its axis. Though it is very simple, the roof does have some potential problems when sunroofs and moonroofs are installed.

Moonroofs and sunroofs may look similar but are very different. A moonroof simply lifts up to allow air to flow into the vehicle. The moonroof sits in a jamb cut into the roof. Beware! The moonroof can fall out when the roof is removed or folded back.

The sunroof is designed to retract out of the way to allow an opening into the roof. This requires a track for the window to follow into the roof lining. The tracks are usually twice the length of the window, giving reinforcement to the roof. The track will prevent any attempt to fold the roof back.

Trunk Areas: The construction of the trunk is much like that of the engine compartment but without the supports for the drivetrain. In incidents involving extrication, the trunk should always be checked. The trunk is a possible danger area that is most often overlooked. Many people carry hazardous materials in the trunk space. Additional victims may also be found here. The latching assembly uses a turning cam to unlock a shaft. The cam is easily exposed by forcibly pushing the cylinder in with a pointed striking tool and hammer.

Interior Components

While the interior of today's vehicle is mainly comprised of plastic materials, the steering column, air bag systems, dash, and seats are important components which may be removed to extricate victims.

Steering Column: The steering column consists of the steering wheel and the column. The steering wheel is constructed of 3/8 in. cold rolled steel covered in plastic or vinyl. The wheel is easy to cut with a variety of hand tools and is not, as some believe, spring loaded. In many extrications, simply cutting the spokes of the steering wheel removes the wheel and provides plenty of room to extricate the driver.

GM cars now use a steering column that was designed to meet a 1960 standard calling for an "energy-absorbing" steering column and rim. These early models collapsed as the driver's chest impacted/compacted the steering wheel. With unit body construction, front wheel drive, and traverse mounting of engines, the column was redesigned to be a split-steering column. This column splits at the fire wall (wall which separates the engine from the occupants). At this split is a plastic universal joint. This joint will fail under pressure exerted by today's rescue tools. The column is mounted to the dash and fire wall by the shear capsule. This capsule is a support whose bolts are designed to shear off under impact. This allows the steering column to freely move about and does not trap the driver. The column itself is a ⅝ in. steel rod covered by a sheet metal shroud. If the column has to be removed, do not cut it off with a reciprocating saw device or hydraulic tool in the event a supplemental restraint system is in place.

The "tilt wheel" is a common luxury found in today's vehicle. The tilt wheel is constructed with a ball-and-knuckle joint in the steering column which allows the steering wheel to move. This is the column's weakest point. Attempts to pull this steering wheel will project the assembly into the lap/legs of the driver.

The pulling-the-column technique raises several important concerns for rescuers and has resulted in this technique no longer being taught in the rescue program:

- The column itself is no longer the problem.
- Pulling the column could lead to sudden movement that could further injure the patient.
- Pulling the column will, at best, cause minimal movement of the dashboard.
- Universal joints and tilt wheels may cause further sudden movement of the column when pulling techniques are used.
- Many electrical components are now mounted in the column, including the supplemental inflatable restraint system (air bag), and movement of the column may result in an electrical short.

Supplemental Restraint Systems (SRSs)

Side Air Bags: A recent addition to the front seat framework of new vehicles such as the 1995 Volvo is the *side impact protection system (SIPS).* This system uses a small air bag to absorb the force of side impact collisions. This system is not a restraint system per se as the occupants are not restrained by the air bag itself.

The system is activated when a sensor mounted in the front seat frame at the level of the floor rail (rocker channel) is depressed by the floor rail. The sensor is much like the firing pin of a gun. When the pin is depressed, a 2 g. smokeless gunpowder charge is ignited. The explosion pushes air through two plastic tubes deploying an air bag located at the top of the seat back. The air bag is approximately 12 in. long and 4 in. in diameter allowing for rapid deployment. The deployed bag absorbs the impact of the B post as it is deflected or crushed inward.

The sensor can be activated with the force of a hammer so disarming the system is important in any extrication. The rescuer can disarm the system by lifting up the plastic molding between the seat and the floor rail. Located under this molding is a red plastic retaining ring. The sensor will be visible at the front of the seat frame. Placing the red retaining ring in the notch of the sensor will prevent the system from deploying.

Front Air Bags: Congress mandated that in the 1990s passenger vehicles must have restraint systems (air bags) that enhance seat belt use in frontal collisions. The first air bag system was placed in Dodge vehicles around 1968. This was a very short production run and air bags were not seen again until 1990.

The supplemental restraint system (SRS), or air cushion restraint system (ACRS), provides passive restraint to front-seat occupants in frontal accidents. A driver cushion is in the center of the steering wheel and a passenger cushion is in the right side of the instrument panel. The deployed driver-side air bag is 28 in. across and fills to about 2.3 cu. ft. The passenger air bag is about 28 ins. × 25 ins. and fills to between 7 to 8 cu. ft. Following inflation, the gas is released almost immediately through vents located on the bottom inner portion of the bags.

Sensors are typically mounted in the front fenders, under the dash, and/or under the driver's seat (Figure 9–5). In order for an air bag to deploy, the sensors must receive energy from an impact equivalent to 8 mph to 14 mph or greater in a frontal collision. It is critical to know that this impact energy is designed to only result from a head-on or near head-on impact, not a side, rear, or roll-over accident. The air bag actually deploys at a speed of 150 mph to 180 mph.

ACRSs contain a gas-generating module that has approximately 75 g. to 80 g. of sodium azide, a flammable solid. Sodium azide is ignited upon sensor contact and the nitrogen gas generated by the ignition fills the air bag. Besides the threat of accidental inflation while working on a wreck, other safety concerns address the chemical itself.

Sodium azide has been used for over 40 years in such diverse applications as explosives manufacture, the treatment of wounds, and as a fungicide. The National Institute of Occupational Safety and Health classifies it, in certain forms, as a "suspected mutagenic," meaning it is possibly damaging to human chromosomes and genes. One part of sodium azide per million parts of air has produced toxic response in test animals: a rapid change in blood pressure, followed by convulsions, and death. The Environmental Protection Agency (EPA) is aware that a number of manufacturers are currently utilizing sodium azide in air bags, however the EPA has made no move to

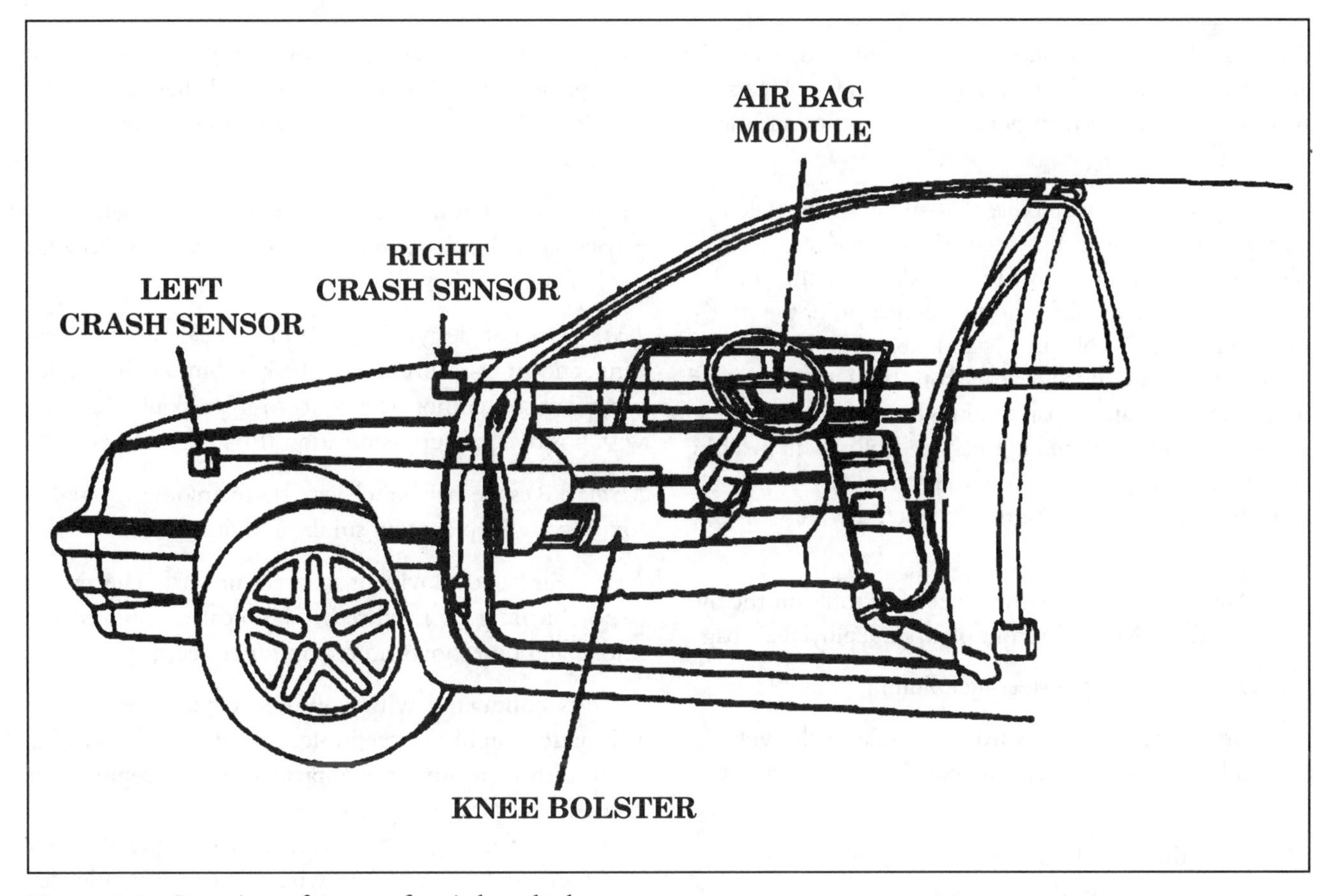

Figure 9–5 Location of sensors for air bag deployment.

restrict its utilization. The sodium azide in an ACRS is in a sealed container and is not exposed.

After inflating, a very small amount of sodium hydroxide powder may be released during the deflation of the air bag. This powder is slightly alkaline and may cause minor irritation to the skin, eyes, and nose, although the powder is considered nontoxic. If the alkaline residue comes in contact with skin, flush the area with copious amounts of cool water. Warning labels have been installed on cars with air bag systems. One label contains following information:

> Contains sodium azide and potassium nitrate. Contents are poisonous and extremely flammable. Contact with acid, water, or heavy metals may produce harmful and irritating gases or explosive compounds. Do not dismantle, incinerate, bring into contact with electricity, or store at temperatures exceeding 200 degrees F.
>
> FIRST AID: If contents are swallowed, induce vomiting. For eye contact, flush eyes with water for 15 minutes. If gases from acid or water are inhaled, seek fresh air. In every case, get prompt medical attention.

If the air bag system has not activated prior to the arrival of emergency personnel, it should be considered an active system. The most reliable visual clue that a vehicle has an air bag system is a large steering wheel hub and an extra thick padded lower dashboard area. An active air bag system is a potential hazard to operating personnel and vehicle occupants.

All air bag systems that operate on electrical impulse have a storage capacitor integrated into their circuitry. The only safe methods to deactivate the air bag system is to disconnect the vehicle's battery and touch the cables together and/or allow time for the stored energy to discharge. The GM service manual for 1989 cars advises to wait 10 minutes after disconnecting the ground cable before attempting to work on the electrical system. Touching the cables together, however, drains the capacitors immediately of their charge without having to wait.

There have been some recommendations made on how to handle ACRS that have not deployed. One is to pry the lid off the ACRS unit and cut the bag with a knife. That way you would not have to worry about it inflating and causing injury to the victims or scaring the rescuer. This misinformation fails to take into account that the output of the gas generator buffing sodium azide is equivalent in energy to ½ cup of gasoline. Besides the heat generated by the burning sodium azide, there is no containment for the residue.

Note: If the ACRS/SRS has not deployed, leave it alone! In any case, *do not* place your body, objects or tools on the air bag trim cover or in front of an undeployed air bag.

There is also the possibility that an intense vehicle fire could also result in deployment. In the rare case of deployment resulting from fire, the deployment will be normal (i.e., there will be no fragmentation of the module or inflator). To obtain a "flammable solid" hazardous materials shipping classification from the Department of Transportation, an air bag module bonfire test was conducted. The test required normal gas deployment in a fire (i.e., without fragmentation of the module).

If the battery cannot be disconnected before working on the steering column:

1. *Do not* place your body, objects, or tools on the air bag trim cover or in front of an undeployed air bag.
2. *Do not* cut into the steering column.
3. Perform rescue efforts from the side of the vehicle and away from the potential deployment path of the air bag.
4. Move the seat of a stabilized occupant back as far as possible or lower the seat back.

Remember: Cutting the steering wheel rim or spokes, or rolling the instrument panel *will not* deploy an air bag if the battery is still connected.

Wear the same gloves and eye protection that rescuers would normally wear. Protective equipment will guard against possible skin or eye irritation from the powdery air bag residue. If gloves are not worn, wash your hands with mild soap and water after handling a deployed air bag.

Avoid getting air bag residue in your eyes or the occupant's eyes or wounds.

Be aware of hot metal parts *underneath* the deployed air bag fabric. These components are located inside the steering wheel hub or behind the instrument panel when there is a deployed passenger-side air bag. These components are somewhat out of the way and should pose no threat.

Push deflated air bags aside for occupant removal. Air bags deflate at once after a deployment. There is no need to cover, remove, or repack the air bag during rescue operations.

Air Bag Myths to Remember

Myth: Air bags contain an explosive solid that can react like a cannon in a fire.

Fact: Today's air bag modules are a flammable solid, not an explosive. Rapid burning of the solid chemical inflates the air bag(s) with nitrogen. Air bags do not explode in a crash or a fire.

Myth: Rescuers must wait 10 to 20 minutes before approaching a vehicle with a deployed air bag, to allow for cooling and venting time.

Fact: Do not delay. The steering wheel rim and column, and air bag fabric *will not* be hot. Smoke from a deployment should not be a concern. If in doubt ventilate with positive pressure ventilation (PPV) fan/blower.

Myth: Rescue personnel may be overcome by highly toxic air bag deployment smoke and dust.

Fact: Air bag deployment smoke is normal. The air bag is not burning or ruptured. Chemical analysis of the smoke and dust shows no reason for concern.

Tests conducted with volunteers who are chronic asthmatics highly susceptible to airborne particles, showed that the atmosphere produced by a deployment posed no respiratory system hazard. Ford has deployed thousands of air bags during its extensive testing. The test engineers and technicians, who regularly handle deployed air bags and test dummies, have not reported ill effects from exposure to the deployments.

Myth: The vehicle interior, air bag, and occupants will be covered in a hazardous residue.

Fact: Any powdery residue consists of corn starch or talcum powder and sodium compounds, mostly sodium carbonates (e.g., baking soda). Very small deposits of sodium hydroxide are also present. The powdery residue may irritate the skin and eyes, but poses no long-term health hazard. The powder is slightly alkaline but is not considered toxic.

Myth: Disconnecting the battery will deploy the air bag in 15 to 20 minutes.

Fact: This is *not true.* Disconnecting the battery deactivates the air bag system by discharging to ground any stored energy in a back-up power capacitor. Disconnecting the battery cable *will not* deploy an air bag.

Dash: In today's vehicles, most of the extrication problems encountered seem to involve the dashboard and fire wall. Rescuers frequently find the steering column loose after impact, and it is not unusual to find the dashboard entrapping the occupant, with the steering wheel and column actually resting on the victim's lap. The unibody constructed vehicle clearly illustrates why this problem has changed.

The dash has become the structure that entraps drivers and front-seat passengers. The dash has very little, if any, structural support and in a frontal impact will collapse downward on the lower extremities of front-seat occupants. Most dash construction consists of plastic, lightweight metal, cardboard, and styrofoam. With this lightweight construction, removal of broken parts can be done manually.

The Side Impact Standard will cause some changes in dash design. A cross-car support is now being added to some models. The support extends between the front posts and supports the dash while adding lateral support to the vehicle. Some designs also add a post from the center of the cross-car support to the floor. With these changes in dash design, the occurrence of the dash trapping occupants may drastically decrease.

Seats: All occupants are seated when the collision occurs and usually stay in the seats after the collision. Therefore any extrication plan involving moving occupied seats should be avoided as this may increase injury to the victim. The front seats are constructed of foam cushions mounted an a metal frame which is mounted to a sliding track on the floor. This track is also bolted to the floor. The rear-seat cushions rest on the floor. Removal of the rear seats may serve as an access to the trunk area.

COMPONENT REACTIONS IN COLLISIONS

Knowing how the vehicle will react allows us to develop an extrication plan. Exterior vehicle components react to a frontal collision in the following ways:

1. Bumper absorbs impact and compresses inward
2. Fenders collapse
3. Hood deflects upward
4. Engine absorbs energy
5. Rails and posts begin to deflect
6. Doors are pushed back and override posts and rear doors
7. Roof deflects as force is transferred via posts and rails
8. Rear quarter panel deflect

Interior vehicle components react to frontal collision in the following ways:

1. Air bags deploy
2. Steering column shear capsule separates at the bolts
3. Dash begins to move
4. Seats slide forward in tracks

The occupants react to impact:

1. Knees stiffen and lock; contact knee bolster
2. Body moves forward until stopped by seatbelts, steering wheel, dash, or windshield
3. Knees may underride dash and become trapped

To extricate the occupants look for strength points. Are hinge points bolted or welded? Is striker bolt visible? Can it be cut?

Look at the striker bolt reinforcement. Can it be forced? Is there a high strength location for hydraulic tool positioning?

Look at the intersection of posts and rails. Can they be cut? Sever the intersection of the A post and rocker panel. Remember, cutting the roof will weaken the entire structure. Be aware of seat belt attachment points and location of mechanism.

Base your action plan on either using or avoiding the strong points of construction. Use strong points to force doors or roll the dash and stabilize when on side or roof. Avoid strong points to remove roof and to isolate dash for roll-up.

DEVELOPING AN EXTRICATION PLAN

Upon arrival on the scene where extrication will be necessary, the rescuer/officer must develop a plan to disassemble the vehicle from around the occupants. The development of this plan must be based on the construction concepts discussed in this session. The plan must embrace use of the points addressed here.

When examining a vehicle, look for its strength point areas. Are the hinges bolted to the posts and are they readily exposed? If so, they may be quickly unbolted and one door connection point defeated. Is the striker visible? Can this be cut or must the door be forced off the striker? When both connection points are removed, the door is free and access to the occupants is available.

There are other parts of the vehicle that may have to be removed to free the occupants. In some cases the entire roof may have to be removed. Cutting the posts above any seatbelt reinforcement will quickly remove the roof and weaken the entire vehicle structure. To remove the windshield at the same time, cut the front posts low at the bottom of the glass; the windshield can then be removed with the roof. Should the windshield not be a problem, cut the posts at the top of the glass and leave the windshield in place. In cases where the windshield glass must be cut, either a flat-head axe, reciprocating saw, Glas-Master, or air chisel may be used.

Extricating occupants in the best-case scenario is based on removing the occupants as quickly as possible while operating in the worst of conditions. Knowledge of the construction of the vehicle will increase the rescue team's effectiveness and reduce stress. Each incident will require its own unique extrication plan. Development of the plan is easier when based on experience, knowledge, and practice. As a company, drill often, and drill a lot! There is *no* substitute for training and safety.

Traditionally the rescue component of the fire service has practiced on vehicles that are in fairly good condition. The reality of this training scenario does not adequately address what the rescue service actually encounters at the scene or a working incident (i.e., damaged/wrecked vehicles involved in motor vehicle crashes).

Rescuers need to practice on vehicles that have actually been wrecked. Current model vehicles involved in accidents react much differently to extrication techniques than old vehicles without damage.

VEHICLE FUEL SYSTEMS

During the assessment or size-up phase of the extrication process, hazardous conditions must be identified. Identifying the fuel system of the vehicle at one time was a simple task, however with modern construction comes different fuel designs. Fuel storage can be located in a number of places. Modern vehicle construction has moved the storage of fuel between the front and rear axles. Storage tanks generally are constructed of metal, however there are also plastic storage tanks. These plastic tanks have shown high failure rates in fire situations. Capacity may run between 10 and 24 or more gallons depending on vehicle.

The most common fuel used in modern passenger vehicles is gasoline. Gasoline is clear to amber in color with an obvious odor of petroleum. The flash point of gasoline is below 0° and its vapor is heavier than air with a vapor pressure of +1.0.

The second most common fuel is diesel fuel. Diesel fuel is straw yellow to dark yellow in color and also has an odor of petroleum. Diesel has a flash point of 100° to 199° and is also heavier than air with a vapor pressure of +1.0.

The fuel vapor control system prevents raw fuel vapors from escaping into the atmosphere. Fuel vapors from the fuel tank and carburetor bowl are collected in a charcoal-filled canister and metered into the intake manifold for combustion.

The filler cap in this system incorporates a two-way relief valve which is normally closed to the atmosphere. The relief valve is calibrated to open only when a pressure of more than 0.8 psi or a vacuum of more than 0.1 ins. Hg. occurs. It is normal to encounter air pressure release when removing the filler cap. At the majority of wrecks and car fires, the fuel system of the vehicle will be pressurized.

The canister used with this system is filled with granules of activated charcoal. Vapors entering the canister are absorbed into the surface of the granules. The canister has two inlets: one for the tank vapor and one for carburetor fuel bowel vapor. The outlet is connected to the intake manifold vacuum. When the engine is running, manifold vacuum draws fresh air through the inlet filter in the canister and purges stored vapors. If the engine is not running after a wreck, the vapors are stored in the canister.

A rollover check valve installed in the fuel system prevents fuel flow from the tank through the vent line in the vent of vehicle rollover.

The check valve consists of a plunger and stainless-steel ball. When inverted, the ball presses the plunger against the valve seat. A properly functioning valve will sustain 3 psi of air pressure on the inlet side when inverted.

Controlling gasoline and diesel leaks or spills during extrications is very important due their potential fire problem. When mixed with other fluids, slip hazards are also present. By using absorbent material both slip and fire hazards can be controlled.

Recently, liquefied petroleum gas (LPG) and compressed natural gas (CNG) have emerged as fuels of choice among utility companies. These after-market additions to the vehicle in conjunction with gasoline establishes a duel-fueled vehicle. With LPG the storage tanks are usually found in the trunk area or the rear of the vehicle. LPG is a colorless gas kept in its liquid state by compressing at high pressure. When released from its pressure container, propane has an extremely high expansion ratio which displaces the air and is easily ignited.

Compressed natural gas (CNG) has the following basic system components:

1. Under hood (injectors/electronics)
2. Regulators

3. Fuel storage cylinders
4. Valves
5. Stainless steel lines

Fuel cylinders are located in vans, under and/or in cargo area. In pick-ups under and/or in bed. In passenger cars, in the trunk (enclosed in box).

Typical CNG fuel storage capacities are:

- Passenger cars–400
- Vans
  BGE (Dodge)–2,400 SCF
  Others–1,200–2,400 SCF
- Medium duty trucks–2,400–4,800 SCF
- Buses (BWI)–7,000 SCF

Rescuers must remember safety points. CNG must meet NFPA 52. Shutoff valves and relief valves include the main valve, which is located under the vehicle, mounted on the frame rail. A label on the rocker panel marks the location. Rescuers should shut the CNG off to the engine from the cylinders.

Cylinder valves and devices are located on the end of each cylinder or inside plastic vent bags if the cylinders are inside the vehicle. Composite type cylinders mounted inside vehicles have a second vent bag for an end plug. Relief devices are located at the cylinder valve. The temperature vents at 212°F. Pressure vents at 5,000° psi. Devices vent via ½-in. line through the floor into the vent bag. Insure that the line is not crushed in the collision.

Properties of CNG include:

- Flame range of 5% to 15% in air
- Stored as a gas at 3,000–3,600 psi; 1,200 ignition temperature
- Odorized–does have an odor
- Asphyxiant–displaces air

Emergency response for responders:

- Position up-wind
- Determine type of fuel
- Remove any source of ignition
- Shut motor off (quarter turn valves)
- Locate main valve and shut off

Identification of a LPG/CNG vehicle is made by a sticker identifying an alternative fueled vehicle. This sticker is usually marked with the identification logo indicating the type of fuel on board (e.g., LPG, CNG).

DEFINITIONS

Composites: Carbon-based synthetic material used as the outer skin of some vehicles.

Full frame: Construction method where vehicle body is assembled in parts on frame rails.

Keeper: Part of the door latching assembly which is attached to the door. The keeper attaches to the striker to keep the door shut.

Posts: Structural members of unit-body construction. Posts are in the vertical position.

Rails: Structural members of unit-body construction. Posts are in the horizontal position.

Side impact protection system (SIPS): Supplemental restraint technology used to absorb energy of side impacts. This system *does not* restrain occupants. Exclusive to the 1995, 900 series Volvo.

Space frame: Construction method where lighter but stronger materials are used. Some unit-body vehicles refer to "space frame" when attaching composite panels. (e.g., Chevy Lumina)

Striker bolt: Part of door latching assembly that attaches to the door post. Commonly referred to as the "Nader bolt." The keeper attaches to the striker to keep the door shut.

Supplemental restraint systems (SRS): Occupant restraint system using bags filled with an inert gas to absorb energy on occupant impact. Commonly referred to as "air bags." Typical systems are the driver's-side air bag. Installation of passenger-side air bags are increasing.

Unit body: Construction method using posts, rails, floors, and the roof as a system to form vehicle structure. No frame rails are used. Commonly referred to as "Unibody."

REFERENCES

Kidd, J.S., and J.D. Czajkowsi. 1991. *Vehicle extrication–A training manual.* Saddlebrook, NJ: Fire Engineering.

Moore, R.E. 1991. *Vehicle rescue and extrication.* St. Louis: Mosby Yearbook, Inc.

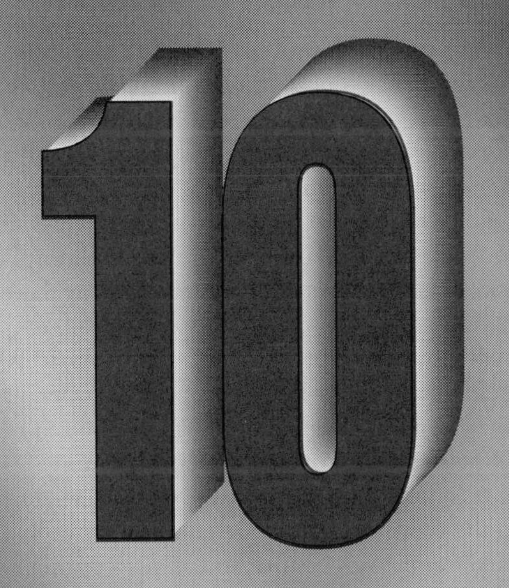

ABCs of Vehicular Rescue

OBJECTIVE

The student will be able to describe the steps necessary to perform vehicular rescue, from memory, without assistance, to an accuracy of 70% and the satisfaction of the instructor.

OVERVIEW

ABCs of Vehicular Rescue

- Preincident Preparation
- Incident Operational Steps
- Postincident Evaluation
- Vehicular R.E.S.C.U.E.

ENABLING OBJECTIVES

10-1-1 List the steps of preincident preparation.

10-1-2 Identify the "ABC" steps of incident operations, the methods to gain access in vehicles, the need for on-going assessment, and the need for a secondary plan of action.

10-1-3 List the steps of postincident evaluation.

10-1-4 Describe the acronym R.E.S.C.U.E. and its application to vehicular scenarios.

PREINCIDENT PREPARATION

Proper preparation is the foundation for operational success during vehicle rescue. The following needs to be considered in preincident planning: personnel, training, equipment, Incident Management System (IMS)/standard operating procedures, and emergency vehicle operator's training. Vehicle extrication revolves around the concept of being time conscious and team oriented.

INCIDENT OPERATIONAL STEPS

Safety is the overriding focus during the entire emergency call from initial response until return to quarters. If the rescue scene is unsafe, make it safe. Otherwise, *do not enter.* This also applies to all EMS personnel.

Use the following mnemonic to recall the steps to use at the vehicle rescue scene:

A - Assess scene

B - Balance vehicle(s)
Begin access (Balance is used interchangeably with stabilization.)

C - Cut roof

D - Do doors

E - Enlarge opening

F - Follow-up

Each rescue requires flexibility and ingenuity. The steps described here may not be followed in this exact order on each response.

Assess the Scene

The first step in scene assessment involves determining the proper place to position the responding apparatus. It is based on personal safety of the response rescuers and achievement of individual tactical objectives of the rescue. Rescuers should consider traffic, roadway, and other obvious hazards. Position apparatus 150 ft. to 200 ft. uphill or upwind of incident whenever possible.

In assessing the problem, circle check and zone establishment (Session 1) should be done. Hazard control requires rescuers to remove dangers or stabilize them. Determine the number of vehicles, patients (triage), and resources needed. Determine any possible hazards such as airbags, animals (K-9 dogs, horses, bees, etc.), bystanders, cargo, downed electric wires, electrical system of involved vehicle(s) (battery acid/electric shock), environmental conditions, fires, fuel leaks, fumes, vapors, smoke, hazardous materials, overexposed rescuers (too many, too close), traffic, underground electrical/gas utilities, unstable vehicles, victims (violent, aggressive), and weapons.

A good scene assessment involves looking completely around, under, over, and inside the involved vehicle(s) for hidden dangers. Don't let "tunnel vision" cause an injury or death to occur. Hazardous materials incidents require specialized resources and training to mitigate the incident. When in doubt, be cautious when approaching involved vehicle(s).

Once on the scene, rescuers must remember that scene assessment is an on-going process. The incident commander (IC) and safety officer must continually reassess the rescue scene as conditions can quickly change.

The narrow-based command concept is very time consuming and makes inefficient use of incident resources. Avoid this approach. Not only is it inefficient, it is nonproductive as well. Many individuals are performing each task, or one rescuer works while two or three others watch.

The broad-based concept is an expeditious process. The IC should utilize broad-based command to obtain a complete picture. Each assigned task is performed. The IC/Safety Officer stays on top of the scene dynamics. Simultaneous task functions can occur. No one has idle time among the crews. The tasks are completed by all.

Multivehicle and mass casualty incidents command philosophy includes implementation of IMS/ICS as soon as possible and use of preincident resources. Large-scale incidents require clear communications and preincident planning. Sectorization is essential to personnel/resource management.

Balance the Vehicle(s)

Balancing is also referred to as stabilization. Rescuers must guarantee vehicle stability *prior* to vehicle access. Vehicles can be found in precarious unstable conditions including on their wheels, on either side, on their roofs, on top of other vehicles, partially into buildings, hanging over/on guard rails or barriers, in gullies/ravines, in between trees, with debris on top of vehicle, and submerged in water or ice. (Refer to session 12 for detailed information and techniques regarding balancing of vehicles.)

Clues for Vehicular Rescue

Impact	*Obvious Damage*	*Common Suspected Injuries*
Front End	Windshield post deformed Dash in and down Steering wheel down Doors compressed	Fractured lower extremity? Abdomen injuries? Chest injuries? Cervical spine (c-spine) injuries Lumbar spine injuries Head-facial lacerations?
Broadside	Door(s) crushed inward Dash/steering wheel displaced	Blunt trauma to trunk? C-spine injury? Dislocated shoulder? Pelvic fracture?
Rear End	Doors compressed Bucket seat back broken Fuel spill	C-spine injury? Lumbar spine injury? Head-facial lacerations?
Roll Over	Roof crushed Fuel spill	Ejected patient? Lacerations? Blunt trauma? Inhalation/contact with gasoline? Breathing compromised?

Rescuers should assume that all vehicles are unstable and should take the necessary steps to assure vehicle stability. The main objectives of vehicle stabilization efforts should include keeping rescuers safe during the extrication process and preventing further injuries to entrapped occupants.

You can stabilize the vehicle by increasing the number of contact points that the vehicle has with the ground or other firm surface. Spread the contact points over as wide an area as possible. The wider the base, the more stable the vehicle.

Rescuers can utilize various devices to stabilize vehicles. Many of the devices and their correct usage described here are described in session 12 "Vehicular Stabilization." Wheel chocks, step chocks, wood cribbing of various sizes, manual or hydraulic jacks, chain come-alongs, jack stands, chains, winches, and tire deflation are all devices that can be used to stabilize vehicles.

Begin Access: Once the vehicle is completely stable, it is time to gain access to the vehicle. Access can and should be done as soon as possible even prior to primary assessment. Primary access is utilized to quickly gain access to the patient and begin emergency care. Secondary or extended access is when rescuers enlarge the opening to perform further care and patient removal. Rescuers can utilize the methods presented below to gain access into vehicles. Normal ingress methods are open doors or windows. Don't forget to try all windows and doors before breaking glass.

Windshields are constructed of laminated glass (contains plastic between two pieces of glass). This type of glass can be cut with hand or power tools and removed. (This is described in a later session.) Tempered glass is usually found in all other windows (side, vent, rear, and roof). It can be punched out quickly with a spring-loaded center punch or other pointed device and removed. When breaking glass, try to break a window away from the patient.

Using forcible entry techniques with doors and vehicle body takes more time and equipment. These techniques are primarily used when rescuers are gaining further access for disentanglement of the patient from the wreckage. Entry techniques through doors and the vehicle body are covered in later sessions. Remember, once access has been gained to the vehicle, the rescuer inside the vehicle should put the vehicle in park, turn it off if it is running, set the parking brake, and take out the keys. The rescuer inside the vehicle must provide protection for the patients inside the vehicle.

Cut Roof

Removing or cutting the roof first allows quick access, gives the rescuer inside the vehicle more room to complete assessment and packaging of the patient, provides more light, and decreases the claustrophobic effect on the patient. Your assessment of the scene will determine your best method/option of gaining access. If necessary, the patient can be quickly removed once the roof is removed.

Removing the roof totally guarantees enough room to work. Folding or flapping the roof, while less desirable, can be done by folding front to back, back to front, or side to side.

Some roof flapping techniques do not provide large enough openings—make them bigger than you think you really need. The method utilized will be determined by the individual need of each extrication.

Do Doors

The first step to gaining access is through the doors, if possible. The second step is to take the door past its normal opening position to allow additional room for patient removal. Various door opening techniques are described in a later session. There are various methods to opening a door: crush and lift, spreading, cutting, and dismantling. Door opening can be accomplished from either the hinge or lock side of the door.

Again, the method used will be determined by the individual need at each extrication. Rescuers must be proficient with different methods using both hand and power tools to accomplish forcible entry into vehicles.

Enlarge Opening

Enlarge the opening involves making an opening around the patient to make removal easier on the rescuers and safer for the patient. Techniques used include: pedal displacement/removal, dash displacement, post displacement/removal, seat displacement/removal, steering wheel displacement/removal (a last resort technique which is not taught in this program), door displacement/removal, third door displacement/removal, and roof removal/flapping. These are techniques described in future lessons.

Follow-up

Follow-up involves having a secondary or backup plan of action in case the primary method of entry and removal is not working or is taking too much time. Always anticipate—have alternative plans ready.

The rescue officer needs to anticipate that changes may be needed and that an alternative method or technique may be needed to accomplish the specific tactical objectives of this particular rescue situation. When Plan A is implemented, the rescue officer has Plan B (the backup plan) ready if he/she needs it. Don't back a loser. The rescue officer need not stay with an initial plan if it's not working. Change it!

In addition to a backup plan, the rescue officer needs enough personnel and equipment to implement his/her plan. The need for additional resources should be determined quickly. It is easier to send personnel back than to have to wait for them. Call for more help early and often. The rescue officer needs to provide the rescue team with rest and rehab as necessary. Following the broad-based command concept allows for a quicker, smoother, and safer extrication.

POSTINCIDENT EVALUATION

This step is where the rescue team can take what it learns from this call and apply it to future emergency responses. Rescuers should continually learn from the calls they respond to.

Stabilize the accident scene. Once the patients are safe, remove and transport them. The rescue scene may need to be further stabilized to prevent any additional injuries from occurring. Continually reassess the scene for on-going hazards that may develop.

Personnel/equipment accountability. Keep track of all personnel at all times. Follow your IMS. Personnel accountability should be maintained throughout the emergency incident. Once the extrication is complete, the sector officer should complete accountability checks for all personnel in their sector.

Safe return to quarters. Arrive and return alive! Many deaths occur while returning to quarters after an emergency call. Don't let your guard down. Drive safety and defensively.

Clean and restock equipment and apparatus for the next emergency response. Follow the Center for Disease Control and Prevention (CDC) guidelines where necessary.

Documentation is extremely important. Accurately complete all required documents and reports related to this response. This data can help in maintaining your quality assurance program. The job is never finished until the paperwork is done! Certain documents are required by law (OSHA exposure reports, etc.). Records may help prevent unwanted lawsuits.

Perform postincident critiques in a positive manner. Critiques are an excellent learning tool for all members of your department. Rescuers should never stop learning.

Critical incident stress defusings and debriefings may be necessary. Know where your department can quickly access a Critical Incident Stress Defusing (CISD) team. On emotionally charged calls, these techniques help providers deal with the emotional issues that can arise in unusual vehicle rescues. The sooner these techniques are used, the quicker they help the individuals who need them. These and other stress management techniques help keep the "players in the game."

Note: Basic concepts of this section used with permission of Rescue Magazine, May/June 1993, Greg Valcourt, *ABCs of Vehicle Rescue.*

VEHICULAR R.E.S.C.U.E.

Six Steps in the Extrication Process

Since all vehicles share some commonality, the tasks required for a proper extrication from various types of vehicles can be identified by the following six steps. They can be remembered by the mnemonic R.E.S.C.U.E.

Reconnaissance Information is essential for the proper planning to complete all the tasks.

Extinguish Putting out or preventing any fires is the first priority.

Stabilize Make sure the scene and vehicle are safe.

Clear an entrance In order to access the victim, an entrance must be used, created, or enlarged.

Untrap Free victims who are trapped.

Exit Once the victims are accessed and disentangled, remove them.

Reconnaissance

The first step in any action is to gather as much information as possible. This ensures that proper decisions can be reached and helps to avoid tunnel vision.

Scene Make sure the scene is safe to work in. Is there traffic, a toxic atmosphere, or live power lines that could injure rescuers or the victims?

Vehicle Is the vehicle stable? Is there any leaking fluids or natural gas present?

Victims Find out where the victims are located, the severity of their injuries, and how many there are.

Resources How many rescuers are available? What type of equipment do they have to use? If you need more resources, where would you get them and how soon would they get here?

Extinguish

The most immediate problem to be handled is fire. Steps need to be taken as quickly as possible to extinguish any fire and to prevent one from starting. Rescuers should wear full personal protective equipment.

When controlling a fire the direction of the attack should ensure that the fire and smoke is not forced into the passenger compartment. The attack should also guarantee a means of egress for victims trying to exit, a fire free path for rescuers to enter, and for ventilation.

Stabilize

Stabilizing the scene is an important step in assuring a safe and effective rescue operation. You need to be proactive in your approach. This may require shutting down a road, using self-contained breathing apparatus (SCBA), or turning off the power in a section of the city.

Traffic: Oncoming traffic is always a hazard but it's much more so at an accident scene. Rubberneckers, or worse yet, those tied up in motor vehicle traffic can cause a second accident. Stabilizing techniques for incidents involving other modes should be considered. For example, aircraft landing on the same runway or a train coming down the track need to be warned or stopped.

Atmosphere/environment: Hazardous environments can be prevented by rapidly sealing any leaks and by the effective use of ventilation.

Care should be exercised in placing power units so they do not contaminate the area with fumes. Consider using nongasoline-driven power units or hose reels.

Power systems: If you want to know what the hazard is, look at how the vehicle is powered. If it's a subway the hazard is electricity; a plane, it's fuel. Land vehicles are now starting to use natural gas liquetied petroleum gas (LPG) or compressed natural gas (CNG).

The vehicle needs to be stabilized so that the rescuers activities do not cause excessive movement of the vehicle and the victims. The wheels should be chocked to prevent horizontal movement. Vertical movement is stopped by the use of cribbing on suitable frame members.

Make sure that the power systems are tuned off to prevent unwanted sparking and movement. The engine should be off and, if there are no electrical devices that need to be used, the battery should be disconnected.

Fuel, radiator fluid, battery acid, and other fluids can

not only be a fire hazard but can also eat through gear. Steps should be taken to reduce leaking fluids and mitigate their effects if leakage has occurred.

Clear an Entrance

Once you know the vehicle is safe to enter, you must determine where to enter and from what point. This is dependant on the condition and position of the vehicle and the location of victims.

A natural opening may be there as a result of the accident. Doors are one of the best entryways because they are designed for that purpose and are wide.

Emergency hatches and exits can be separate openings like in the roof of a bus or special-opening windows.

Windows are usually the third most easily accessed entrance on a multipassenger vehicle. On buses and trains the mounting mastic can easily be removed and the window taken out, leaving a wide opening in the vehicle. The entire frame should be cut out. One of the advantages of working around the window area is that you can see inside the vehicle to ascertain if there are any victims near where you are about to cut.

The sides and roof can also be opened sufficiently to be used as an entrance or exit. Care should be exercised to make sure there is no victim or hazard on the other side.

The floor should be used only as a last resort because it is often the most difficult part of the passenger compartment in which to create an opening.

If the vehicle is on its side or roof the order of entry may change.

Untrap

Once you have gained access to the victims, the untrapping stage begins. Rescuers should first concentrate on removing simple unattached debris. Try to remove entire assemblies when possible. For example, cutting away the four posts of a seat is more effective and faster in the long run than trying to just bend away a section.

Disentangling the victim can be as easy as removing a seat but may involve pushing away a floor section or cutting out extraneous metal.

Exit

After the victim is freed from the wreckage, the exiting process begins. The goal is to have enough room to remove the victim without adding to his/her existing injuries by manipulating him/her into comprising positions.

One of the bottlenecks in moving rescuers and equipment in and victims out is the sharing of one opening. This leads to gridlock and a general slowing down of the operation. To speed up the removal of victims, have one entrance where rescuers and equipment enter the vehicle and another on the opposite side for removing victims. This can help ensure one-way traffic through the vehicle and improvement in resources and equipment flow.

This R.E.S.C.U.E. process provides a different perspective for your consideration. The ABCs and this new acronym will assist you in looking at the big picture when addressing vehicular extrication regardless of the size of the vehicle(s) involved.

REFERENCES

Fire Protection Publications. 1990. *Principles of extrication,* 1st ed. Stillwater, OK: Oklahoma State University.

Maryland Fire and Rescue Institute. 1989. *Rescue technician course.* Berwyn Heights, MD: MFRI.

Moore, R. E. 1991. *Vehicle rescue and extrication.* St. Louis: Mosby Yearbook, Inc.

Valcourt, G. 1993. ABCs of vehicle rescue. *Rescue magazine* 6 (May/June).

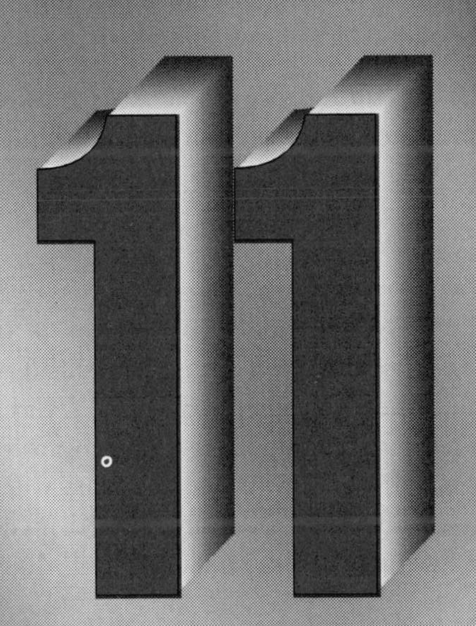

Vehicle Extrication Tools: Hand, Hydraulic, Electric, and Pneumatic

OBJECTIVE

The student will be able to describe the maintenance and inspection procedures and the basic rules for safe operation of each piece of rescue equipment provided, from memory, without assistance, to an accuracy of 70% and the satisfaction of the instructor.

OVERVIEW

Vehicle Extrication Tools: Hand, Hydraulic, Electric, and Pneumatic

- Hand Tools
- Hydraulic Powered Rescue Tools
- Electrically Powered Rescue Tools
- Pneumatic Rescue Tools

ENABLING OBJECTIVES

11-1-1 Identify the various hand tools and describe how they are used in vehicle rescue operations.

11-1-2 Describe the care and maintenance, basic operating, and safety procedures for hydraulic powered rescue tools.

11-1-3 Describe the basic operating and safety procedures for electrically powered rescue tools.

11-1-4 Describe the basic operating and safety procedures for pneumatic rescue tools.

HAND TOOLS

The automobile, as a unit, is made up of individual components and subassemblies. As such, these items are fastened together using welds, screws, bolts, and other assorted fasteners—and can be disassembled with hand tools.

Most of these tools can be packaged and transported in a carry-around toolbox. All of the tools mentioned in this chapter can easily be carried by two rescuers. With proper planning, hand tools need not take up valuable compartment space on fire/rescue apparatus. With the advent of larger emergency care/transport vehicles, even some ambulance companies now carry an abbreviated selection of these tools. Thus, patient access can be accomplished while awaiting assistance from a more thoroughly equipped piece of support apparatus.

The hand tool package ensures that if power rescue tools fail, an alternative means to accomplish the task is immediately available. Hand tools can also be used in conjunction with power tools, and in some instances, disassembly by hand may be a better alternative. Keep in mind that application of power tool technology may result in additional discomfort or pain to the patient involved in an accident.

Hand tools can be subdivided into six categories: striking, cutting, prying, lifting and pulling, disassembly, and miscellaneous. Some of these tools are multifunctional and are discussed under each category. Many tools are probably already in fire department inventory.

Striking Tools

Flat-head axe The flat side of the axe's head can be used for driving some cutting tools. Rubber sleeves are available for the handle so that overstrikes do not damage the handle.

Pry-axe The application is the same as the halligan tool, but is a physically smaller tool.

Halligan tool Like the axe, the flat side of the tool head can be used to deliver a striking blow. The pick can be used for driving out locks or puncturing metal for starter holes when a cutting operation is needed.

3 lb. drilling hammer Used for driving cutting tools. This hammer is superior to a carpenter's hammer or ball-peen hammer because of its weight and large striking surface. The short handle on this hammer makes it more maneuverable and less cumbersome than an axe or maul.

8 lb. maul For heavy driving and cutting, the maul has the necessary weight. For extended operations it may wear out the user.

Center punch or spring-loaded center punch Used for breaking tempered auto glass.

Cutting Tools

Schild panel cutter This is an autobody shop tool. The tool is designed to cut sheet metal and is struck with a hammer.

Leaf-spring cutter The spring cutter does the same task as the Schild panel cutter. It is fabricated from an automobile leaf spring or an old lawnmower blade.

Flat-head axe Use the cutting edge of this axe to cut sheet metal. Strike the flat head with another axe or maul.

Pry-axe The pry axe can be used the same way as previously discussed cutters.

Hacksaw These saws usually come in 10 in. or 12 in. lengths. The shorter length usually has less flex in the blade. The hacksaw works well in cutting windshield and door posts because the construction is several layers of sheet metal formed into a hollow tube. Cutting of the roof and rocker panels can also be accomplished with a hacksaw. Quality, bimetallic blades are a good investment because of flexibility and durability.

Glas-Master This tool is designed to cut safety glass. It uses a large toothed blade that is supported on one end. It cuts very rapidly, but makes a lot of glass dust and throws shards of glass everywhere. Protection of the patient and EMS provider is a must.

Knife, linoleum knife, and seatbelt cutter Many emergency services personnel carry some form of lock blade knife on their belt (buck, leatherman, etc.) These, as well as a linoleum knife, can be used to remove the rubber mounting from the rear window, some side windows, and windshields. The glass can be taken out intact with little effort and there is no mess from broken glass. The seatbelt cutter, which was developed for aircraft rescue, can be used for freeing a patient when the release cannot be accessed. Additionally, when the roof of a vehicle is removed the belt may have to be cut at a mounting point on the door post.

Chisel Used for cutting fasteners. The chisel can also be driven through sheet metal. The end or head of the tool is struck much like the leaf-spring cutter.

Can opener Several tools have this feature incorporated into their design. The K-bar is a slide hammer with the can opener cutter on its end. The Biehl tool is a variation of a pry-axe with this feature. This cutting arrangement can also be found on a halligan-style tool.

Bolt cutter As its name implies, this tool is used for cutting round stock (not hardened fasteners). Some import vehicles use a U-shaped device to which the door lock hooks. Spreading the jamb wide enough can give access to this component and it can be cut with the bolt cutter. If the door is removed from the hinge side, the door limit stop can be cut so that complete removal is possible.

Prying Tools

As the name implies, these tools are used as simple levers. When given a choice, and workspace permits, use a tool with the greatest length (a 36 in. halligan tool verses an 18 in. multitool). Thus, more mechanical advantage (MA) can be achieved.

Tools in this category are a pinch bar, crow bar, halligan bar, pry-axe, and even large, massive screwdrivers. This is just a sample of a wealth of possibilities of prying leverage tools available.

Lifting and Pulling Tools

Chain or cable come-along This MA device uses a ratcheting handle through a gear arrangement to compound force exerted and increase it for pulling power. The design is such that the handle should not be extended with a pipe to decrease the force needed for it to operate. To do so is courting mechanical failure of the come-along. Units with single or double runs of chain or cable seem to be easier to manipulate on an emergency incident. Chain is probably safer than cable because if it breaks it will drop. Cable has a tendency to whip toward the drum and hence toward the operator. Emergency service/rescue units favor 1½ ton capacity come-alongs because they are simple to put into operation and are compact for storage.

A high capacity steel mechanical jack is also known as a *Hi-lift jack* or *Handyman jack*. These mechanical jacks range in height from 36 ins. to 48 ins. and can be purchased for $50 or less at an agricultural supply store or quality hardware store. Vehicle stabilization, lifting, pulling, spreading, squeezing, and clamping can be accomplished with these jacks. This tool has a rated lifting capacity of 7,000 lbs., a rated pulling capacity of 5,000 lbs., and a 750 lb. squeeze or clamp capacity rating.

Hi-lift jacks are designed to be used as a solitary, in-line adjustable pole, to provide support to an unstable load—*not to lift the load during stabilization efforts*. The jacks contribute a more stabilizing contact point with the ground. To provide this stabilizing factor, the force applied to a jack should be only the amount needed to put pressure between the jack's base and the vehicle.

Disassembly Tools

Auto extrication need not always be of a violent nature with cutting, pounding, and prying, generating bent and twisted metal. Sometimes the end result can be accomplished by simply disassembling the vehicle from around the accident victim. Hand tools come into play because of their reliability and the constraints placed on the rescuer because of available workspace.

Combination wrenches Both Standard Automotive Equipment (SAE) and metric sizes can be used to remove the fasteners from many automotive components. Where workspace is limited, 12-point box wrenches work best when small movements of the tool are all that is possible. Six-point wrenches give more contact surface with the nut or bolt for the stubborn, frozen threaded fastener.

Ratchet wrench When the nut or bolt can be addressed straight on, the ratchet wrench works very well. In addition to 6- and 12-point sockets, extensions, and universal joints are handy accessories.

Lug wrench tool Using an inexpensive lug wrench and a 6 in. long by ⅜ in. drive extension, this tool is relatively simple to fabricate. Using a socket on one leg of the lug wrench, fit the ⅜ in. drive extension into it and pin through both components. This configuration can also be welded or brazed into place.

This tool, using ½ in. for SAE or 12 mm for metric, can be used for removal of bolted hinges on car doors. The door can be removed and pivoted on the Nader bolt to provide access and removal of the patient.

Valve Stem Removal Tool: Purchased at automobile stores, this tool is used to remove the valve stem from the tires. Used in conjunction with stabilization, the tires deflate giving a firm foundation on which to work. The positive aspect of this procedure is that the stem may be reinstalled, the tire inflated, and the vehicle more easily towed away. Accident reconstructionists prefer this method over complete stem unit removal as they may need to reinflate certain tires pursuant to their investigations.

Pliers There are a variety of tools in this category. Essentially pliers are used for gripping irregular-shaped or deformed components. Types of pliers include: slip joint, needle nose, electricians, and vise grips. An assortment of several pliers is advantageous to the rescuer.

Screwdrivers Straight tip in sizes ¼ in., 5/16 in., ⅜ in., and larger are appropriate. Phillips tip in sizes #2, #3, and maybe larger provide a good selection. Torx head in size #10 through #35 can usually be obtained in prepackaged kits.

Functional fixity is using a tool for only the purpose for which it was designed. As previously mentioned, screwdrivers of large dimensions can also be used as lightweight pry bars and cutting tools.

Miscellaneous

Anything and everything not mentioned in the broader categories falls into this catch-all.

For maintenance purposes, the tools discussed can often be used on each other to perform this task. Add a quality metal file for sharpening cutting edges and your hand tool package is complete.

Hand Tool Maintenance

Hand tools should be inspected as described below:

- Check hammers for broken handles, mushroomed heads, loose heads, or other damage. Repair or replace as required.
- Check chisels for mushroomed heads, cracked, or chipped blades or burrs on the shanks. Hone to proper configuration or replace if needed.
- Check screwdrivers for loose, broken, or cracked handles. Repair or replace as necessary.
- Check ratchets for proper operation; make sure rachet locks in desired position without slipping. Check for burrs on all exposed surfaces. Repair as needed.
- Check extensions and sockets for twisted, bent, or otherwise damaged parts. Look for burrs on each piece. Repair or replace as needed.
- Check wrenches, pliers, and other like tools for spread or damaged jaws, bent or distorted handles, and burrs. Repair or replace as required.
- Check handsaws for distorted, bent, or broken handles; bent, broken, dull, missing, or improperly installed blades. Repair, sharpen, or replace as needed. Oil blades on handsaws to prevent rust.
- Clean and oil as required and restore inspected tools to their proper place on the squad where they are secured against movement and damage.

HYDRAULIC POWERED RESCUE TOOLS

Principles of Powered Tools

The concept of a hydraulic or power plant pump is that its primary function is to produce a flow of pressurized fluid. It produces pressure only as a secondary function and only when a load or restriction is placed against its flow. Then it produces only sufficient pressure to overcome the resistance so it can produce its rated flow. This rated flow, depending on the brand/manufacturer, ranges between 5,000 psi and 10,500 psi and is usually positive displacement in nature.

In Figure 11–1 a load of 9,600 pounds is to be lifted. Since the cylinder piston has 12 sq. ins. of surface area, the pump must build up to 800 psi on every square inch to develop a total of 9,600 lbs to equal the load resistance:

$9{,}600 \div 12 = 800$ psi.

In a practical situation the pump or power unit will also have to build up some additional pressure to force the fluid through connecting lines. The amount of additional pressure required depends entirely on the flow resistance of the piping or tubing.

Conversion of Mechanical Force into Fluid Pressure

In any fluid system the fluid force on one side of an output piston is equal to the mechanical opposition force. This was true in Figure 11–1. It also works in reverse as shown in Figure 11–2. The pressure generated in the fluid by a load weight on the output piston is equal to but no more than the load weight.

Standard catalog cylinders are designed only for thrust loads; the rod bearing is too small to handle heavy side loads and this is not required on most applications. For applications where a heavy side load must be supported, this can be handled in one of several ways:

- If space permits, a double-end-rod cylinder can be used. It has a rod bearing on each end of the cylinder and can handle a moderate amount of side loading.
- An outboard bearing can be installed on a standard cylinder, but this must be done by the user.

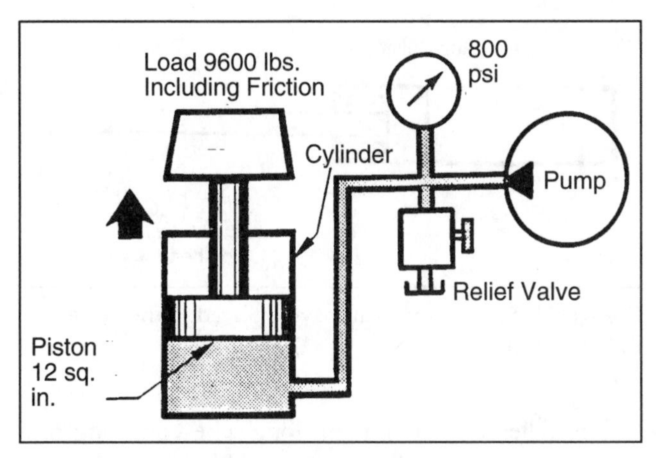

Figure 11–1 Primary function of hydraulic power is to produce a flow of pressurized fluid.

- A custom cylinder may be necessary and can be ordered from a number of specialty-building cylinders companies.

To avoid side loading (Figure 11–3), the cylinder should be carefully and accurately mounted in alignment with the load, and the alignment should be checked in two planes at right angles and at both closed and fully extended positions. During alignment, a hydraulic cylinder, if unloaded, can be extended by compressed air to check the alignment, or can be extended by a hydraulic hand pump if it is connected to a heavy load. Binding at any point in its stroke means that a side load is being transmitted to the rod bearing and the barrel. If the cylinder cannot be perfectly aligned with the load throughout its stroke, it may be necessary to use a hinge-mounted cylinder with a linear alignment coupler attached to the end of its piston rod.

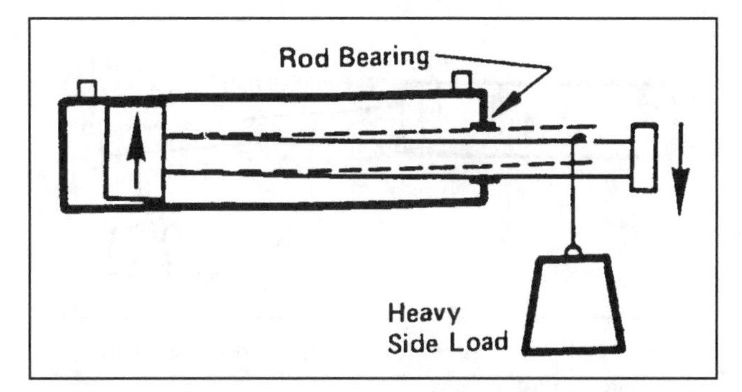

Figure 11–3 To avoid side loading the cylinder should be carefully and accurately mounted in alignment with the load.

Side load may produce several undesirable results. The piston rod can be permanently bent. Usually a bent rod cannot be satisfactorily straightened. It should be replaced with a new rod ordered from the cylinder manufacturer. The rod bearing can become worn to an oval shape. The side clearance thus opened can cause the rod seals to be distorted or deformed, extruded, or blown out. Fluid leakage around the rod seal can become excessive. The entire rod bearing or cartridge should be replaced; new sealing rings installed with a worn bearing will not last. Finally, a heavy side load can cause the barrel to be scored, resulting in a loss of power and speed, and short

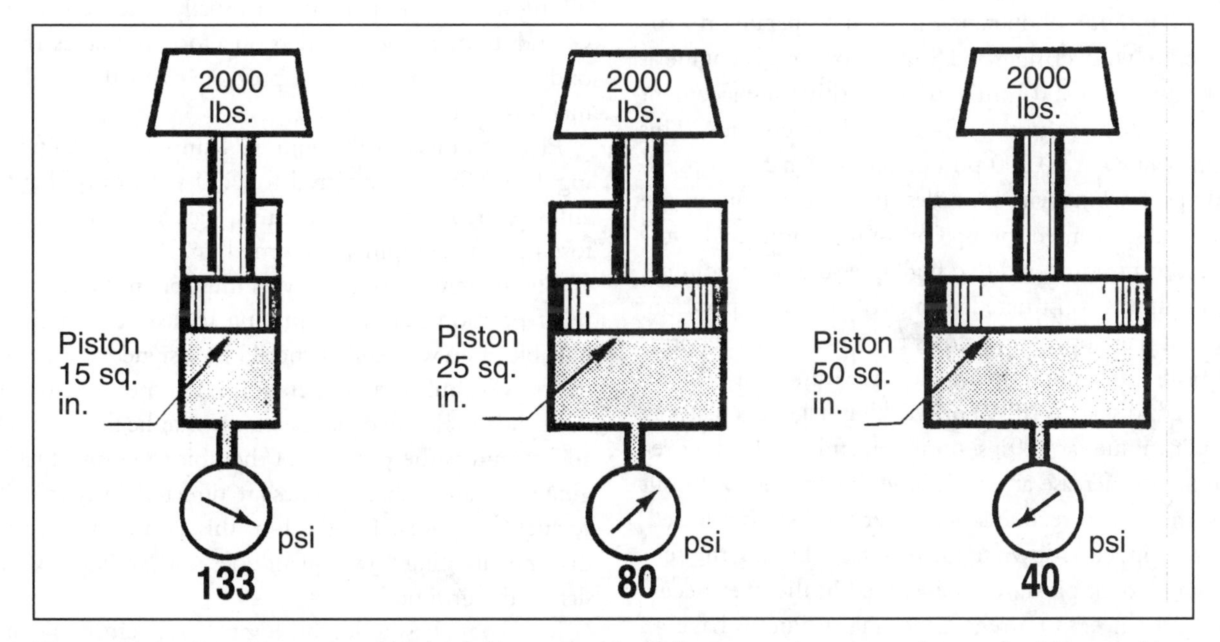

Figure 11–2 Pressure generated in the fluid on one side of the output piston is equal to mechanical opposition force.

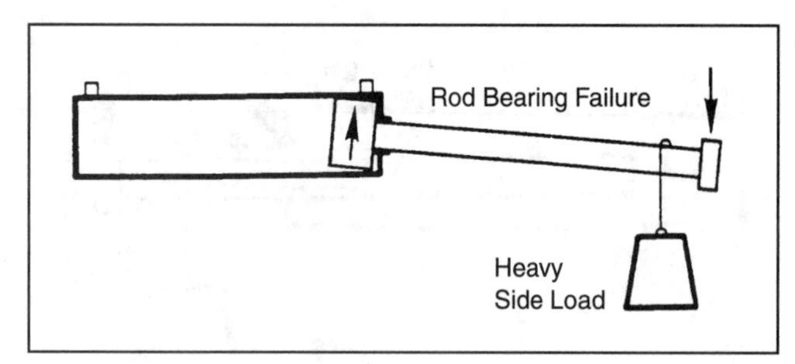

Figure 11–4 A heavy side load on the rod may damage the cylinder at full extension.

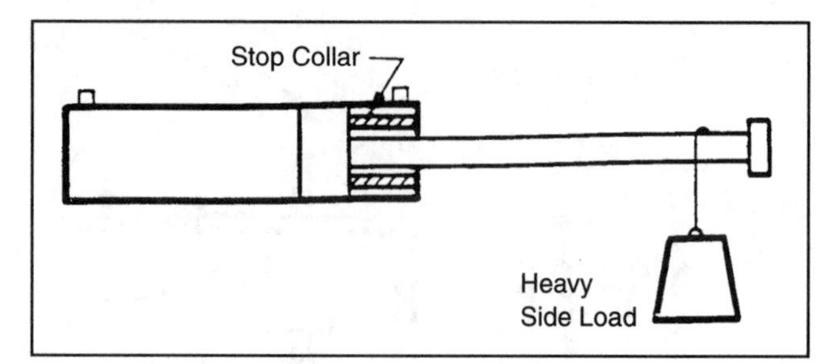

Figure 11–5 A stop collar may be placed in the cylinder to limit its stroke.

piston seal life (Figure 11–4). A stop collar may be placed in the cylinder to limit its stroke (Figure 11–5).

Power Rescue Tools

There are over 15 different brands of power rescue tools on the market today with distinctive differences as well as similarities. This discussion focuses on the similarities of rescue tools generally, therefore it is the responsibility of each student to become familiar with the specifics of the equipment used by his/her company/department.

Hydraulic rescue tools have four basic components: the power plant, spreaders, cutters, and rams.

The Power Plant: The power plant is the means through which the system pressurizes the fluid. Power units, which are the prime mover of hydraulic fluid, are powered by gasoline engines, diesel engines, electric motors, or compressed air. Gasoline-powered units provide 20 to 60 minutes of operating time, and operate on a rotary action with a Briggs and Stratton or Honda engine at 3,000 rpm to 3,400 rpm and are positive displacement pumps. They are usually 2- to 4-cycle engines. This pump is rated at 10,500 psi but operates at 5,000 psi to 5,500 psi for longevity purposes. It has six pistons in the positive displacement pump consisting of four high-volume, low-pressure, and two high-pressure, low-volume.

This unit is constructed with two stages for operation. The first stage opens and closes the spreader/cutter arms and blades. It will pump 1.5 gals. per minute at 800 psi. The second stage (HPLV) or working stage, circulates .5 gals per minute at 800 psi until demand and loading requirements increase at which time the pressure will shift from the first to second stage. After the load is released, the psi drops back down to the first stage. During this second stage, back pressure is developed in the lines necessitating the need for a relief mechanism. Pumps have 4½ in. suction tubes on their ends to facilitate movement of fluid found in the reservoir.

The relief valve is a 1½ in. long tube consisting of a popit-spring-screw set screw assembly that essentially regulates/controls pressure in the operating system. This assembly operates at 250 times/second when the system is operating. As a result, this unit must be pressure-tested yearly. If it is allowed to go untested, over time this unit will experience a 20% loss of power (e.g., units rated at 5,000 psi may only develop operating pressures of 4,000 psi). This can be a significant factor in operational efficiency on a working incident.

Hydraulic dump valves are directional control valves that regulate the fluid flow from the reservoir to the cutter/spreaders/rams. Internally, a spool valve diverts the flow. The positive displacement pump is situated ½ in. off the bottom of the reservoir. The bottom of this pump is protected by a circular screening device to secure the components of the pumping mechanism. As fluid levels drop, air/dust are drawn into the screen, clogging it, resulting in slowed operation. It usually takes less than 18 seconds to open the spreaders on a tool. If it takes 18 seconds or more, you have a problem with the screening mechanism being clogged.

Electric units usually require 84 amps on start-up if using 110 volts. Units wired for 220 volts only draw 42 amps. When using electric units, start and run them before lighting equipment is turned on.

The hydraulic control levers must be in the neutral or relief position before attempting to start the engine. If possible, a crew member should be assigned to stay with the power unit during operations. This person stops and starts the unit as needed, operates hydraulic flow controls, and monitors the position of the unit to ensure that engine noise and exhaust fumes are directed away from the rescue work area. In addition, this person also ensures that the vibrating power plant does not "walk away" as it sits on the ground.

It is always best to let the engine cool before refueling, however this is not always possible in rescue situations. If hot refueling (unit runs awhile, is hot, then fuel is added) is necessary, certain precautions need to be taken. Be downwind from the operating area, don full protective gear, use an approved safety can and a wide-mouthed funnel. A firefighter with either a hose line or extinguisher should also be standing by.

Many different hydraulic fluids are used in power rescue tools. Some, such as phosphate ester, can cause skin inflammation and burning, respiratory irritation if inhaled, and gastrointestinal problems if swallowed. Many systems pose the danger of pressure-penetration injuries in the event there is a leak or rupture to any component of the system. Rescuers should be in full protective clothing when operating any component of a system; this includes even the simple task of making and breaking couplings. Never mix hydraulic fluids. Always use the fluid specified by manufacturers for their equipment to prevent damage.

In an emergency situation (out of fluid), Hurst tools are designed to run on water. There is a common misconception associated with the use of ethylene glycol as a substitute for phosphate ester fluid. Hurst says not to use it in its tools. It will work as a substitute for one year at which time evaporation sets in and ruins the tool.

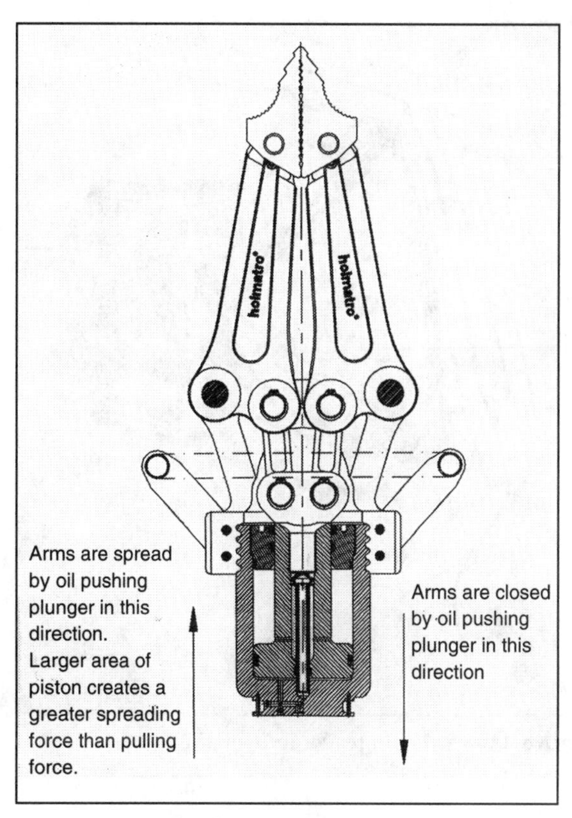

Figure 11–7 Hydraulic spreader actions and functions.

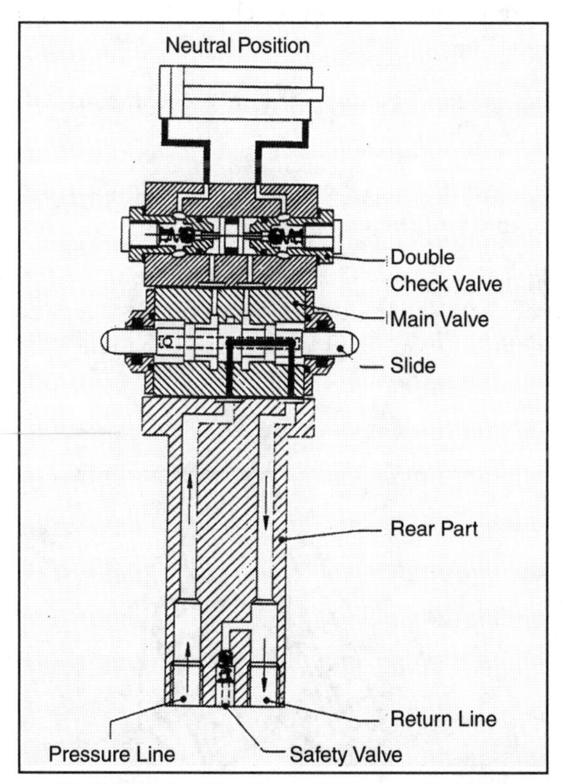

Figure 11–6 Hydraulic valve schematic of a Holmatro spreader.

Maintenance of the power plant includes checking all fluid levels, spark plugs, starter cords, electrical cords, hoses, and hose connections. Check for dirt, damage, and operation. Consider regular preventive maintenance. See manufacturer's recommendations. Store a hydraulic tool with the piston/cylinder retracted as this protects the shaft from dirt and contaminants.

The Spreader: The spreader consists of a piston connected to metal arms that open and close as the piston moves. Depending on the brand and the model, spreaders can weigh from 45 lbs. to 72 lbs. when filled with hydraulic fluid, and can open to as wide as 32 in. In addition to spreading, this tool can also be used for lifting, pushing, pulling, and clamping or squeezing by exerting 10,500 lbs. of pressure at 5,000 psi. (Figures 11–6, 11–7, 11–8)

The actual operation of a spreader is typically handled by one person, however, it may be necessary to have two rescuers move, place, and operate the tool. Rescuer height, weight, and personal conditioning factor into whether or not a hydraulic spreader is operated by one or more persons. If this is the case, then the *control operator* is the person responsible for the operation of the tool while the *assisting operator(s)* simply supports the weight of the

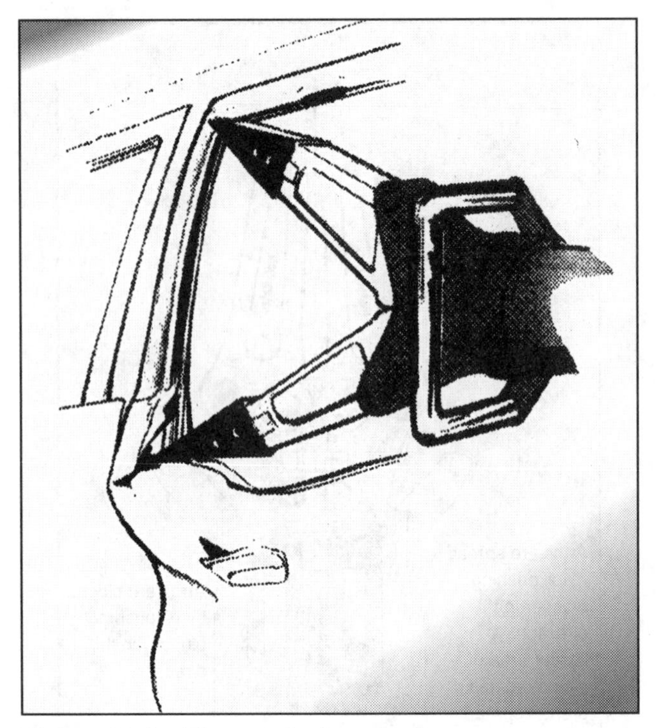

Figure 11–8 The spreader in operation.

tool. The unit is controlled by thumb pressure from either hand at any angle. Operators should be in full protective clothing and wearing wrap-around eye protection (safety glasses with side panels or safety goggles). *Never* place hand(s) on/or between the arms of the spreader or position your body between the vehicle and the tool.

Several different accessories may be used with spreaders. The most common are the automotive tips found on all spreaders and used for most operations. The automotive tip is a wedge-shaped tip with serrations or ridges on its working surfaces and is used for spreading and lifting. Another set of tips, available for many tools, are the aircraft tips. These consist of a narrow tip and a companion wide-shaped tip which are used together to rip or tear sheet metal. These tips have a tendency to tear the aluminum shell rather than spread and grab. A third tip is the grabber jaw; used for auto extrication and spreading jail bars (Figure 11–9).

The most common accessories are those used for pulling, usually a chain-and-shackle system. There are several designs, including some with pins permanently attached to the shackle. When using the standard chain-and-shackle system (such as Hurst), there are four critical safety procedures to follow:

1. Use only chains provided by the manufacturer.
2. Position the hooks so that the open sides are facing out.
3. Insert the pins that secure the shackles to the unit from the bottom side of the arms. In this way any load applied to the pins from underneath forces the pins to seat themselves rather than be forced out.
4. Attach the chains to the hooks so that the free end remains accessible from the top. If one chain were to be inserted from the bottom and the other from the top, a serious imbalance could occur which can cause spreader arms to completely fracture suddenly and violently.

Spreaders should be inspected on a regular basis and after each use. Check:

- *Cracks or dents.* These are critically important signs of possible tool failure.
- *Alignment of arms.* The tips should close and meet each other evenly. If there is a noticeable difference in alignment, you should suspect that the unit has been

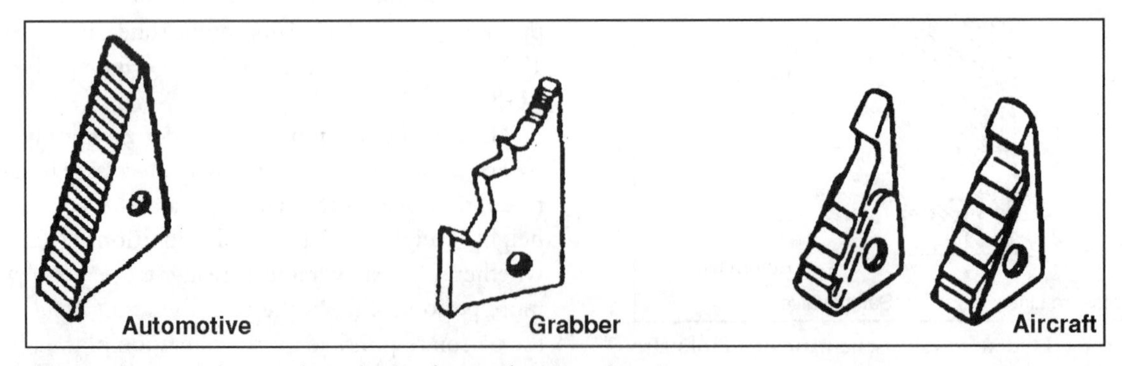

Figure 11–9 Selecting the right tips for purchasing points.

subjected to overload and needs factory inspection and service.

- *Nuts, bolts, screws, retainer rings, and pins.* Be certain they are in place and secure.

Safety: The tremendous power of hydraulic spreaders requires strict compliance with the following safety precautions:

1. Members using this tool should wear full fire protective equipment and safety eye goggles (wrap-around type; flip down shields are not safe for this operation).
2. As a force of approximately 5 tns. is exerted at the tips of the jaws, extreme caution must be observed while operating the tool. Only trained members, under close supervision of the officer in charge, should use the tool.
3. Couplings should be made up carefully (Figure 11–10). The hydraulic fluid is under high pressure and an improper connection, allowing fluid to spray, can cause injuries to eyes and exposed skin surfaces.
4. When necessary, proper shoring should accompany openings made by the tool.
5. Officers/rescuers supervising operations should utilize rescuers not using the tool to carefully and constantly observe overall areas to warn of possible collapse, car flipping over, or any other dangerous situation developing (safety officer).
6. Spreaders provide a small bearing area and must be opened and closed slowly in order to prevent the tool from shifting or slipping.
7. Never substitute chains or other materials on this tool.

Caution: Personnel must, at all times, use extreme caution where hands are placed on the arms of the tool. Never place hands or arms on spreader arms because the tool could easily close on them resulting in severe crushing injuries.

The Cutter: Power cutters are equipped with blades specifically designed to cut certain metals, such as the sheet metal found on vehicle door and roof posts. When the cutter is used to sever solid metal objects such as concrete reinforcing bars, unwanted tool stress and blade damage can occur. On the typical automobile, problems may be encountered if you attempt to cut:

- Cold rolled steel, ¾-in. steering columns
- Torsion bars
- Solid cast brake pedal or clutch pedal shafts
- Cast metal door hinges
- Seatbelt mounting bolts and reinforcing plates
- Hardened steel Nader bolts and reinforcing plates

Some cutters have a recess designed into the throat of the blade where the cutting power is at its greatest. These are commonly called *round stock cutters.* Manufacturers make different claims as to what their cutters will and will not cut. Check with your tool distributor or manufacturer before attempting to cut any heavy steel material.

Inspection of the cutter should be done routinely and after each use.

- Clean and visually inspect the unit to see that all nuts, bolts, retainer rings, screws, and pins are in place and secure.
- Visually inspect the blades for signs of obvious flaws or hairline cracks.
- Check the flatness of the blade with a straight edge.
- If possible, have the blades x-rayed or magnafluxed periodically to check for interior faults.

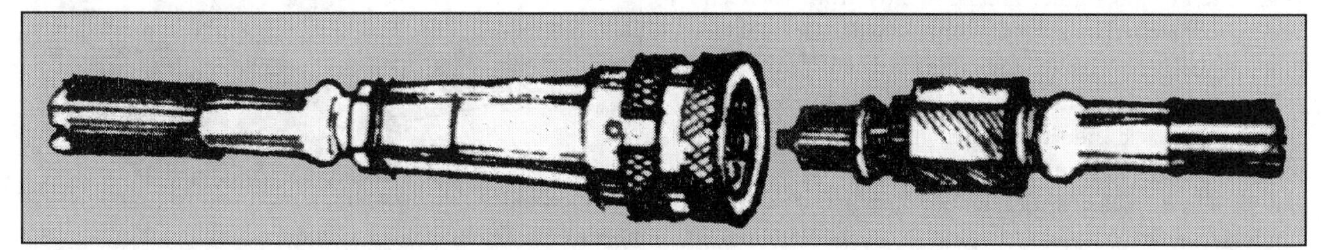

Figure 11–10 Hose connections must be made up and checked.

- Store the cutter with the blades closed just enough so that the outer edges touch each other. This protects the cutting edges and reduces the hydraulic pressure that can build up if the blades are closed too tightly.

When operating the cutters, be in full protective gear, including eye protection. Protect patients and attending medical personnel. Position the blades as close to perpendicular as possible to the object being cut. If, during operation, the blades shift any appreciable amount, reposition the cutters to prevent blade damage. Make every effort *not* to cut unsupported or "free" ends of objects. The force developed can launch the cut end with enough force to cause serious injury. There are cases in which portions of metal roof posts weighing from 4 lbs. to 5 lbs. have been launched more than 20 ft.

The Power Ram: The ram is the last component of the power rescue system. Rams range in length from 22 ins. to 65 ins. fully extended. Capabilities of rams differ from manufacturer to manufacturer. Some rams have pulling as well as pushing capabilities and are most frequently used for dash displacement, roll-up maneuvers, spreading, and third-door evolutions. These, however, on the average will develop only one-half of their total capacity in pulling operations.

Regardless of the make/model/manufacturer, rams generally consist of three basic components:

- Hydraulic hoses, couplings, control valves
- Tool casing that houses the hydraulic piston(s) and plunger
- Ram base, plunger head, and accessories that are interchangeable (e.g., B-post tool/rocker panel tool; Figure 11–11).

Most hydraulic power rams are single plunger units consisting of a stationary base at one end and a movable plunger on the opposite end. The plunger is the movable piston that travels in and out of the hydraulic cylinder that makes up the body of the tool itself. Holmatro and Viking Rams are examples of twin plunger units with two independent plungers incorporated into one tool. Both extend and retract independently from each end and are controlled by a single-control hydraulic valve located at the center of the rams (Figure 11–12).

The latest generation power rams, presented first by the F. M. Brick Industries, Inc., now use a two-piece telescoping plunger unit. Hydraulic power rams are also classified as a single- or double-acting hydraulic unit. A single-acting ram extends its plunger by hydraulic fluid pressure. The return of the plunger is generally accomplished by means of mechanical springs. The double-acting ram, the most prevalent and reliable type, uses hydraulic fluid to both extend and retract its plunger.

Another important difference between power rams is whether they are direct-control or remote-control types. Direct-control rams, which are the most common, have their hydraulic control valves mounted directly on the ram itself. In addition, grip handles are located directly on the tool body. The Phoenix Ram, a remote-controlled power ram, has its control valve situated on a short hydraulic hose attached to the tool. One advantage of this style of remote-control ram is that its lower tool profile allows it to be positioned in more restricted spaces than conventional direct control rams. Rescue personnel can also situate themselves in a somewhat safer location when operating the remote control ram under actual rescue situations. One disadvantage is that it may require two hands to operate the ram's remote control.

Power rams come in various shapes and sizes and are designed for specific tasks based on their length of extension. In general, ram lengths are:

- *Short*—Retracted lengths of 12 ins. to 24 ins.
- *Medium*—Retracted lengths of 24 ins. to 35 ins.
- *Long*—Retracted lengths in excess of 35 ins.

Depending on the manufacturer, rams can extend to lengths of 65 ins. as featured by Holmatro, Inc. Regardless of the manufacturer, all power rams are more power-

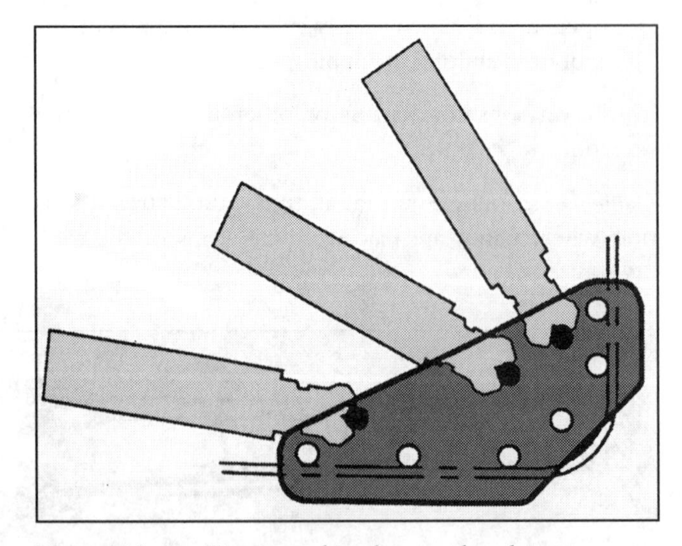

Figure 11–11 B-post tool/rocker panel tool.

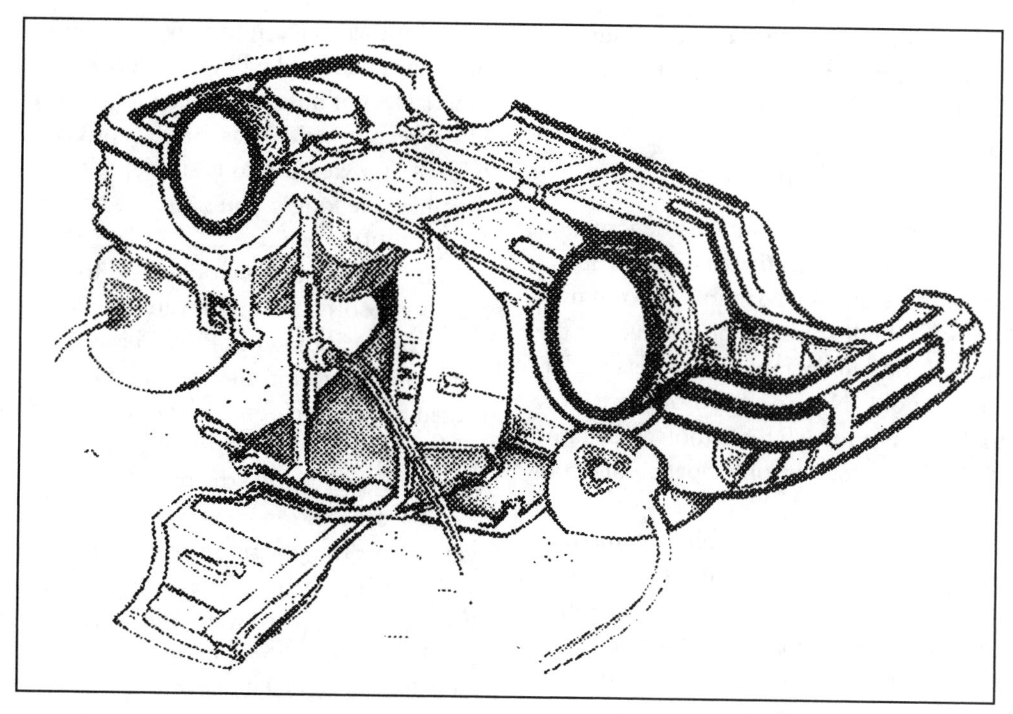

Figure 11–12 Twin-plunger unit.

ful while extending or pushing than when retracting. To extend the ram, the rescuer/operator diverts hydraulic fluid under pressure against the full side of the disk situated at the bottom of the plunger rod inside the body of the ram (A side). The available hydraulic fluid pressure is multiplied by the available surface area of this piston disk to create a given force rating for the ram. During the retraction phase of operation (B side), fluid is diverted against the other side of this disk, or the side with the rod attached to it. Even though the fluid pressure remains the same, there may be up to 50% less surface area, which is the reason why rams cannot retract or pull with the same force as when they extend/push. As a rule, rams develop only half of their maximum power during their retraction phase of operation.

Because of the inherent dangers associated with hydraulic tools, rescuers should always don personal protective gear. This is especially true when using hydraulic rams. When you use rams to lift, push, pull, or stabilize, there is also an element of unpredictability as to how these tools will operate. Occupants and rescuers must be protected as best possible in the event a ram suddenly dislodges from its intended object or breaks loose some component of the dash, rocker panel, etc.

In the interest of safety, rams should only be held or maneuvered by using the grip handles or by the body of the tool itself. Hands should never be placed on the moving plunger as this may contaminate the plunger surface with dirt and/or subject the operator to pinching injuries.

Power/hydraulic rams have the least structural integrity when fully extended. Extending the ram moves the plunger out from the body of the tool, diminishing contact between the plunger and the cylinder. Heavy loading or stressing of the ram during a long spread or push can deform the tool. Operating personnel should be alert for long reaches or off-center loading that can cause undue stress and affect the integrity of the tool as it extends.

During pulling operations, rams *can* be damaged if they are subjected to bending. To prevent this, the operator must ensure that all loads applied to the tool/ram run parallel to the tool. Having a completely solid base under the ram or having the ram suspended without any contact under it will ensure a safe, parallel pull.

Power/hydraulic rams are also vulnerable to damage when used in the conventional pushing mode. Rescuers/operators must be certain that both the base and the plunger ends of the ram are properly positioned before any load is applied to the tool. Most ram designs locate the grip handles and any hydraulic lines clear of the extreme ends of the tool. Rams should be stored with the plungers extended by ¼ in. to ½ in. to prevent overretraction into the body of the tool and excessive pressure on the tool's hydraulic system. Visually inspect the tool and plunger ends for damage. Clean as necessary.

Manifolds

Rescuers over the years have experienced a phenomenon known as *lock-up* caused by *intensification.* This problem begins with the use of a manifold. Manifolds are not used as they were intended. Some rescuers operate under the false assumption that you can operate three tools simultaneously with a manifold. Not so! Manifolds are only management tools. You can attach three tools at the same time to the manifold, but you can only operate one tool at a time.

There are three positions on a manifold system: 1, 2, and 3. Spreaders should occupy the #1 position, cutters, #2; and ram, #3. Sequential operation simultaneously can create the problem of intensification which generates pressure spikes of 10,500 psi, causing the tools to lock up. This mathematical property occurs when you attempt to operate these tools together. The 5,000 psi is channeled into the A side of a spreading tool which displaces fluid under pressure. This intensifies into the second tool whereby you now have approximately 6,540 psi into the cutters, then the rams (third tool) intensify by 1,400 psi to a maximum pressure of 7,800 psi.

To prevent lock-up, follow this sequence to relieve pressure after operation.

1. Retract the piston/cylinder (B side closes).
2. Throw the dump valve after working the trigger mechanism twice. This bleeds the entire system (power unit).
3. Disconnect the supply line (pressure side) all the way around.

Another factor that contributes to lock-up is failing to hook up a tool to all manifold ports. It can not function properly without all props hooked up to a tool. You will also need to purchase an in-line dump valve if you are going to use a manifold system. Don't deadhead this system. If you deadhead an Amkus system, it will crash the system.

Hurst hydraulic systems are designed to operate with 25 ft. to 30 ft. of hose. Lock-up and associated manifold problems occur more frequently when added hose lengths are used. For example, some rescue units have 100 ft. hose reels. Remember, it takes three seconds to pressurize 16 ft. of hose, utilizing 1 qt. of hydraulic fluid. Thus, 100 ft. of hose will utilize 6 qts. to 7 qts. of fluid. You must also take into consideration that each attachment on a manifold will yield approximately 25 to 30 additional feet of hose for a total footage of 175 ft. to 190 ft. Hurst recommends that 100 ft. cord reels only be used with 30 ft. extension to ensure optimal functioning. Remember, the longer you stretch it, the longer it will take for the tools to operate.

With all extensions hooked up to a manifold system and three tools operating at various intervals, the reservoir will drop by as much as 40%. This low fluid level can result in fluctuation in the tool head on a spreader. This is caused by air developing in the system and expands when it hits the reservoir. To prevent this problem, add hydraulic oil and recycle the tools.

If for some reason you reverse the hydraulic hoses, you will reverse the operation of the tool. Tools operate on an A and B principle. The A side of the piston/cylinder (bottom up) is the power stroke that pressurizes (opens). The B side (top-down) closes. The A side is designed to fail 9,400 psi as a safety factor.

Safety

As with any hydraulic rescue tool, do not attempt to mix and match various parts of the hydraulic systems with any components other than the ones specified by a particular manufacturer. Read these fact sheets carefully and when in doubt, call the equipment representatives directly.

Porta-power Rescue Tool

The porta-power is a hydraulic rescue tool operated by a hand pump rather than a power-driven pump. It was designed as an autobody shop tool and has been adapted for rescue work. The tool serves well in rescue situations when operated properly.

With the advent of the power rescue tool, the porta-power has, in many cases, been put aside during training or even removed from the rescue unit. Rescue companies should recognize the value of this tool in their rescue arsenal and continue to maintain and train with it.

The porta-power consists of several different components. The pump unit may be single-, two-, or three-stage. It pressurizes the fluid to a maximum of 10,500 psi. The pump should be operated in the horizontal position or with the hose end of the pump held below horizontal. Holmatro has a three-stage hand-operated pump that generates 10,500 psi and operates cutters, spreaders, and rams.

The ram is the only part of the porta-power kit that can achieve the full kit rating, generally 4 tn. or 10 tn.

The ram can be used by itself or with any of a variety of extension tubes, heads, bases, and adapters. With these adapters the ram can be used to lift, push, pull, spread, or clamp objects.

The spreader, wedge, and duck bill accessories allow the porta-power to be used in the same basic way as the power spreader. The large spreader will typically open to 12 ins; the wedge to approximately 3 ins. to 3½ ins. The duck bill, which is used in conjunction with the ram, has an opening distance of 6 ins. Remember, these tips will not develop the full power rating of the kit. Generally the spreader and duck bill heads will have a maximum rating of 1,200 lbs., while the wedge has a maximum rating of 600 lbs.

There are a variety of head attachments which provide a contact point between the tool and an object: smooth, serrated, crowned, vee, wedge, and rubber.

Bases increase the contact area between the tool and an object and extension tubes increase the reaching capabilities of the ram. Remember, the longer the ram (column), the weaker it is.

Connectors and locking pins connect the extensions and adapter attachments are used to make connections between the ram, tubing, or other components. The cylinder and plunger toe attachments are used together to allow the porta-power ram to be used in small areas for lifting or spreading.

When operating the tool, wear full protective gear. Be fully aware of the power ratings of the particular attachment you are using and work within these ratings. When the pump and handle can no longer be squeezed together, the capacity of the tool has been reached.

Inspection and maintenance of the tool consists of visually inspecting all components for loose items, missing parts, and physical damage. Fluid levels should be checked and topped off if needed. Clean and properly store all tools and accessories. Never interchange components or accessories between manufacturers brands or equipment. Serious damage or injury could result to the equipment and to the rescuer.

ELECTRICALLY POWERED RESCUE TOOLS

Many gasoline-powered tools can also be powered electrically. Electrically powered tools are quieter than gasoline powered and require less maintenance. Some disadvantages may be that tools such as spreaders and cutters will operate at a slower speed and may not develop as much power. Also, generator and electrical cords may pose problems in situations where the rescue unit can not be pulled in close enough to the working area.

Reciprocating Saw

The reciprocating saw is an extremely versatile tool which can be used to cut through roof posts, brake and clutch pedal shafts, steering wheel rings, steering columns, and more. Generally a 6-in. blade, 18 teeth per inch, is sufficient for use on standard automobile extrications, however, you will need 8-in. blades to perform some tasks on a bus rescue.

When operating the saw, wear full gear with eye protection. Keep the foot of the saw in contact with the surface of the object being cut. Lifting the foot off the object eliminates the efficiency of the reciprocating action of the saw and will stress the blade to the breaking point. Move the saw along with a gentle rocking motion. This rocking motion allows the saw to work at its best. Keep the blade lubricated. Use soapy water or lightweight lubricating oil in a spray bottle. If you do not have this available, use the compressed air from an SCBA bottle. Keep the blade clean. Lubricating cools and cleans the blade and minimizes the likelihood of sparks being produced.

Additional tools which may be of use are an electric drill and an impact wrench. Among other uses, the drill may be used with a ¼-in. bit to vent the hydraulic piston of a shock-absorbing bumper. The impact wrench can be used to remove a door at the hinges.

PNEUMATIC RESCUE TOOLS

Air Chisel

The air chisel is a cutting tool with many uses on the rescue scene. The air source of the air chisel is usually an SCBA bottle, however, you may also use larger storage cylinders, compressors, or the air brake system of the apparatus. Several departments have used inert gases such as nitrogen in place of compressed air to power the air chisel.

Note: Never use oxygen to power the air chisel or any other pneumatic tool. Oxygen will react with the oil used to lubricate the tool and may cause the tool to explode in your hand.

The air regulator reduces the pressure from the air source to the working pressure of the tool. Standard regulators are designed to accept pressures of up to 2,216 psi. Newer regulators are designed to accept up to 6,000 psi, making them compatible with the 4,500 psi SCBA cylinders.

Air hoses are generally ⅜-in. diameter and have working pressure ratings of 250 psi. Standard lengths are from 15 ft. to 20 ft. Longer lengths reduce the ability of the air to flow through the hose thus reducing the efficiency of the tool.

The air chisel is a pistol-grip tool with a trigger. A piston operates the chisel bit. The retainer device on the tool is used to hold the bit in place. There are several types of retainers available. The best, the pull-back swivel collar, is generally referred to as the safety retainer.

Note: The older coiled-spring beehive style retainer is unsafe. The blade may unexpectedly fly out of this retainer during use. Also, it does not meet OSHA safety requirements for retainer systems. Air chisels can be retrofitted with approved safety retainers.

The more common types of chisel bits for the air chisel are described below.

Flat chisel Has a rounded shank end with a curved, half-moon cutting edge. It is used to cut heavy-gauge material and multiple-layer material such as vehicle roof posts, firewalls, bolts, and nuts.

Cold chisel Has a tapered, pinch-point working end resembling a standard cold chisel. It is used to cut through solid-stock material such as rivets, bolts, and nuts.

Single-panel cutter This bit has a working end resembling a "T" with the bottom of the T forming a cutting tooth. The top portion of the T acts to control the cutting depth. The single-panel cutter is used to cut light-gauge material such as vehicle roofs.

Double-panel cutter Has a wide flare at the working end. Each corner of the flared end forms a small metal cutting tooth. One tooth cuts the sheet metal and is guided by the thicker center portion of the tip. The second tooth serves as a backup in case the first tooth fails.

Air chisels consume approximately 7 cu. ft. of air per minute at a working pressure of 90 psi. This means that the average 45 cu. ft. SCBA bottle will provide about 6.5 minutes of effective cutting time. After this time the efficiency of the tool will decrease. Standard low-pressure bottles will yield lower operational times depending on consumption rates of 90 psi to 110 psi.

To put the tool into operation, first attach the regulator to the air source—*hand tight only.* Place the cutting blade in the tool and put several drops of lubricating oil into the air inlet at the bottom of the tool handle. Connect the air hose to the tool and make a quick safety-check, then pressurize the tool. At this point the tool should be treated as a loaded gun. In addition to standard body and eye protection, hearing protection should be used by the operator and rescuers working inside the vehicle. Identify a standard method for stopping the operation in the event of a problem. A physical signal should be used since verbal communication will be difficult.

The most important preventive maintenance for the air chisel is lubrication. A new tool should be lubricated before it is used. Tools should also be lubricated after each use or once for every hour of operation. Place a few drops of lubrication oil such as SAE No. 5 or 10 into the air inlet and then operate the tool under a load to blow the excess oil out of the exhaust ports. Wipe the tool clean.

Tighten any loose parts, paying particular attention to the set screws which hold the retaining collar in place. Clean and inspect the tool, making sure there is no dirt or foreign matter at the air inlet, exhausts, or between portions of the tool. Blades should be sharpened periodically, taking care not to overheat.

Air Gun—Paratech Airgun 40

Problems can be encountered when rescue units attempt to cut through heavy-gauge metal like that found on school buses or structural frame areas of trucks or trains. In these cases a larger, more powerful tool is needed. In 1984 Paratech Incorporated developed the Airgun 40 specifically for rescue applications.

The Airgun 40 goes beyond the limits of the standard air chisel. It operates at a pressure of 250 psi, yet has an air consumption rate of approximately half that of the standard air chisel. This low air consumption rate is achieved by using a spring return for the operating piston rather than an air-powered return. The tool operates with a distinctive cycling sound like a jack hammer. The Airgun 40's estimated 600 blows per minute enable it to cut through thicker and more solid materials than possible with the standard air chisel. Operation, safety, and maintenance are the same as the standard air chisel.

Pneumatic Impact Wrench

Also available with electric power, the impact wrench is a valuable tool to the rescue company. It can be used in disassembly operations such as door removal. It is crucial to have a complete set of both standard and metric sockets available. So that the socket will be able to withstand the hard use of rescue operations, only case-hardened sockets should be used.

Air-lifting Systems

The air bag and air cushion systems have four components:

1. Air source Typically comes from SCBA cylinders,

but may also be compressors, manual pumps, or the air brake system of the rescue vehicle.

2. Controller The piece of equipment that allows air to flow into and out of the air bag. It contains gauges to monitor the pressure in the bag, and relief valves to prevent overpressurization of the bags. In addition, the control switches are deadman-type switches which require constant intervention to allow air to flow. When the switch is released, it returns to the neutral position.
3. Air hoses Air hoses are usually 16 ft. to 32 ft. long and usually come in different colors in order to avoid confusion when using more than one bag at a time. The couplings are designed with safety systems to prevent accidental disconnection. The two most popular are the safety lock ring (Paratech), which can be screwed forward to hold the release collar of the female connector in position, and the double-locking coupling (Vetter), which requires that the female connector be forced forward to release the first lock and then pulled backward to completely release the coupling from the male nipple.
4. Air bag Exerts force measured in pounds. The capabilities of the air bag range from 1 tn. to 75 tns. maximum lifting force. Sizes range from 6 ins. × 6 ins. to 36 ins. × 36 ins. The coupling on the bag has a small diameter opening which causes the bag to deflate slowly. This is a safety feature since rapid collapse of the bag could endanger rescue personnel. Another type of air bag is the leak-sealing type. It is designed for use in haz-mat incidents involving the application to cracks, open-end pipes, and holes in low-pressure liquid storage containers. They inflate from minimum pressures of 5 psi to 7 psi to maximum pressures of 25 psi.

There are three categories of air lifting systems: low-, medium-, and high-pressure air cushions.

Low-pressure Air Cushions: Low-pressure cushions provide vertical lift over a large surface area. These cushions perform especially well when thin-skinned, light-walled vehicles such as aluminum truck trailers, tank vehicles, buses, or aircraft require moving or lifting. Lifting capacities range from 3 ins. to 30 tns. with air consumption requirements ranging from 2 cu. ft. to 42 cu. ft. Inflation height is generally accepted at 24 to 60 ins.

Low-pressure air cushions are constructed of a strong reinforced fabric material (up to 7 ply) forming the top and bottom plates of the cushion. The internal composition is engineered with nylon strapping supports. The low pressure cushion itself is constructed of a simple canvas of eremite/Kevlar impregnated and bonded to neoprene. These cushions are designed to function at 7 psi. This low pressure enables the cushion to mold itself to uneven surfaces and/or objects. Maximum lifting capacity is only achieved when the cushion is fully inflated.

Rescuers should use caution when using these cushions because they are more susceptible to physical damage than high-pressure air bags/cushions.

Medium-pressure Air Cushions: Medium-pressure cushions are designed to operate at 15 psi, although most tasks can be accomplished with pressures of 8 psi to 12 psi. Air cushions designed to function at 15 psi have bursting pressures of between 58 psi and 100 psi depending on manufacture size and style. Medium-pressure cushions generally have thicker sides than lower pressure cushions. From a safety standpoint, it is important to remember that when working with air cushions on slippery/wet surfaces, or in mud, ice, or snow conditions, rescuers should place a sand or gravel material under the cushion for increased traction.

High-pressure Air Bags: High-pressure air bags are constructed with neoprene/nitrate rubber outer layers, with the inner layers made of Kevlar fiber and/or steel wire. They are designed to lift 1 tn. to 75 tns. to heights of 7 ins. to 20 ins. depending upon the size of the bag. High-pressure air bags should always be used with cribbing, with a protected surface as a base.

High-pressure cushions are designed to accommodate inflation pressures of 90 psi to 145 psi, depending on the manufacturer's make and design. With high-pressure cushions there is a direct relationship between lifting capacity and inflation height. All high-pressure air bags have ratings for both the maximum force in pounds that they can exert and the maximum height they can achieve when fully inflated.

To calculate the theoretical lifting capacity of a high-pressure air bag, the following formula is useful. This example features the dimensions of a 30 × 30 in. air bag.

L × W × Internal air pressure of bag

30 ins. × 30 ins. = 900 sq. ins. working area

900 sq. ins. × ★118 psi = 106,200 lbs. or 53 tns. rated lifting capacity

★118 psi provided air

The maximum inflation height would be 18 ins. This would reduce the lifting capacity to 27 to 28 tns. because a high-pressure air bag maintains its theoretical 100% capacity only until the center is approximately 2 ins. in height. Continued inflation diminishes this capacity. Higher inflation means lower capacity, hence, maximum height yields one-half maximum capacity. This is because as the bag continues to expand, the contact surface area begins to diminish, thereby reducing the total lifting capacity to the point that at full inflation height the bag generally has only 50% of its original working surface area still in contact with the surface below.

Lifting capacities of a two-bag configuration (stacked) are dependent on required inflation heights. Useable height of both bags can be added together to estimate the total lifting height. When stacking air bags, always place the largest air bag on the bottom and the smaller air bag on top. *Never stack more than two air bags in height.* Remember, the higher the lift, the more unstable stacked bags become because of their susceptibility to shifting/kicking out of position. Stacking air bags versus simultaneous lifting from two separate locations on an object does not allow you to add the lifting capacities of the bags together to get an estimate of their lifting capacity. This means *the smallest capacity bag that is inflated is the maximum that the stacked bags will lift.* A 10-tn. capacity bag placed on top of a 26-ton capacity bag will lift a maximum of 10 tns.

Depending on which bag is inflated, stacking configurations can lift either 10 tns. of weight or 26 tns. Heavier weights, up to the sum of two lifting bags, can be lifted when bags are positioned at two separate locations and inflated simultaneously. The safe total lift with stacked bags is a judgement call made by the rescuer based on the scenario encountered. This limit is achieved when the contact area between two bags is diminished, to the point at which the stacked bags become unstable.

If both stacked bags were to be inflated fully, it would be like trying to balance one basketball on top of another. The hard, crowned surfaces of the bags actually become like wheels, allowing the load to roll or shift. Full inflation of stacked bags pose a safety threat of "kick-out" to the rescuers operating near them. Maintaining the bags at less-than-full inflation pressure/height allows the surfaces of the two bags to bond themselves together, thereby increasing stacking configuration.

Safety in operation is as important in using air bags as it is with any other tool. Standard protective clothing is required for all operating personnel. Keep the area clear. Visualize the path the air bag would take should it slip or be kicked loose, and clear that "strike zone" of all persons for over 25 ft.

The rescuer controlling the air bags should be in a position where at least one bag can be seen. This control operator accepts commands from *only one* person. Commands should refer to the color of the hose supplying the bag to be operated, such as, "Up on red" or "Down on yellow."

Maintenance of air-lifting systems requires cleaning of the bags, hoses, and controller and visually inspecting for damage. Inflate the bag or cushion to 50% of its working pressure, wash it with a mild soap, and rinse with water. While wet, inspect for leaks. High-pressure bags must be returned to the manufacturer for repair or replacement. Small tears and punctures in medium- and low-pressure cushions can be repaired by using a patch kit supplied by the manufacturer. Any cushion which has been field repaired should be tested at 50% of its operating pressure for five minutes after the patch as properly dried. During this test the cushion should not lose any pressure. Additional information on air-lifting systems and bags is presented in session 12.

Jimi-Jak

The Jimi-Jak is an air-shore pneumatic vehicular stabilization device. This device has an enclosed cylinder with a perforated piston sealed on one end with a rubber diaphragm cover. A variety of attachments are available.

SUMMARY

It is important that rescue companies assess their needs and acquire the tools and equipment they need to perform the types of rescue operations to which they may be called. Rescue tools, however, do not operate by themselves. The true measure of a rescue company is its ability to perform on the scene with whatever tools and equipment it has available. This requires well-trained personnel and well-maintained tools.

DEFINITIONS

Disassemble: To take apart with small hand tools (e.g., pliers, wrench, ratchet or screwdriver). *Example:* To unbolt door hinge from A pillar.

Displacing: To move an object from its original position. *Example:* Lowering, lifting, pushing, pulling, rotating.

Distorting: To change shape without severing or

parting. *Example:* Spreading, bending, enlarging, prying, squeezing, compressing.

Severing: To divide into two or more parts. *Example:* Cutting, piercing, splitting, penetrating, breaking.

Stabilization: The use of wooden cribbing and wedges for stabilizing unstable vehicles and loads.

Important: Stabilize before attempting to gain access, and when you raise an inch you must also crib an inch to ensure safety.

HIGH-PRESSURE AIRBAGS

A 53-year-old Takoma Park, Maryland, city employee can be thankful for the skills of fire and rescue workers, particularly in the use of air bags.

This rescue incident began when the employee, Kenneth L. Jones, city superintendent of streets, was called to Piney Branch Road in Takoma Park, where an 11-year old refuse truck developed brake problems.

The truck driver had pulled over to the side of the southbound lane and was outside the vehicle, waiting for a city mechanic. But the emergency brake failed and the loaded truck, grossing about 40 tns., began rolling backwards.

Jones saw the vehicle moving and he also saw several cars approaching it from behind. He jumped on the right running board of the right-hand drive truck. After the truck had struck a car parked at the curb, Jones steered it into the northbound lane, which was clear of traffic. Jones then attempted to steer the powerless vehicle into a vacant lot. Just short of the lot, however, it left the road, Jones was thrown, and he landed on a concrete culvert. The truck flipped over and landed on top of him, pinning him just below the hips.

The Takoma Park Volunteer Fire Department received the report of an overturned truck, with someone possibly pinned beneath it, and dispatched an initial assignment of Takoma Park Engine 21, Truck 2, and Ambulance 29, Silver Spring's Medic 5, and Wheaton Rescue Squad's Rescue 29.

I monitored the dispatch and responded to take command. Upon arrival, I asked Montgomery County Communications to contact the nearest heavy equipment dealer for a crane capable of lifting 35 tns. to 40 tns. A unit was sent from neighboring Prince George's County.

Chief P. Sterling, a Montgomery County police officer and a member of the Wheaton Volunteer Rescue Squad, was being cleared from a SWAT call several miles away. He and a fellow police officer responded. En route, they commandeered a Potomac Edison Power Co. (PEPCO) utility truck and crane.

The initial size-up described a truck cab lying on a culvert with its body in adacent soft ground, and a man, who was conscious and able to move his upper body, pinned under the truck.

First-in Ambulance 29 crew members went to aid the pinned man, making primary and secondary surveys. Next-in Truck 2 personnel concentrated on shoring the overturned truck. They secured lines from its front and rear axles to a bridge abutment, then placed planks and jacks under the top of the truck body, which was lying on soft ground. The crew of Engine 21 established fire protection.

Takoma Park and Montgomery County police established traffic control. Also on the scene was City Manager A. Nichols. He coordinated a supply of heavy planks from Public Works.

Paramedic R. Stephan, a lieutenant with the Chevy Chase (Maryland) Fire Department, who was riding with Medic 5, arrived and reviewed the incident status with Ambulance 29 personnel. He confirmed the victim's vital signs, and consulted by radio with the trauma unit at Suburban Hospital. Preparing for a worst-case scenario, Stephan requested a doctor with additional equipment. Then he returned to the patient to establish an intravenous line.

Rescue 29, manned by Lieutenant R. Weber, Paramedic M. Collins, and Squadsman T. Williams, arrived. After consultation with this rescue crew, it was decided to use air bags to lift the truck. The PEPCO crane was used to establish a support line to the top of the truck body, thus preventing the vehicle from rolling farther onto Jones.

On three occasions Jones pulled the IV from his arm; each time Paramedics Stephan and Collins reestablished a feed. Because of the victim's high blood pressure reading, they were worried about shock. Other personnel readied a backboard, or Stokes, a litter, and a MAST suit, so that, when the truck was lifted, the victim could be put on the board to be carried up a short 15-ft. grade and placed into the litter and MAST suit.

As personnel supplied additional support to the truck and began to place the air bag, Bethesda–Chevy Chase Rescue Squad personnel arrived from Suburban Hospital with a doctor. After a consultation with everyone involved in the operation, Wheaton personnel began to lift the truck with an air bag. They had placed planks on the ground and had set the air bag between the truck body and the planks.

As the vehicle lifted, crews shored it more. A second air bag was required to get the several inches needed to free Jones. Once freed, he was placed on the backboard, or Stokes, moved up the grade, and placed on the litter. The MAST suit was put in place, although it was not required.

Jones was transported to a trauma center in Washington, D.C. His injuries included bruised legs and a bruised kidney. He spent several days in the hospital, followed by weeks on crutches.

The city impounded the refuse truck and requested the Maryland State Police to conduct an investigation.

Cooperation between the three fire and rescue departments was excellent. With each unit's officers reporting its status step by step, command was well coordinated. Each step was reviewed carefully to ensure the safety of the patient and the fire and rescue personnel. Once again, well-trained crews coordinated command of multiple companies and the use of innovations in tools proved invaluable in handling an emergency successfully.

Wheaton personnel got their air bags less than a year before this incident. They had used them in training and in automobile accidents, but this was their first use with a large vehicle. In his comments during a critique held in Takoma Park, Chief Sterling said, "Training squad personnel in the use of air bags had paid off in this incident."

Note: Reprinted with permission, R. A. McGary: *Fire Engineering*/March 1987. Chief Roger A. McGary began his fire service career in Pennsylvania in 1956 and served nine years as fire protection engineer and fire chief of the Merck & Company chemical facility in Rahway, New Jersey. He became career chief at Takoma Park in 1979.

METRIC CONVERSIONS FOR THE FIRE SERVICE

These metric conversions are particularly useful to firefighters:

To convert gallons per minute (gpm) to liters per minute (lpm):

(3.79)(gpm) = lpm

A 1,500 gpm pump would equal a 5,685 lpm pump.

To convert lpm to gpm:

(.264)(lpm) = gpm

A 3.790 lpm pump would equal a 1,000 gpm pump.

To convert ft. to meters (m.):

(.3048)(#ft) = #m.

An 85 ft. aerial ladder would equal a 25.9 m. ladder.

To convert m. to ft.:

(3.28)(# m.) = ft.

A 30 m. aerial ladder truck would equal a 100 ft. aerial ladder truck.

To convert ins. to millimeters (mm.):

(25.4)(# ins.) + # mm.

2 in. fire hose would equal a 63.5 mm fire hose.

To convert mm. to ins.:

(.039)(# mm.) = ins.

90 mm. would equal 3 ins.

To convert mph to (kph):

(1.609)(mph.) = kph

55 mph. would equal 88.5 kph.

To convert kph. to mph:

(.62)(kph) = mph

90 kph. would equal 55.8 mph.

To convert lbs. to kilograms (kg.):

(.4536)(# lbs.) = kg.

A 6 lb. sledge hammer would equal a 2.72 kg. sledge hammer.

To convert kg. to lbs.:

(2.205)(# kg) = lbs.

An 8 lb. pick-head axe would equal a 3.6 kg. pick-head axe.

To convert degrees F to degrees C:

(# degrees F − 32)(5/9) = degrees C

A 75° Fahrenheit day would equal a 24° Centigrade day.

To convert degrees C to degrees F:

(degrees C)(9/15) + 32 = degrees F

A 27° Centigrade day would equal an 80° Fahrenheit day.

Water freezes at 32° Fahrenheit and at 0° Centigrade.

Water boils at 212° Fahrenheit and at 100° Centigrade.

Metric Conversion Chart (Approximations)

	Symbol	*When You Know*	*Multiply by*	*To Find*	*Symbol*
Length	mm	millimeters	0.04	inches	in
	cm	centimeters	0.4	inches	in
	m	meters	3.3	feet	ft
	m	meters	1.1	yards	yd
	km	kilometers	0.6	miles	mi
Area	cm^2	sq centimeters	0.16	sq inches	in^2
	m^2	square meters	1.2	sq yards	yd^2
	km^2	sq kilometers	0.4	sq miles	mi^2
	ha	hectares (10000 m^2)	2.5	acres	
Mass weight	g	grams	0.035	ounces	oz
	kg	kilograms	2.2	pounds	lb
	t	tonnes 1000 kg	1.1	short tons	
Volume	mL	milliliters	0.03	fluid ounces	fl oz
	L	liters	2.1	pints	pt
	L	liters	1.06	quarts	qt
	L	liters	0.26	gallons	gal
	m^3	cubic meters	35	cubic feet	ft^3
	m^3	cubic meters	1.3	cubic yard	yd^3
Temp exact	°F	Fahrenheit temperature	5/9 (°F-32)	Celsius temperature	°C
Length	in	inches	°2.5	centimeters	cm
	ft	feet		centimeters	cm
	yd	yards		meters	m
	miles	miles		kilometers	km
Area	sq inches	6.5	6.5	square centimeters	cm^2
	sq feet	0.09	0.09	square meters	m^2
	sq yards	0.8	0.8	square meters	m^2
	sq miles	2.6	2.6	square kilometers	km^2
	acres	0.4	0.4	hectares	ha
Mass weight	oz	ounces	28	grams	g
	lb	pounds	0.45	kilograms	kg
		short tons (2000 lb)	0.9	tonnes	t
Volume	tsp	teaspoons	5	milliliters	mL
	tbsp	tablespoon	15	milliliters	mL
	fl oz	flu ounces	30	milliliters	mL
	c	cups	0.24	liters	L
	pt	pints	0.47	liters	L
	qt	quarts	0.95	liters	L
	gal	gallons	3.8	liters	L
	ft^3	cubic feet	0.03	cubic meters	m^3
	yd^3	cubic yard	0.76	cubic meters	m^3

Pressure is more complicated to convert since some countries measure pressure in atmospheres or Pascals.

One atmosphere is 14.696 psi, or average barometric pressure at sea level. One atmosphere is also equal to 760 mm., or 29.92 ins. of mercury (Hg.). Also the unit called "tan" is equal to 1 mm. of mercury.

REFERENCES

Fire Protection Publications. 1990. *Principles of extrication,* 1st ed. Stillwater, OK: Oklahoma State University.

Hurst/Hale Fire Pumps. 1995. *Operator inspection program.* Conshocken, PA: Hurst Company.

Maryland Fire and Rescue Institute. 1989. *Rescue technician course.* Berwyn Heights, MD: MFRI.

Moore, R. E. 1991. *Vehicle rescue and extrication.* St. Louis: Mosby Yearbook, Inc.

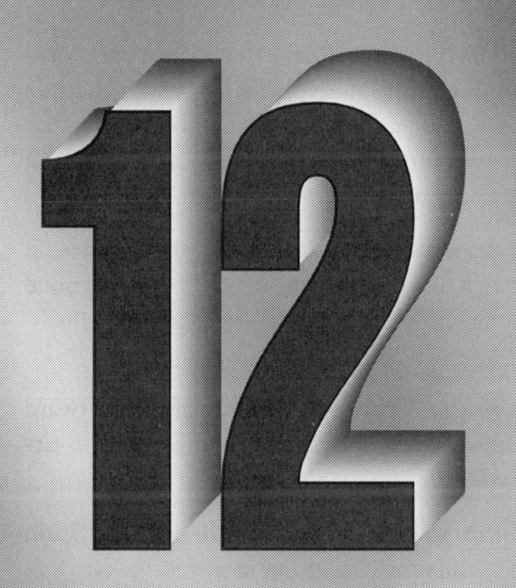

Vehicular Stabilization

OBJECTIVE

The student will be able to identify and demonstrate, as a member of a rescue team, wearing appropriate personal protective equipment (PPE), the principles and application of basic vehicle stabilization techniques, from memory, without assistance, to an accuracy of 70% and the satisfaction of the instructor.

OVERVIEW

Vehicular Stabilization

- Purpose of Vehicular Stabilization
- Devices and Tools
- Methodologies and Principles

ENABLING OBJECTIVES

12-1-1 Identify and describe the purposes of vehicular stabilization.

12-1-2 Demonstrate the various devices and tools used in the vehicular stabilization process.

12-1-3 Demonstrate various acceptable methods of vehicular stabilization given different scenarios.

PURPOSE OF VEHICULAR STABILIZATION

The process of vehicular stabilization is part of the overall concept of incident readiness. This involves preplanning, training for task-specific scenarios, response (to and from), size-up (initial, sustained, and response), safety, accountability, and effective utilization of resources.

One of the most overlooked and often ignored factors associated with the process of vehicular stabilization is ensuring that the necessary safeguards are positioned and the obvious hazards controlled. Whether the incident involves one or more vehicles including large trucks, buses, construction equipment, etc., an attack line, staffed by suppression personnel in full protective equipment, should be charged and in place prior to any rescue crews advancing into the inner circle of the incident. This does not mean a booster line! It means a 1½ in. to 1¾ in. attack line for rapid intervention should something unplanned or unexpected occur that poses a serious threat to firefighter safety and survival. Booster lines do not provide adequate fire protection in the event an unanticipated emergency occurs.

Once the proper safeguards are in place, the process of vehicular stabilization can begin. The cardinal rule is: *If you respond to a vehicular/mobile conveyance incident, stabilize it* before *you commence extrication/disentanglement activities.* Obvious fender-bender type crashes generally do not require extensive stabilization. If you suspect spinal injuries to the occupants, however, it certainly can't hurt to go the extra mile and stabilize the vehicle(s) in question. Always opt on the side of occupant safety.

Position and stability of the vehicle(s) must be determined prior to entry. Personnel operating within the inner circle would look awfully bad having to explain why a vehicle rolled backwards or forwards down an incline, or rolled over because it wasn't properly stabilized. Practice makes perfect! Get in the habit of reaching for step chocks or cribbing as a matter of routine when you exit your rescue vehicle.

Vehicular stabilization addresses vehicles found on all four wheels, their side, or their roofs. To understand why stabilization is important, let's examine the dynamics associated with five directional movements of a vehicle. These directional movements are identified and described below.

Conceptualize a series of lines drawn through a vehicle where all of the lines pass through an imaginary point that approximates the centerpoint of the passenger compartment. This centerpoint will differ according to various makes and models of vehicles.

Each imaginary line corresponds to an axis. *This is a straight line about which the entire structure of a vehicle will rotate or can be expected to rotate.* These axes are:

Longitudinal (horizontal) axis line A horizontal line drawn from the rearmost point of a vehicle toward the front that runs parallel to its sides and passes through the imaginary center point of the passenger compartment.

Vertical axis line A vertical line drawn from a point above the roof that passes through the imaginary center point of the passenger compartment and terminates at ground level below the undercarriage area.

Lateral axis line A horizontal line drawn from a point outside the passenger's side of a vehicle, to a point outside the driver's side, that runs parallel to the front/rear of the vehicle, and passes through the imaginary center point of the passenger compartment.

Using these three axis lines as a point of reference, it is easy to see that an unstabilized vehicle can now move in five basic directions: horizontal, vertical, roll, pitch, and yaw.

Horizontal movement Vehicle moves forward or rearward on its longitudinal axis or moves horizontally along its lateral axis.

Vertical movement Vehicle moves up or down in relation to the ground while moving along its vertical axis.

Roll movement Vehicle rocks side to side while rotating on its longitudinal axis and remaining horizontal in orientation.

Pitch movement Vehicle moves up and down on its lateral axis causing the vehicle's front and rear portions to move left/right in relation to their original position.

Yaw movement Vehicle twists or turns about on its vertical axis causing the vehicle's front and rear portions to move left/right in relation to their original position.

Proper stabilization increases the contact between the vehicle and the ground contact areas, and relieves the existing vehicle suspension system of its load or tension, minimizing unwanted vehicle movement. This is why it is extremely important to remember that all accidents or fire-involved vehicles, regardless of size, shape, condition, or position, must always be promptly stabilized in the position first encountered.

DEVICES AND TOOLS

Vehicular stabilization devices and tools include:

- Cribbing, wedges, and step chocks
- Air-lifting systems
- Load spreader
- Cables and chains

Cribbing, Wedges, and Step Chocks

Wooden cribbing (constructed out of 2×2s, 4×4s, 2×6s, and 6×6s), wedges, and step chocks (Figure 12–1) work best for vehicles found in most any position. They are used to secure an object in its position. They may also be used in conjunction with hi-lift jacks and jack stands to save cribbing material. These devices also work best when a vehicle is found resting on flat, even surfaces.

Cribbing is inserted or positioned where the load presented is perpendicular to the plane of the cribbing "box" (Figure 12–2). A box crib is a crisscross pattern of equal size wood pieces, arranged as a column to support the weight of an object. The box crib, by design, has a hollow center. Wedges are inserted or positioned between the box/load when the load presented is not perpendicular to the cribbing box (Figures 12–3 and 12–4). Step chocks are inserted or positioned in the back of both front wheels, and in front of the rear wheels, flush to the body of the vehicle. In certain situations, it may prove more effective to raise the step chocks up to contact the underside of the vehicle. This can be accomplished with wedges inserted or positioned under the step chock base.

Lowering a vehicle to the step chocks and/or cribbing may be accomplished by one of several methods. The most common is to remove the valve stem with a pair of pliers or valve stem remover and deflate the tires. State/local police accident reconstructionists often prefer that just the snifter valve itself be removed from the stem to deflate the tires. The reason behind this is that in investigating serious accidents, they may need to reinflate the tires to take certain measurements of tread depth and design characteristics.

Air-Lifting Systems and the Use of Cribbing

As you recall, box cribs, described earlier, have hollow centers. While this is acceptable for cribbing supporting an object, *it is totally unacceptable for use under an air bag. Whenever wood is used in contact with an air bag, it must be a solid layer of wood. If a box crib is necessary to lift an air bag closer to an object, the crib can be hollow, but the top layer must be doweled. Without a complete layer of wood under an air bag, the pillow-like shape of the bag will push the wood outward when inflated.*

Ronald C. Moore, author of *Vehicle Rescue and Extrication,* expounds on this issue for cribbing and air bag use:

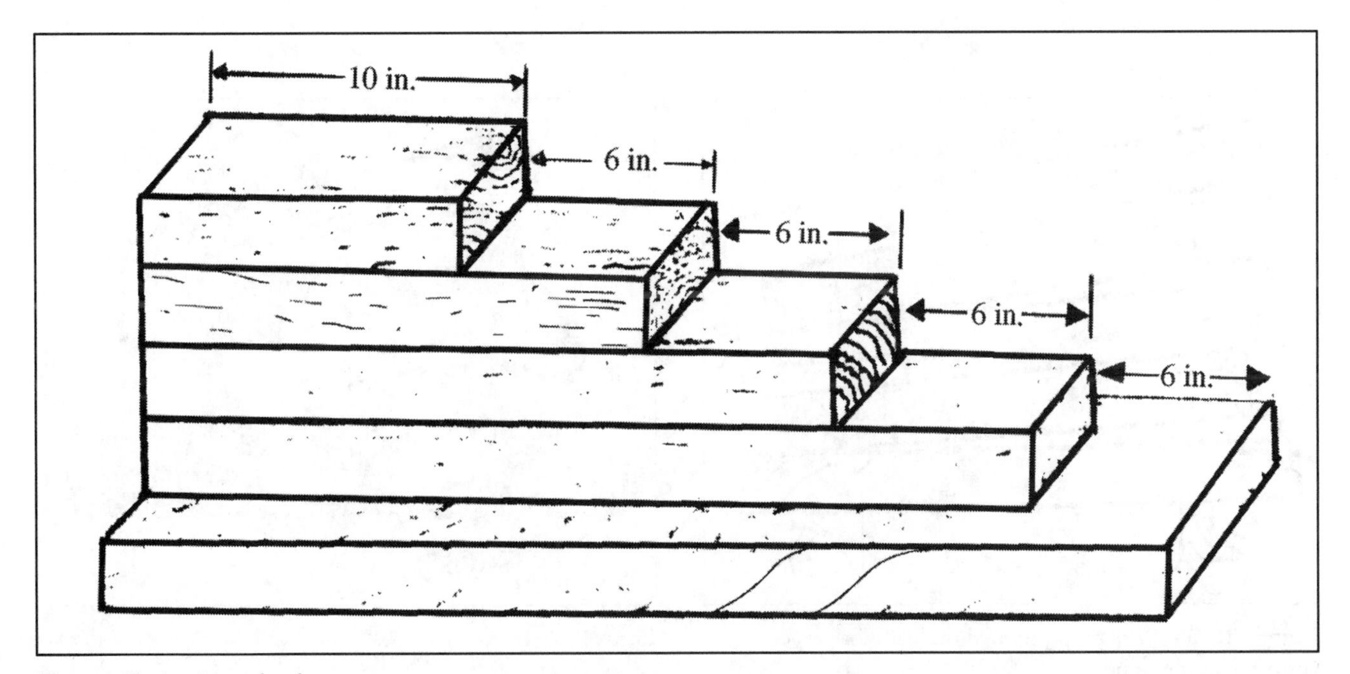

Figure 12–1 Step chocks.

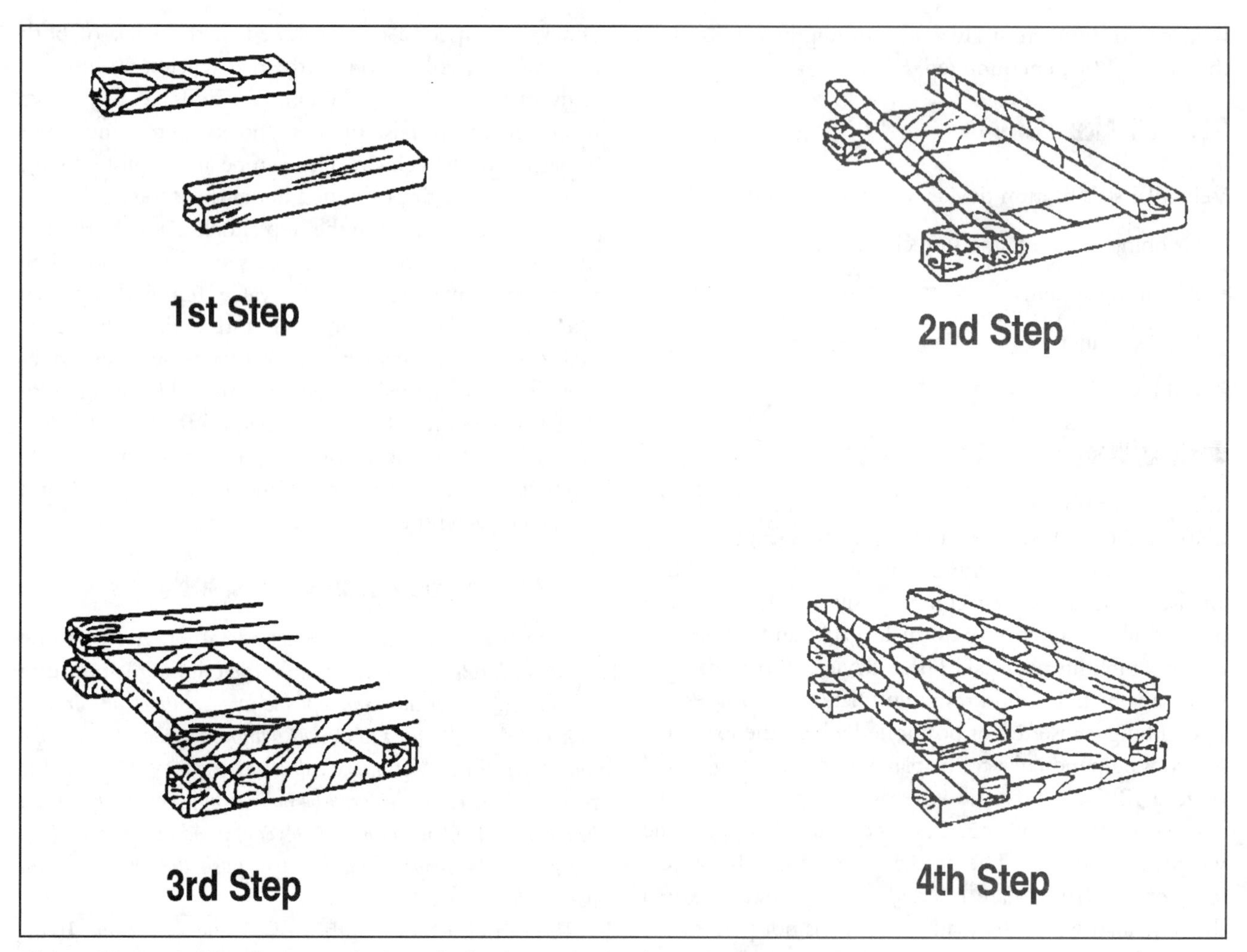

Figure 12–2 Cribbing is inserted where the load is perpendicular to the plane of the cribbing box.

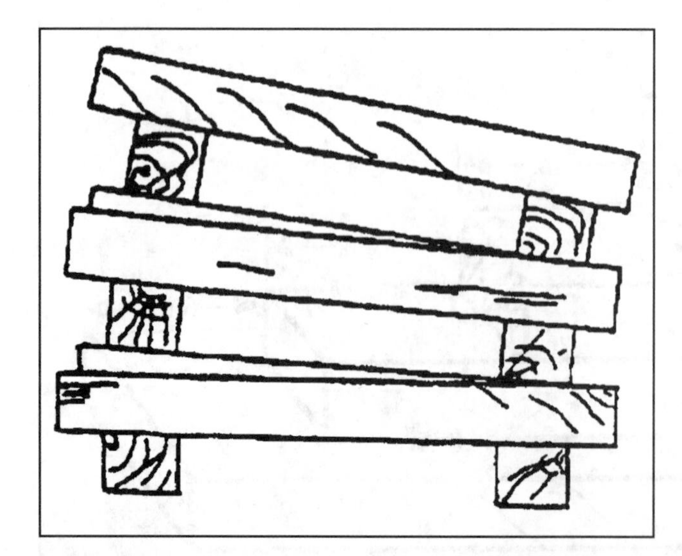

Figure 12–3 Wedges positioned on load not perpendicular to the cribbing box.

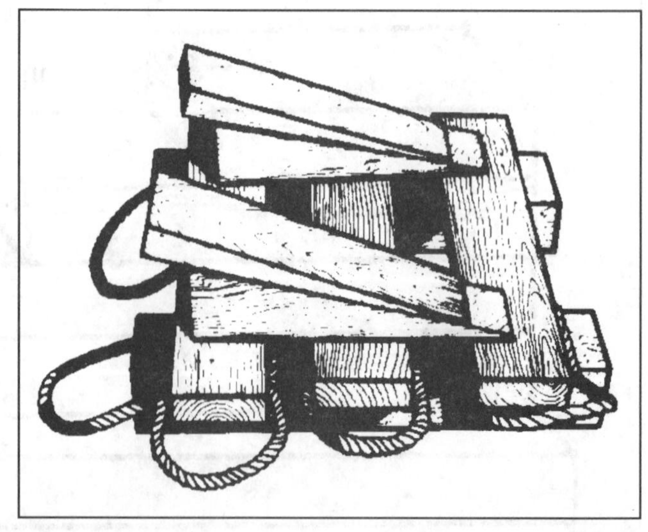

Figure 12–4 Wedges positioned on load not perpendicular to the cribbing box.

To further ensure safety, personnel should avoid placing wood on the top and the bottom of the same air bag. The top surface of the bag functions most effectively when it is placed directly in contact with the surface of the object being lifted or spread and allowed to mold itself to the shape of that object.

Load Spreader

When using any device or combination of devices for vehicle stabilization on nonpaved surfaces, particularly dirt and sand, use a load spreader to aid in preventing the device from sinking into the surface and thus losing its stabilizing effect. A load spreader is a wide plate, usually constructed of wood, and of sufficient thickness placed on the ground under the device to spread the load out. Like snowshoes or skis, it spreads the body's weight over a much larger area. This spreading of weight or load prevents the skier from sinking down into the snow.

Cables and Chains

The most positive way of accomplishing stabilization with chain and cable come-alongs is by securing both sides of the vehicle. For example, where a vehicle is on its side, chains may be looped around the front axle and each one attached to chains or cable come-alongs located and anchored on the opposite sides of the vehicle. The same maneuver is repeated on the upper rear tire. Be certain the object providing the anchor point for each securing system will restrain the load being applied, and will not become a hazard to traffic moving in the vicinity.

In an emergency, another vehicle could be used by securing it to the unstable vehicle. If at all possible, the securing vehicle(s) should not be a piece of emergency equipment. Such use may result in loss of equipment, personnel, and victims. For example, a pumper is used to stabilize the crash vehicle. A flammable liquid becomes ignited. The pump operator is driven away from the pumper, resulting in the loss of victims, perhaps some fire and rescue personnel, as well as the destruction of the lost pumper and other vehicles.

METHODOLOGIES AND PRINCIPLES

Regardless of the devices selected and used, care must be taken that the securing devices do not impede the efforts of those attempting to extricate the victims from the vehicle, nor by their location, induce additional hazards to the rescue scene.

A vehicle resting on its roof must be stabilized to prevent the roof from collapsing onto the victims and those emergency personnel who may be working inside the vehicle. This can occur when there is a structural change made to the vehicle. Such change occurs when doors are opened, windows broken, roofs cut, etc., not to mention the change that occurred as a result of the incident.

Stabilization of vehicles that are on their roofs may be accomplished by placing cribbing between the hood and trunk areas and the ground or roadway surface, by installing hydraulic/hi-lift jacks, backed up with cribbing, at various points around the vehicle, or by inserting air bags under the hood and the trunk.

When installing stabilization devices, be certain that the installation does not move the vehicle in such a manner as to induce or increase injuries to those entrapped. As far as possible, without entering the vehicle, determine that all those entrapped are totally inside the vehicle and do not have arm, legs, or heads under door posts, etc. Opening the trunk lid and hood as far as possible will provide some stabilization when a vehicle is on its side and there is not any equipment available. In some instances, a spare tire, depending on its size and the size of the vehicle, may provide stabilization when placed under the lower wheels. A spare may also be used as a wheel chock. Using tires may induce a hazard should any of the tires go flat. A hi-lift jack should be used as required on either side of the vehicle.

Air bags designed specifically for use in vehicle extrication are available and can also be used. As with cribbing, they should be placed where they will provide maximum stability. Care must be taken that the load does not roll off the bag causing the vehicle to shift.

There may be instances when it is necessary to stabilize one vehicle in order to gain access into another vehicle. These incidents occur when one vehicle has run up and over the rear of another vehicle, or the load shifts in a tractor trailer going around a corner and the trailer topples onto the vehicle running beside it.

When first sizing-up an incident of this type, the natural inclination is to pull the first vehicle off the other. This is not a very good idea. In almost every instance such efforts can cause additional, often fatal injuries to those entrapped. It is better to stabilize the upper vehicle and its load in its present position, gain access to the lower vehicle, extricate the victim(s), then attempt to disengage the vehicles. Efforts to disengage vehicles involved in such incidents often result in uncontrolled, sometimes violent, movement of both vehicles and their loads. Remember this basic principle: stabilize the vehicle in the position in which found. Do not try, at this time, to raise or reposition the vehicle.

Stabilizing a vehicle resting flat on its wheels to a hard surface is probably the easiest evolution to carry out. It requires that step chocks/box cribbing be inserted or positioned behind the front wheels, and in front of the rear wheels on both sides of the vehicle. Deflate all four tires to enable the vehicle to rest on its stabilization supports, or raise the step chocks to the underside of the vehicle by wedging the base of the step chocks/cribbing.

REFERENCES

Fire Protection Publications. 1996. *Fire service rescue,* 6th ed. Stillwater, OK: Oklahoma State University.

Fire Protection Publications. 1990. *Principles of extrication,* 1st ed. Stillwater, OK: Oklahoma State University.

Moore, R. E. 1991. *Vehicle rescue and extrication.* St. Louis: Mosby Yearbook, Inc.

National Fire Academy. 1993. *Rescue systems I.* Washington, DC: United States Fire Administration and California State Fire Marshal's Office, Fire Service Training and Education System.

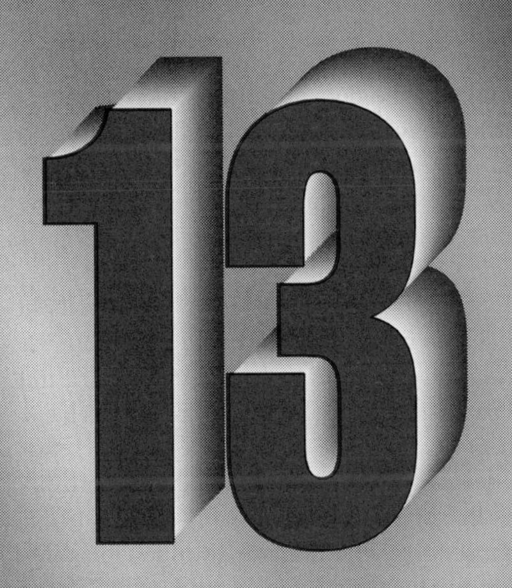

Hand Tools and Vehicular Extrication

OBJECTIVE

The student will be able to demonstrate appropriate techniques associated with basic hand-operated tools during a practical application scenario, addressing vehicular extrication, from memory, without assistance, to an accuracy of 70% and the satisfaction of the instructor.

OVERVIEW

Hand Tools and Vehicular Extrication

- Entrapment and Disentanglement
- Gaining Access Through Doors
- Gaining Access Through Windows
- Gaining Access Through the Body

ENABLING OBJECTIVES

13-1-1 Describe the entrapment and disentanglement process associated with vehicular extrication.

13-1-2 Demonstrate gaining access to entrapped victims through doors.

13-1-3 Demonstrate gaining access to entrapped victims through windows.

13-1-4 Demonstrate gaining access to entrapped victims through the body of a vehicle.

ENTRAPMENT AND DISENTANGLEMENT

Disentanglement is the release of trapped victims from the mechanisms of entrapment. The process involves making a pathway through the wreckage that will allow emergency services personnel to reach the victims with additional extrication tools of various sorts. It also entails removing wreckage that entraps the victims. It can involve a long and complex extrication operation often resulting in overlooking the condition of victim(s) (EMS personnel should monitor patients). Those first on the scene should conduct an inner/outer circle process along with a proper size-up and assessment of incident hazards and general layout of resources.

The objective is to make an opening in the wreckage just large enough to allow a rescuer to crawl though or to be moved through the wreckage on a long backboard. Once inside the rescuer can secure the ignition and remove keys, place the vehicle in park/gear, unlock the doors, roll down the windows, and unlatch the hood. It is very important that appropriate personal protective equipment, (PPE) be worn by EMS personnel. Personal safety is your responsibility.

The first step is to initiate life-saving activities with a basic life support (BLS) kit. Evaluate the victims' situation in regard to further extrication activities. Check for pinning and entrapment. Victim protection must be done during extrication and victims must be packaged after all other duties have been performed. All of these are to be carried out once inside the vehicle.

Once the trapped victim has been reached by qualified rescue personnel, and the victim has been stabilized and protected, disentanglement and removal operations can be undertaken at a relatively unhurried and safe pace.

To determine the status of victims, first determine where they are all located. They can be almost anywhere. Stop and look at the big picture! Pause and take all factors observed into account. *Don't overlook obvious things.* Check inside the vehicle—even in the trunk. Look along the roadside in natural coverings. Check inside adjacent buildings or vehicles; underneath the dashboard (infants and small children are often found there). Check underneath crushed seats.

The physical appearance of a vehicle can provide clues as to the probability of victim entrapment. Is there structural damage? Major structural damage can include jammed doors, displaced steering columns, overturned vehicles, etc. Determine the degree of entrapment. Check the windows and doors. Gaining access should not be attempted until the vehicle is stabilized. Access points should be considered in the following order: through doors, through windows, and through the body of the vehicle itself. *Try before you pry!*

GAINING ACCESS THROUGH DOORS

If the door is undamaged and unlocked, it should open in a normal manner. If the victim is conscious, ask him/her to unlock and open the door from the inside. Utilize a locksmith's tool if available (Lock Joc, Half Moon, S Hook, Leoko-unlocker, Z-tool, and Slim Jims) to unlock the car in an expedient manner. It is helpful to know whether or not the locking mechanism is a vertical or horizontal lock.

To unlock doors with framed windows, use a small pry bar or other lever to move the door frame away from the body of the vehicle. Utilize an L-shaped wire to snag and pull up mushroom-shaped locks. If no wire is available, a wire stand from a flare can be used. Use a coat hanger or commercial devices, if available, for opening horizontal/vertical locks.

For unlocking doors with unframed windows or thin-chrome frames, pry the outside of the window and lift the mushroom head lock with a flat-blade screwdriver, point of key-hole saw, or a windshield wiper arm. With antitheft locks, use an improvised wire and washer that can be dropped over the smooth shank of the lock while the window is pried open. As the wire is pulled up, the washer digs into the shaft and the locking mechanism is unlocked.

With the new construction of 1990 models, cutting door panels to access locking mechanisms may be required. The rescuer can insert a Halligan-type bar or other heavy-duty forcible entry tool between the door handle (surface mounted) and the body. The tool is pulled sharply down so that the locking mechanism and handle are broken and pulled away. The lock operating rod should be exposed and can be tripped with a screwdriver or needle-nose pliers.

Use a dent puller or slam hammer to pull a lock cylinder out of the vehicle and then a screwdriver to trip the locking mechanism. Utilize a leaf-spring cutter or a panel cutter for making a three-sided cut. A short-handled sledge hammer and the cutting tools are used to start the cut close to the edge of the door and above the lock. With the three-sided cut complete, the handle can be pulled exposing the lock paddle, rods, and levers. Pushing or pulling the rods and levers opens or releases the locking mechanism. Pushing the paddle plate opens the door. A cold chisel, screwdriver, heavy-duty case, hardened cold chisel, and K-bar can be utilized to expose the locking mechanism.

Safety latches are designed to withstand 4,000 lbs. of force, making entry through jammed doors more difficult. Prior to attempting any forcible entry evolutions, the locking mechanisms should be released as previously discussed. Vehicles from 1973 and up will have double safety locks (Nader), and the type of equipment that can force them are high-performance hydraulic, mechanical tools, or saws.

Vehicles built prior to 1965 do not have safety locks and the doors often fly open on impact. Conventional forcible-entry hand tools can be used to spread the door open and gain easy access to such vehicles. Vehicles from 1975 on have reinforced box-beam members for collisions/additional protection of occupants.

Once the locking mechanism is released, a prying tool or lever can be inserted with the flat edge at the midpoint of the door. Using the pillar as a fulcrum, apply force to the end of the bar. *Glass must be removed from the door areas prior to forcing.* If two bars are available, the effort is usually much more effective. With the force of one bar forcing the door away from the frame, the second bar is inserted deeper into the frame. As the second rescuer applies force to the bar, the first rescuer takes a better bite until the door is forced open. If a gap is needed, any tool with a flat-tapered edge can be utilized to widen a gap between the door and pillar (e.g., pry-axe, Halligan tool).

Use chain come-along to open the back door. When assessing door hinges, consider the use of ratchets to unbolt hinges after you have cut the fender(s) away. The door should then pivot and open easily. Pivot pins may have to be driven out.

GAINING ACCESS THROUGH GLASS

Types of Glass

Laminated glass is used in automobiles as safety glass. It is manufactured by bonding a piece of transparent plastic between two pieces of glass at high temperatures. When struck during impact, the shards of fractured glass are held together by the plastic laminate. All windshields are made of laminated glass and generally will hold the victim inside the vehicle even when they impact with great force.

Tempered safety glass is plate glass that has been specially tempered and hardened. It is used on side and rear windows of automobiles. Some foreign autos utilize laminated safety glass on the rear windows and/or all windows. When the glass fractures, it shatters into small squares resulting in injuries, usually superficial. Particles of glass fragments can create severe complications for a victim when they enter an open wound. Consequently, removal, rather than breaking, of the glass is recommended.

Removal of Windshields and Rear Windows

Prior to 1965 all windshields and rear windows were set in U-shaped rubber channels. Beginning in 1965 and by 1969, all automobiles manufactured had windshield and rear windows set in a mastic or thermosetting material. Today many trucks and vans are constructed with rubber-channel windshield mountings. It is easier for rescuers to break those windows than to try to cut the rubber or plastic mountings.

Breaking Windshields

If the windshield must be broken, make every effort to protect the victim(s). Select a window and make the cut as far away as possible from the victim. If the victim can be reached, try to provide some type of eye protection (safety goggles) and protect open wounds from glass particle contamination.

When using an axe to break windows, the rescuer should have full PPE donned during the evolution. The rescuer stands on the side of the vehicle and carefully drives the axe blade into the upper midpoint of the windshield. Use only enough force to just penetrate the glass. Chop downward until you reach the bottom of the glass. Then cut across the top of the glass from the center to the upper corner. Chop downward in the next step until you reach the lower corner. When cutting the glass, once an opening is made, the strokes in the cutting action should be parallel with the surface of the glass, thus limiting the dispersal of glass fragments on the victims. This is an alternative method used in the absence of more modern resources.

Using a bailing hook, force the point of the tool through the upper midpoint of the windshield. Use a shoring block or hammer to drive the tool through the glass and forcefully move the hook in and out of the glass with a sawing motion. Follow the same travel route as used with the axe. Pull the broken segment out and put it aside.

When using a Glas-Master saw, make a *purchasing point* first. Force the point of the tool through the windshield. Insert the saw and pull the tool to cut the glass. Make sure you protect the occupants and yourself from fragments/slivers (wrap-around eye protection and PPE). For a reciprocating saw, repeat the same steps as used with the Glas-Master.

Breaking Windows

When breaking side windows of tempered glass, the sharper the tool used, the less glass dispersed. A sharp-pointed tool (punch or spring-loaded center punch) can be utilized with a relatively light tap or just enough force to break the glass and not disperse it. The punch is held against the glass in the lower corner closest to B-C posts. Force is applied to knock out a very small hole in the glass. A gloved finger can be inserted in the glass and shattered pieces can slowly and methodically be pulled out into a salvage canvas or debris bucket. There are other methods available such as a screwdriver, flat-headed axe, spanner wrench, or Halligan bar.

Removing A Victim from A Windshield

A victim on the passenger side of the front seat may have his or her head driven through the windshield in a high-impact collision. Glass shards may be pressing against the victim's carotid arteries, therefore, the victim should not be immediately pulled back through the opening. Removing the victim is best accomplished by a minimum of three emergency services personnel with an EMT, CRT, or EMT-P, who has gained access into the inside of the vehicle. The person on the inside will provide body stabilization. BLS will be administered by the second rescuer on the outside of the vehicle if available. The third rescuer supports the victim's head during the activity. A fourth rescuer slowly and methodically places protective dressings around the victim's head. Then, using a sharp-pointed knife, cut the plastic laminating layer from the glass. The knife is gently forced down through the cracks in the glass. Pieces are slowly removed, thus enlarging the hole in the windshield. At the direction of the rescuer on the inside, a multitrauma dressing/collar is placed between the victim's chin and the glass. This rescuer guides the head back through the opening, while rescuers on the exterior support the victim's head. This method addresses a victim whose head has passed through a windshield, but whose body is still entrapped. It is only one method that can be used.

It is important to don the appropriate PPE including wrap-around eye protection when conducting glass removal operations. The inherent dangers associated with breaking or removing glass far outweigh any other factors. *Remember,* you only have one pair of eyes. Does it make any sense not to protect them? Rescuers who rely on helmet shields solely to protect their eyes are courting disaster. All it takes is a fine sliver of glass propelled by a saw, striking, or pneumatic tool to require an unwanted trip to one of several eye centers for treatment.

Safety Pointers

Here are several pointers to consider when working with, in, or around glass hazards at the scene of a rescue incident:

1. Always wear PPE clothing, including head, eye, hand, and foot protection. Heavy canvas gear or other approved cut-resistant clothing is a must. The requirement applies to all rescuers near the operation.
2. Always, without exception, protect the occupant when you are breaking glass.
3. When practical, control the glass as you break it.
4. Keep your mouth closed when breaking glass.
5. Strike the glass nearest the A-B-C post corners to prevent the tool from accidentally entering the passenger compartment.
6. When you break a passenger window, strike or center punch the glass on the corner near the occupant. This will direct the veins/patterns of glass breaking away from the victim(s) rather than towards them.
7. Warn the interior rescuer before you begin breaking glass.
8. Pull the glass outward when it has broken.
9. Roll the window down until approximately 1 in. to 1½ in. of the glass is showing. When you break this glass, the majority of it will break inside the door panel itself.

GAINING ACCESS THROUGH THE BODY

Roof

When a rescue team makes the decision to flap or remove a roof from any mobile conveyance, the end result is the same. You now have a convertible on your hands that will either enhance the underwriters assessment that the vehicle is totaled, or create additional damage to a vehicle that will be very costly to repair or replace. The end result, which does not really concern rescue providers, is none the less a necessary evil. What dictates the dynamics of roof removal or flapping? Several factors influence the decision-making process:

1. What is your tactical objective?
2. Type and size of mobile conveyance.
3. Number of occupants, size, and positioning within the conveyance.
4. Complexity of the extrication scenario.
5. Size of rescuers.
6. Type of extrication devices to be used.
7. Position of the conveyance and logistical support required to mitigate the access process.
8. Is this procedure actually necessary in light of your objective?

An argument can be made in support of the premise of why flap when you can totally remove? Removal en-

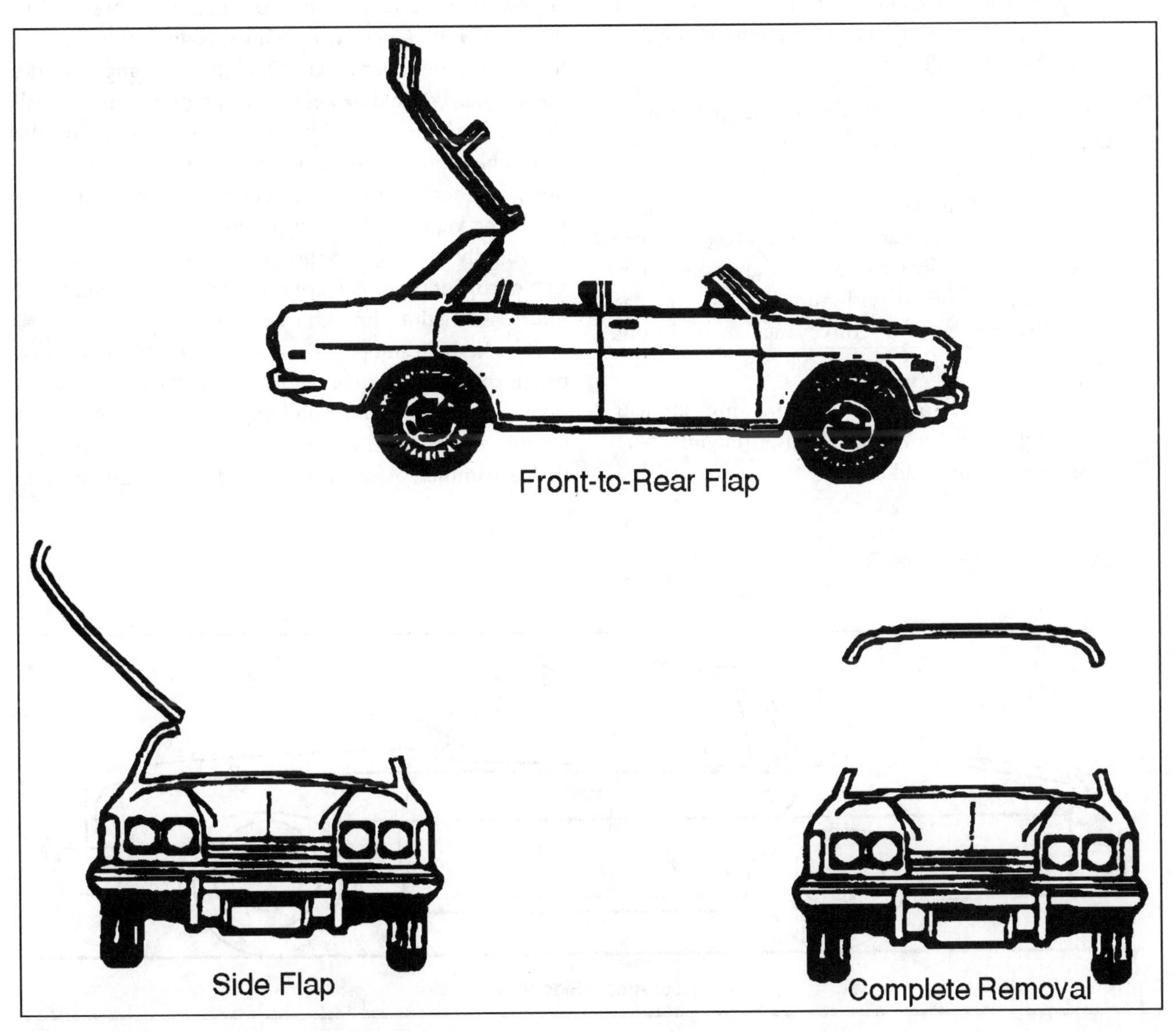

Figure 13–1 Three basic roof flap configurations.

hances your sphere or scope of operation and affords greater mobility and flexibility within the working/occupant environment.

Removal is safer in the long run because there are less hazards to contend with. Rescuers can have a clear and unobstructed ingress/egress point by removing driver and occupant doors and/or conducting third-door cuts in the rear side panels of sedans. It also affords the safety officer a clearer picture of incident dynamics.

When you are using hand tools exclusively for an extrication scenario, the decision to flap or remove a roof must be made very quickly for several reasons:

1. When using hand tools, rescuers will find it more difficult and time consuming to open and displace a jammed door. Therefore, it is essential to flap or remove the roof early in order to provide a means of vertical egress for the occupants/patients in case their conditions suddenly deteriorates.

2. It is usually best to flap or remove the roof in order to provide more room for EMS personnel to assess, treat, package/immobilize, and remove an occupant/patient. With the current trend of decreasing the size of domestic cars today, the size of the rear passenger seating area has greatly diminished. This reduction, combined with the decrease in head room that results from conveyance streamlining, makes roof removal more sensible.

There are three basic roof flap configurations: side flap, front to rear flaps, and complete removal (Figure 13–1). They are discussed in detail below.

Vehicle on Its Side

With a vehicle on its side, use the roof as an ingress/egress point. One rescuer should be assigned to each end of the vehicle to stabilize and prevent movement and to function as a safety observer.

Remember: Always stabilize the vehicle *first* before attempting access/extrication.

Appoint a safety officer to oversee the rescue operation. The location of the victims/occupants must be ascertained prior to cutting operations. Usually access is made by making a three-sided cut with the skin folded over on the place where the victim will be removed. The cut should be made in the following manner. Cut along the top. On compact cars this separates the roof from the B post. Cut the edge of the roof behind A post and in front of C post. Cut down the sides, connect the cuts, and fold down the sheet metal. Once the opening is made, the axe head should be kept parallel with the metal. Half the axe is in the sash and half is out. At the final cut, the roof is bent down, exposing the roof supports and headliner. The headliner should be cut with a sharp knife from inside the vehicle whenever possible. Roof supports can be carefully broken from spot welds with a hammer. Victim/occupant position is critical—do not cause additional injuries to victims through carelessness.

A makeshift can opener tool or K-bar tool can be used to cut the roof in a manner similar to the above operations. Schild panel cutters and improvised leaf-spring cutter can also be used for roof cutting when struck by a sledge hammer. A screwdriver and cold chisel are also

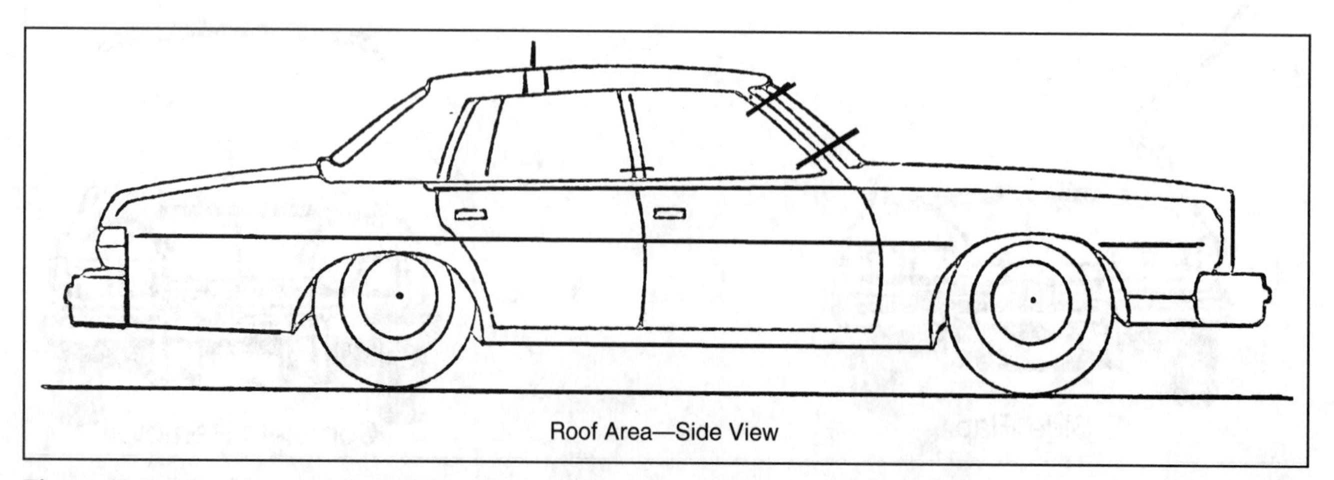

Figure 13–2 Cutting points for roof flapping.

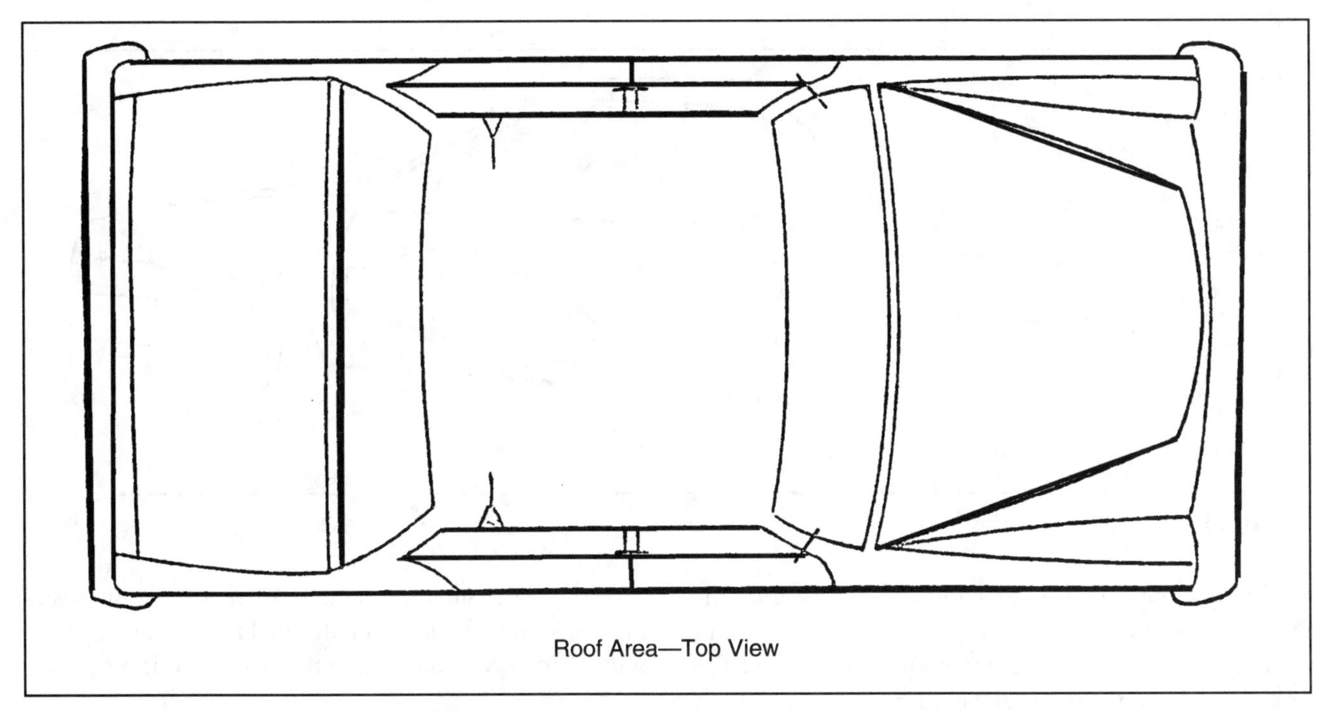

Figure 13–3 Cutting points for roof flapping.

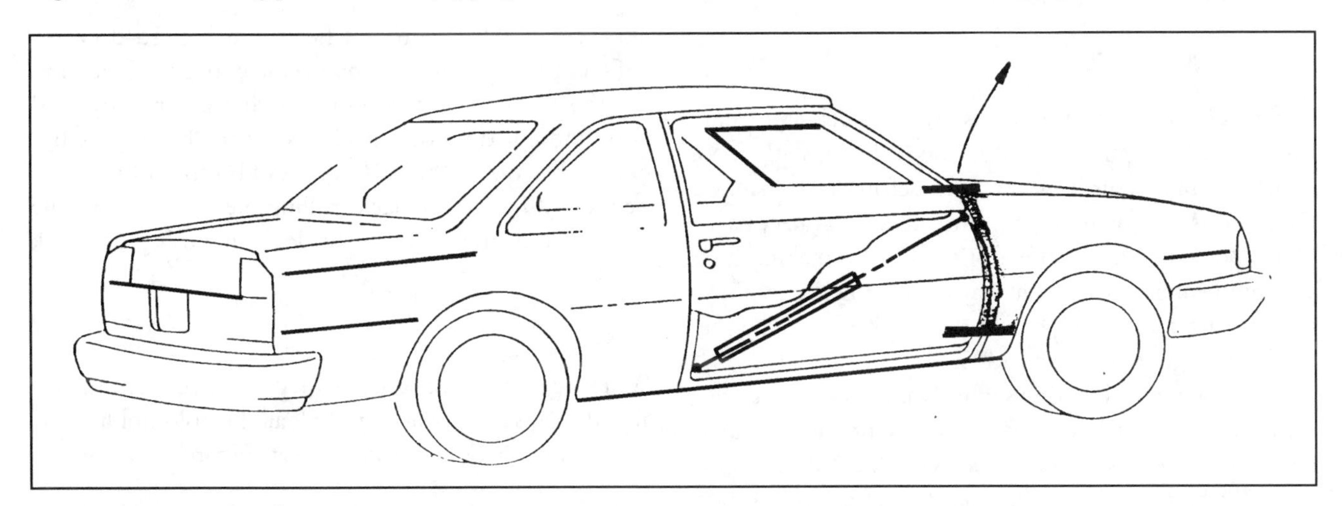

Figure 13–4 Dash roll-up maneuver.

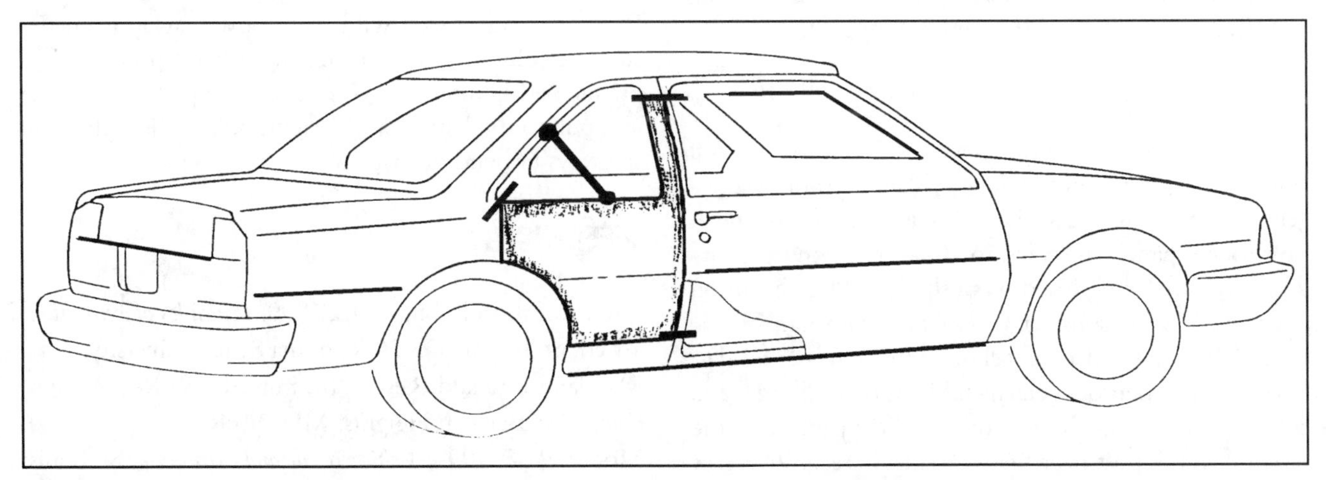

Figure 13–5 Third-door relief technique.

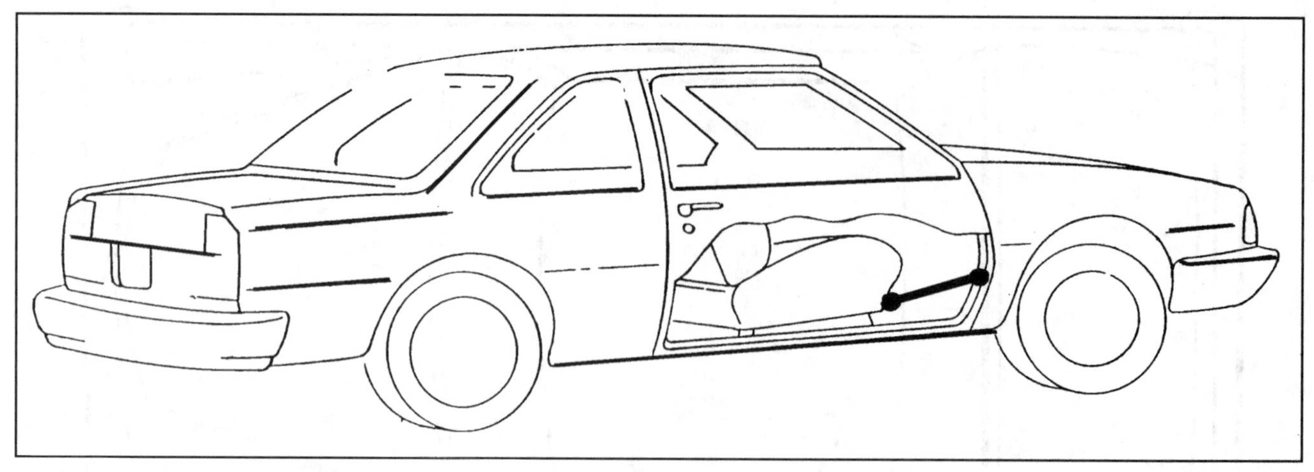

Figure 13–6 Seat displacement.

available for the task in conjunction with the sledge hammer. Always cover jagged A-B-C posts with some form of protective cover to prevent injuries. Discarded fire hose (split down the side) can be utilized to protect both the victims and rescuers from injuries.

Vehicle on Its Wheels

When accessing a vehicle that is on its wheels and using roof access/flapping, stabilize the vehicle with step chocks, cribbing, air bags, etc., and deflate the tires. Cut the A posts; cut or remove the windshield as necessary. Cut B posts. Cut the roof in front of C posts making sure you cut through the roof rail. Lay a bar across the roof between C post cuts (long backboard on its edge). Flap the roof. (see Figures 13–2 and 13–3.)

When the vehicle is on its wheels and you want to remove the roof, stabilize the vehicle. Cut the shoulder belts, then cut A-B-C posts and windshield at the bottom. Lift high and move the roof forward. Do not pass the windshield over patient/occupant. All glass should be broken and removed prior to removal of roof.

Dash

In a dash roll-up maneuver, sever the A posts on both sides of the vehicle and remove or flap the roof. Make a relief cut 5 ins. to 6 ins. above the intersection of the A post rocker panel, and 8 ins. to 10 ins. back on the horizontal rocker panel. Insert sill push plate. Place beam on appropriate step (consider B post tool with ram operation). Without sill plate, install moveable spreader head to base of jack. Insert or attach hi-lift jacks on both sides and push upwards with the *base* on the door jambs and the *head* on the A post near the windshield area. Wedge or block relief cuts as necessary (Figure 13–4).

Note: In some situations cutting or removing the steering wheel may be appropriate. Pulling the steering column is not advocated within the scope of this program.

Third-Door Access

To access a vehicle on its wheels with a third-door relief technique on a two-door vehicle, begin by stabilizing the vehicle. Cut B post, cut the lower body at B post, and cut the body at C post. Place hi-lift jack between the roof, behind B post, and bottom of window opening. Operate the jack, rolling the body toward the ground. Pull the body metal down exposing the back seat (Figure 13–5).

Seats

When accessing past seats, first try to move them manually. If that is not possible, unbolt all the bolts holding the seats or use a jack to move the seat (Figure 13–6).

Pedals

Pedals can be moved with hand power away from the steering column. Use rope, chain, or hand-powered hydraulic pedal cutter to move or remove pedals. If on the left, pull to the left; if on the right, pull to the right. Pull sideways to bend or snap.

REFERENCES

Fire Protection Publications. 1990. *Principles of extrication,* 1st ed. Stillwater, OK: Oklahoma State University.

Maryland Fire and Rescue Institute. 1989. *Rescue technician course.* Berwyn Heights, MD: MFRI.

Moore, R. E. 1991. *Vehicle rescue and extrication.* St. Louis: Mosby Yearbook, Inc.

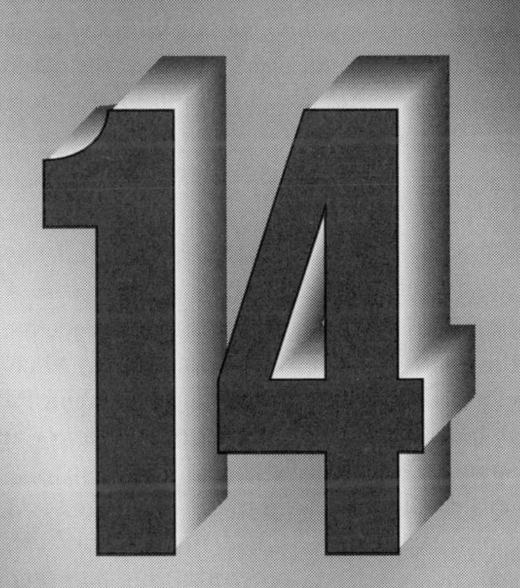

Power Tools and Vehicular Extrication

OBJECTIVE

The student will be able to demonstrate safe methods of gaining access into vehicles via roofs, doors, and enlargement of openings, and accessing occupants utilizing power tools/equipment, from memory, without assistance, to an accuracy of 70% and the satisfaction of the instructor.

OVERVIEW

Power Tools and Vehicular Extrication

- Safety Perimeter/Scene Assessment
- Stabilization/Balancing Techniques
- Gaining Access Through Roof Area(s)
- Gaining Access Through Door Area(s)
- Enlarging Access Points

ENABLING OBJECTIVES

14-1-1 Demonstrate the methods associated with establishing a safety perimeter around the scene of a rescue incident.

14-1-2 Demonstrate stabilization/balancing techniques on a vehicle scenario.

14-1-3 Demonstrate the proper methodologies associated with gaining entry through the roof of a vehicle.

14-1-4 Demonstrate gaining entry through the door(s) of a vehicle utilizing power equipment.

14-1-5 Demonstrate the proper enlargement techniques on the following areas utilizing power tools and equipment appropriate for the evolution:
a. Windshield(s)
b. Body of vehicle
c. Front seat displacement
d. Pedal displacement
e. Dash displacement/roll-up

SAFETY PERIMETER/SCENE ASSESSMENT

The first step in scene assessment involves determining the proper place to position the apparatus. Conduct a circle check and establish the operational zones consistent with session 1. Determine the number of vehicles involved and the immediate/secondary factors that pose life safety hazards to/for rescue personnel. Establish command and control.

STABILIZING/BALANCING TECHNIQUES

Place the step chocks but do not crawl under unstable object. Hydraulic jacks can also be used to lift objects and place cribbing. Coordinate movement if using more than one jack, making sure a matched pair is always used. Place a wooden buffer or barrier between the jack head and the material being lifted.

Use air bags to stabilize and/or balance in the position found. Set up the air bags with low-pressure hose connections facing out, making sure the hose is not kinked and the pressure relief valve is functioning. As the object is lifted, construct cribbing for stabilization and/or balancing and safety. Inflate the air bags slowly and evenly and deflate the same way.

GAINING ACCESS THROUGH ROOF AREA(S)

Use a flat chisel for posts and bolts making a circular motion around the material severed. If the vehicle is lying on its side, it only requires three cuts on the roof. ("Enlarging Access Points" "Body of the Vehicle" in the section following.)

With a hydraulic cutter, hold the shears perpendicular to the material being sheared. Cut at the roof line near the shoulder harness mount, avoiding shoulder mount(s) by 3 ins. Cut the A post at the roof line or at the base, then cut the B post. Repeat this procedure on the other side. Crease and lift the roof, remove or flap backwards or forwards. The windshields are generally cut at the roof line.

Remember: Total roof removal is preferred when the circumstances dictate. Removal is safer than flapping when rescuers are working to treat, package, and remove occupants.

GAINING ACCESS THROUGH DOOR AREA(S)

To gain access through door area(s) using the porta-power, select the ram and attachment to best perform the task. Do not overextend the rams. Make sure attachments, such as the Spee-D-Coupler, are correctly attached. Check the jack oil level. Close the pressure release valve in a clockwise direction to commence operation. Hold the pump in a vertical position with the hose end down and pump the handle for application of force. Turn the pressure relief valve counter-clockwise for lowering the load.

When using the power spreaders, make sure you follow the techniques for safe operation/handling. With the hydraulic spreaders, pinch, pry, or crimp the doors to locate purchase/access point(s). The spreader can also be placed inside the window area to create a purchase/access point(s). The operator should be familiar with the hoses and the various types of connectors to be used and avoid locking-up the system. Activate the dump valve before disconnecting the lines.

ENLARGING ACCESS POINTS

Windshield

Before commencing operations, think about *why* you are removing this glass. We no longer do steering wheel pulls. Therefore, in situations where windshield removal is warranted, in all probability removal of the roof or at minimal, flapping, should be considered. Make sure occupants are protected from glass particles. A salvage cover or impermeable cover should be used, not hospital sheets or blankets. An air chisel or reciprocating saw can be used to enlarge the access area of the windshield.

Body of the Vehicle

To access the body of a vehicle use the air chisel on low pressure at 90 psi to 100 psi and on high pressure at 200 psi to 250 psi. A high-pressure chisel utilizes 10 cu. ft. of air per minute. A 45 cu. ft. bottle will be used up in approximately 4 minutes. Secure the chisel bit with the retainer. Start with the low pressure and work up to the higher pressure. Use panel cutters for flat sheet metal and flat chisel for door posts and bolts. Place the chisel in contact with the metal before operating. When cutting sheet metal, after starting, the barrel should be parallel to the material being cut. When cutting heavy metal, such as bolts or door posts, a circular motion should be made around the material being severed. Bleed-off air prior to disconnecting the lines. A reciprocating saw, either electric or air, and a sheet metal nibbler can be used.

Front Seat Displacement

Displacing the front seat can be done by using porta-power, power rams, or jaws/spreaders. First, however, attempt to release the seat latch and push the seat back or unbolt the seat. Any movement of the seat requires careful consideration with respect to aggravating the occupants' injuries.

Pedal Displacement

Pedal displacement can be done with the porta-power using the duck bill spreaders. Assorted hydraulic rescue tools such as cutters are also suitable for the task. Think about *why* you are displacing the pedals? Have you considered a dash roll-up and roof removal? Seat displacement implies there is difficulty in extricating an occupant. Just remove the obstacles around your occupant if the situation dictates.

Dash Displacement/Roll-Up

The preferred method for disentanglement and dash displacement/roll-up is to relief-cut the A post door jamb 5 ins. to 6 ins. above the rocker panel after the roof has been removed or flapped and the doors removed. Place a relief cut in the rocker panel 8 ins. to 10 ins. back from the A post door jamb. This cut keeps the floor from buckling and subsequently lifting or moving the occupant's legs. Next place the B post tool against the B post door jamb (rocker panel) and place the butt plate or ram on the tool. You may also create a purchase point in the rocker panel with jaws or cutters to anchor the butt or the ram in the absence of the B post tool. Place the operating tip of the ram firmly against the upper portion of the A post door jamb. When the ram is extended, the dash will lift up and away from the victims (Figure 14–1).

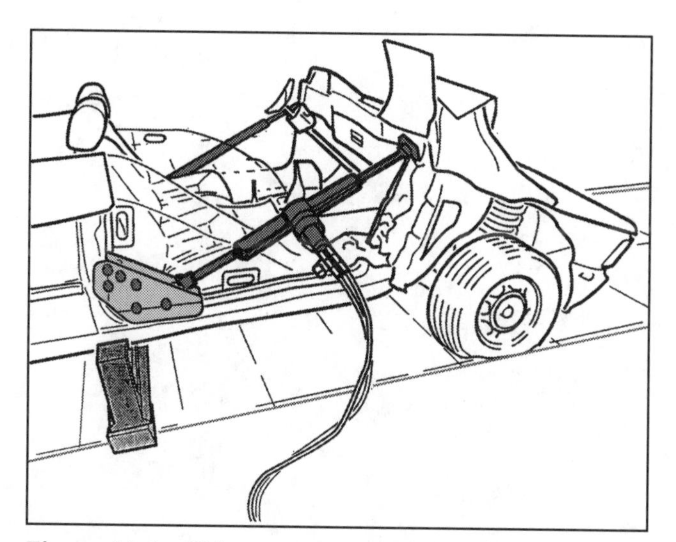

Figure 14–1 Using a ram to extend the dash.

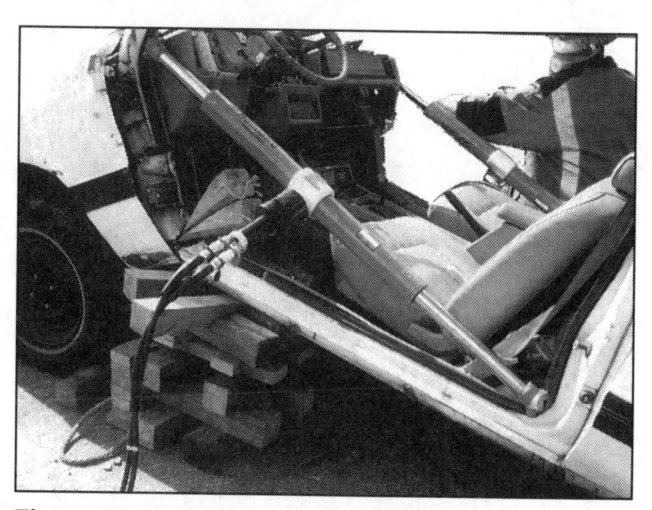

Figure 14–2 Using a ram to extend the dash.

When the dash displacement/roll-up is completed and the tool is still in place, put chocks or wedges in the relief cuts in the door jambs as necessary. Build the cribbing as you go (Figure 14–2). The dynamics may require additional post roll-up stabilization due to movement.

Remember to employ power rams and equal relief cuts to both sides of the vehicle at the same time.

With the proliferation of front-wheel drive vehicles, and the difficulty of identifying these vehicles, treat *all* cars as front-wheel drive vehicles and perform a dash displacement/roll-up. We are no longer teaching to pull/displace the steering columns because the potential for further injury to the occupants is very prevalent.

REFERENCES

Fire Protection Publications. 1990. *Principles of extrication,* 1st ed. Stillwater, OK: Oklahoma State University.

Hurst/Hale Fire Pumps. 1995. *Operator inspection program.* Conshocken, PA: Hurst Company.

Maryland Fire and Rescue Institute. 1989. *Rescue technician course.* Berwyn Heights, MD: MFRI.

Moore, R. E. 1991. *Vehicle rescue and extrication.* St. Louis: Mosby Yearbook, Inc.

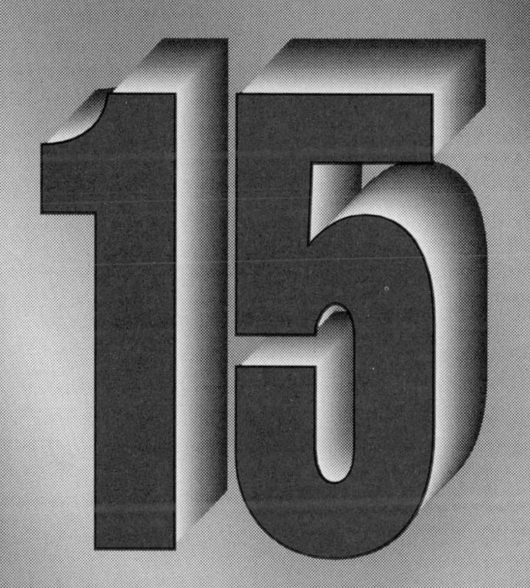

Skills Proficiency Evaluation: Vehicle Extrication and Exam #2

OBJECTIVE

The student will be able to demonstrate knowledge and understanding of the skills learned in sessions 9 through 14, on a written exam and skills proficiency evaluation, from memory, without assistance, to an accuracy of 70% and the satisfaction of the instructor. **This is a pass/fail point in the program.** Satisfactory completion permits the student to continue in the program.

OVERVIEW

Vehicle Extrication

- Vehicle on Its Side
- Vehicle on Its Roof
- Vehicle on Its Wheels

ENABLING OBJECTIVES

15-1-1 Demonstrate vehicle stabilization for a vehicle on its side and access occupants using hand and power tools.

15-1-2 Demonstrate vehicle stabilization for a vehicle on its roof and access occupants using hand and power tools.

15-1-3 Demonstrate vehicle stabilization for a vehicle on its wheels and access occupants using hand and power tools.

Skill Station 1
Vehicle on Its Side (Team Evaluation)
Correctly demonstrate the following:

19. Circle check
20. Stabilization
21. Gain access via removal of window glass using hand or power tools specified by the evaluator
22. Gain access via through a roof flap using hand or power tools specified by the evaluator
23. Safely remove all equipment

Skill Station 2
Vehicle on Its Roof (Team Evaluation)
Correctly demonstrate the following:

24. Circle check
25. Stabilization
26. Gain access via removal of window glass using hand or power tools specified by the evaluator
27. Gain access via removal of doors using hand or power tools specified by the evaluator
28. Gain access via removal of roof using hand or power tools specified by the evaluator
29. Safely remove all equipment

Skill Station 3
Vehicle on Its Wheels (Team Evaluation)
Correctly demonstrate the following:

30. Circle check
31. Stabilization
32. Gain access via removal of window glass using hand or power tools specified by the evaluator
33. Gain access via removal of doors using hand or power tools specified by the evaluator
34. Gain access via removal of roof using hand or power tools specified by the evaluator
35. Dash displacement using hand or power tools specified by the evaluator
36. Seat displacement using hand or power tools specified by the evaluator
37. Safely remove all equipment

REFERENCES

See Session 9–1 through session 9–14.

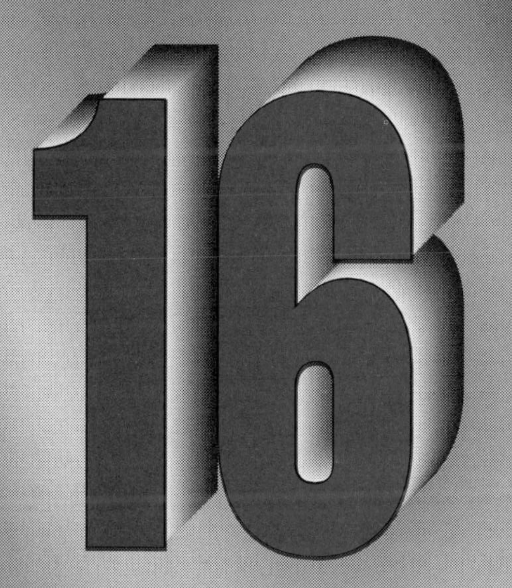

Principles of Passenger and Commercial Conveyance Rescue—Buses and Trucks

OBJECTIVE

The student will be able to identify and describe the basic components of vehicle construction relating to buses and trucks, along with special rescue problems presented, from memory, without assistance, to an accuracy of 70% and the satisfaction of the instructor.

OVERVIEW

Principles of Passenger and Commercial Conveyance Rescue—Buses and Trucks

- Issues in Truck Extrication
- Truck Construction
- Large Vehicle Stabilization
- Large Vehicle Access
- Occupant Handling and Removal
- Issues in Bus Extrication
- Bus Construction
- Bus Stabilization
- Bus Access
- Occupant Handling and Removal

ENABLING OBJECTIVES

16-1-1 Identify and describe the points involved in truck extrication as they relate to mobile conveyance extrication and large vehicle rescue.

16-1-2 Identify and describe heavy/large truck construction characteristics and their impact on rescue operations.

16-1-3 Identify the issues in large truck stabilization and the most appropriate alternative to accomplish effective stabilization.

16-1-4 Identify the most appropriate area for victim access in large vehicles based on the situation presented and the proper techniques to deal with vehicle doors, exterior panels, roofs, and dash.

16-1-5 Identify why occupant removal from large vehicles is more difficult than from an automobile.

16-1-6 Describe the points involved in bus extrication as they relate to mobile conveyance extrication and large vehicle rescue.

16-1-7 Identify and describe bus construction characteristics and their impact on rescue operations.

16-1-8 Identify the principles in bus stabilization and the most appropriate alternative to accomplish effective stabilization.

16-1-9 Identify the most appropriate area for victim access in buses based on the situation presented.

16-1-10 Identify why occupant removal from buses is more difficult than from an automobile.

ISSUES IN TRUCK EXTRICATION

The command and control of a heavy vehicle extrication scenario requires an effective strategy. Rescuers must focus on the fact that an extrication is an extrication regardless of the size of the vehicle(s) involved. The fire/rescue service devotes a great deal of time and effort to small vehicle extrications involving cars, minivans, and all-purpose vehicles. The occurrence of a large commercial accident involving a bus or tractor trailer often overwhelms the responder's perception of the incident because of size alone and the resulting devastation encountered.

Remember, as vehicle size and components increase, the complexity of the resolution process increases proportionally. A rescuer, having the basics of extrication principles, can address these larger scale incidents with calculated planning. The big difference being, larger scale vehicles will take longer to mitigate.

Rescuers must maintain this perspective as they approach extrication incidents involving big rigs. These rigs may cost in excess of $100,000 and provide the means by which contract/independent operators earn their living. Closely evaluate the necessity of dismantling a rig by traditional methods such as those used on passenger-type vehicles. Removal of a roof may render a rig out of service for months and severely impact the owner's ability to generate revenue. This does not in any way discourage proper occupant care and removal efforts. Rather, it implies that if a windshield area could be used as an egress point safely, consider it first.

In developing an effective strategy to address these incidents, it is important to establish priorities. Consistent with the principles of vehicular rescue found in session 9, the rescuer's *first priority* is scene assessment and hazard control. The circumstances often dictate the means. The variety of hazards encountered in heavy rescue scenarios pose serious threats to rescuer safety and survival. Your hazard assessment must include a careful scrutiny of:

- Types of fuels and associated volumes
- Batteries
- Generators/alternators/electrical systems
- Height/weight/cargo/pressurized systems
- Tools

Types of Fuel and Associated Volume(s)

Fuels of the 1990s include diesel, gasoline, kerosene, propane/compressed natural gas, and electricity. Volume can involve as small a quantity as 20 gals. to literally hundreds of gallons. It is not uncommon to encounter some fuel tanks on tractor trailers containing 175 gals. Some larger trucks may carry three to four tanks (saddle tanks) situated on the sides of the cab, behind the cab, and/or under the trailer.

Batteries

Batteries are normally found under the cab area with outside access, but, depending on the manufacturer's design and type of truck involved, may be found anywhere including the trailer. Large trucks and fire apparatus often have dual battery banks. Consequently, the number and size of the batteries increases the potential hazard to rescuers. It is very possible for batteries to explode. Massive short circuiting could result from a surge of electrical current hitting the battery or from exposure to heat. Rescuers must be alert to the possibility of multiple battery cables because cutting or disconnecting just one cable may not completely interrupt the electrical circuit, thereby leaving an unsuspecting crew member/rescuer with an electrical system that is still energized. You may find a shut-off with the battery bank.

Generators/Alternators/Electrical Systems

Rescuers must be fully aware of the operating characteristics of a typical vehicle electrical system and be able to anticipate potential hazards during extrication activities. A typical tractor trailer, depending on the make, model, and year, will have either a generator or an alternator to power the electrical system and maintain a charge to the battery. These systems are not without risk when operating in, around, or near them. It is not uncommon to come across an older tractor trailer with a 110 converter system (A/C to D/C). If for some reason one of these vehicles is involved in an accident and the converter grounds to the body, a sizeable shock is possible to a rescuer coming into contact with it.

This basic problem with electrical systems in general is the electrical current being generated. Multiple battery banks for instance may produce 1,500 amps to 2,000 amps for cold cranking power. The risk here lies in the fact that inadvertent contact with a component of these batteries may cause severe burns. Extreme caution must be exercised when approaching big rigs loaded with accessories and large amounts of electrical wiring. Rescuers should be cognizant of additional electrical hazards that may be present in recreational vehicles and over-the-road (sleeper) trucks. These units may be equipped with inverters that will supply 110V AC 60-cycle current to operate various household appliances such as microwaves, TVs, etc. Because many of these units are driver installed (directly wired to battery), it is necessary to disconnect the vehicle batteries to remove electrical potentials.

Height/Weight/Cargo/Pressurized Systems

The height of tractor trailers pose a serious challenge to rescuer's efforts to extricate. Remember that occupant's feet sit at the 5 ft. level while their heads can easily be at the 10 ft. level. Overall height can be 12 ft. or more which may require folding ladders, platforms, and backboards to help create a work surface to improve access

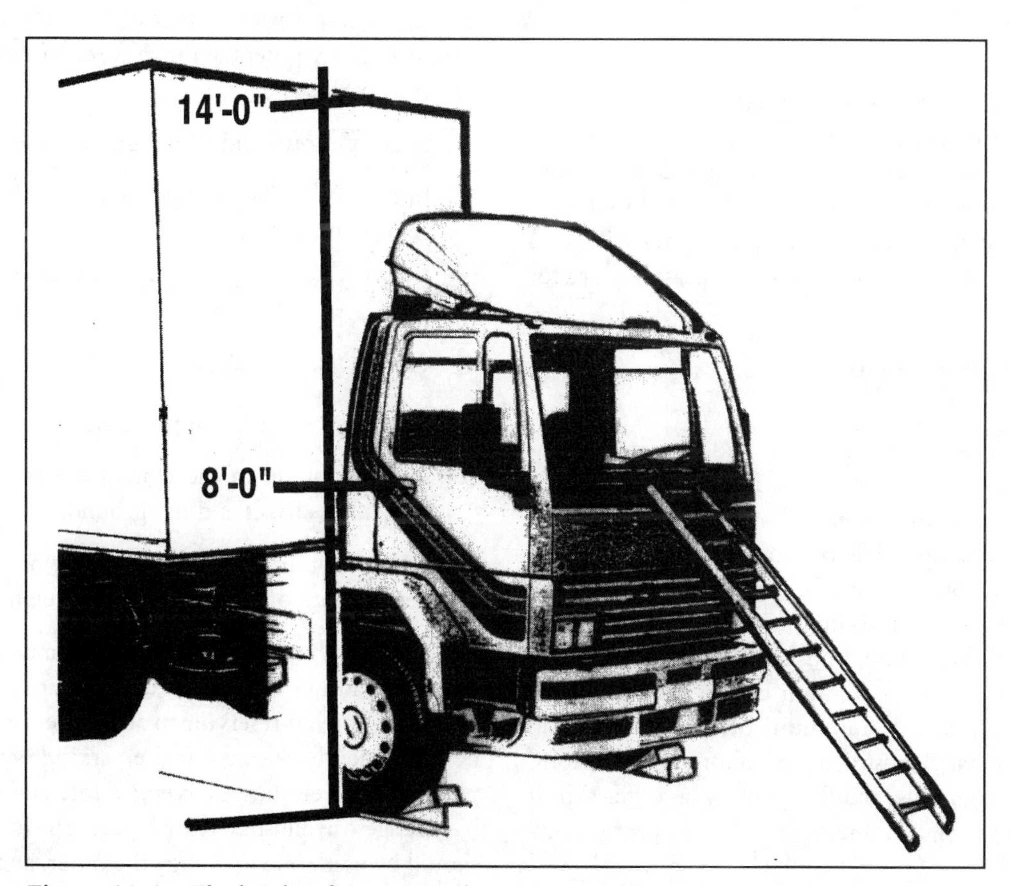

Figure 16–1 The height of a tractor trailer poses serious challenges to rescue efforts.

(Figure 16–1). Additionally, a tractor trailer may typically measure 45 ft. or more in length. Consider the stability of an access platform if an accident is situated over an embankment with difficult terrain.

The weight of a tractor trailer may be a significant factor to rescuers attempting to lift these vehicles—the maximum allowable weight is 80,000 lbs. (40 tns.). Stabilization efforts could be adversely impacted, because cargo can run the gamut between hazardous materials to livestock, creating specialty considerations.

Trucks carry various cargos. There may be hazardous materials on board which should be identifiable through placards and bills of lading. Consideration should be given to the amount, weight, and type of cargo containers. Some trucks may require special consideration; they may be carrying livestock or be equipped with refrigeration units. The stability of the cargo is of importance to rescuers.

Pressurized systems (air) may be situated throughout the vehicle including the A posts and small lines running to the seats. Fuel lines are pressurized systems as well as coolant/refrigerant lines. These are typically found in the cab, especially in the area referred to as the "dog cage." This is the area protecting the occupants from the engine.

Tools

Traditional extrication tools will work on tractor trailers, however, there will be slower operational times and more effort on the rescuer's part. Be prepared to use more blades, fuel, air, and everything else associated with tool operations. For the most part, the procedures with tool operations are the same for tractor trailers as they are for automobiles.

TRUCK CONSTRUCTION

Trucks are generally referred to, and constructed, as cabover or conventional in design. In either case, general cab construction is the same. A cabover has the cab situated over the engine, while conventional designs feature the engine in front of the cab. Trucks consist of a full frame with independent components (e.g., drivetrain and frame, suspension system, and cab configuration). Cab mounts usually have a minimum of four mounts, while sleeper models have a minimum of six mounts. Cab frames are generally constructed of aluminum extrusions, tubular steel, roof rails, and floor rails. The outer skin is typically sheet steel, aluminum, fiberglass, or plastic composites.

Doors are flush in a door frame and consist of frames, exterior panels, window mechanisms, and an inner surface of vinyl over cardboard. There are usually no collision bars or Nader bolts because no uniform standardization exists. Door hinges are described as piano, automotive, or hinged.

Safety glass comprises the windshield and is set in rubber. Some models do have tempered glass windows while others may have something different. It is not uncommon to find dangerous shards of glass in and around these vehicles. Seats are usually comprised of air ride and/or mechanical suspension systems. Rescuers must know how to operate these types of seats to their advantage during an extrication process.

Rescuers should be aware of how the cab is connected to the load: by fifth wheel, king pin, electric, air, or return.

LARGE VEHICLE STABILIZATION

A rescuer's *second priority* in establishing control at the scene of a rescue incident is the process of stabilizing a tractor trailer. Rescue teams must maintain the perspective that the vehicle must be stabilized before they begin the activity of occupant stabilization. The following steps should become a routine part of a rescuer's approach to minimizing any potential for movement during an extrication scenario:

1. Shut off motor and deenergize the electrical system.
2. Engage or apply any mechanism on board used for parking immediately.
3. Chock or wedge the wheels in both directions (Figure 16–1).
4. Stabilize the cab mounts.
5. Stabilize the seats, if appropriate.
6. Apply cribbing to the rear of the front wheels between the chassis and the ground.
7. Ensure stabilization of the load whenever possible being aware of the potential for weight to shift.

If large vehicles must be moved or separated, the parking brake should not be applied unless there is sufficient air pressure in the air reservoir to allow the parking brake to be subsequently released. If the parking brake is not applied, the wheels must be wedged fore and aft with double wedges, as illustrated in Figure 16–1. Two wedges should be used: one to wedge the other, and tapped with a hammer to provide a purchase/contact point between the road and the ground. On level ground, wedge the wheels in both directions.

LARGE VEHICLE ACCESS

The *third priority* essential to the safe mitigation of a rescue incident focuses on accessing the occupant(s) via the door and roof area(s). A jammed door may prove difficult to force open by conventional spreading with hydraulic tools because of the thickness of the panel, metal used in the construction of the truck cab, and also the height of the cab off the ground.

Unless the accident damage lends itself to the insertion of the spreader, it will be necessary to work from ladders or a platform when forcing doors. When gaining access to the door post for hydraulic cutting, spread or cut door hinges to remove the door. Considering the height of the cab, cutting door hinges offers an easier solution with more control over the door removal process.

When using a door area for initial occupant access, remember:

- Safety first! "A safety person always has his/her feet on the ground, and is touching the rescuers who are off the ground."
- Always try before you pry.
- Conduct an assessment of the cab area for possible tool purchase points.
- If possible, avoid using heavy tools in an elevated position.
- Use several rescuers if you must use tools in an elevated position.
- Work with hand tools and reciprocating saws first, and resort to hydraulic spreaders/cutters last.
- Forcing the door from the hinge side will, in most cases, be difficult.
- If you use hydraulic tools, force the door from the bottom if you can obtain a purchase point.

Rear cab panels are more advantageous access points for occupant removal, because the area behind the cab normally provides a platform or stand to work from, the panel is easy to remove, and work may be accomplished with less impact on the patient.

In addition to interior patient care personnel, interior personnel should be assigned to assess the cab construction and to direct exterior operation. Interior personnel should strip the interior finish of the cab to make cutting easier and to assist in guiding exterior personnel. Utilize a utility knife, straight blade screwdriver, and a pair of dikes. Strip the vinyl, cardboard, insulation, low voltage electrical lines, and other interior finishes. Direct exterior cutting operations.

Exterior personnel should try to place planking (or a long back board) across the chassis frame behind the cab to stand on.

At the direction of the interior person, exterior personnel utilizing a reciprocating saw, an air chisel, or other cutting tool should cut an opening the appropriate size to allow patient removal. A hydraulic cutting tool can be used to cut the ribs encountered while cutting the panel. Three sides should be cut with the bottom area left uncut and folded down to provide a relatively safe work area.

In many cases the front windshield becomes the primary, initial occupant access point because windshields are frequently not in place after impact. Occupant removal through the windshield area is not recommended because it may result in twisting an occupant's c-spine as he/she is lifted over the steering wheel/column and dashboard.

When you consider roof removal or flapping to afford better occupant access, remember that the complete roof assembly of a truck may weigh in excess of 500 lbs. This will pose a labor-intensive challenge to the overall extrication effort. Where the availability exists to quickly remove the roof structure, it will offer rescuers and EMS personnel a sizeable advantage in conducting critical care management, particularly with the flatbed or tractor unit (Figure 16–2).

The roof can be made of aluminum, fiberglass, sheet steel, or plastic. A roof can also be made of a combination or materials including fiberglass and aluminum. When two materials are used, the split will normally be across the cab between the driver and the rear of the cab.

Removing an entire roof is a labor intensive operation. Personnel are required at the roof level as well as on the ground to receive the heavy material. If the vehicle is on its side, roof removal may be an excellent patient removal access.

When conducting an assessment of the accident scene, a rescuer must satisfy himself/herself as to the most realistic and practical plan of attack and convey this to the EMS personnel on location. Your discussion should address partial or complete roof removal, the tools suitable for the task, placement of rescue personnel, and the actual removal technique to be employed.

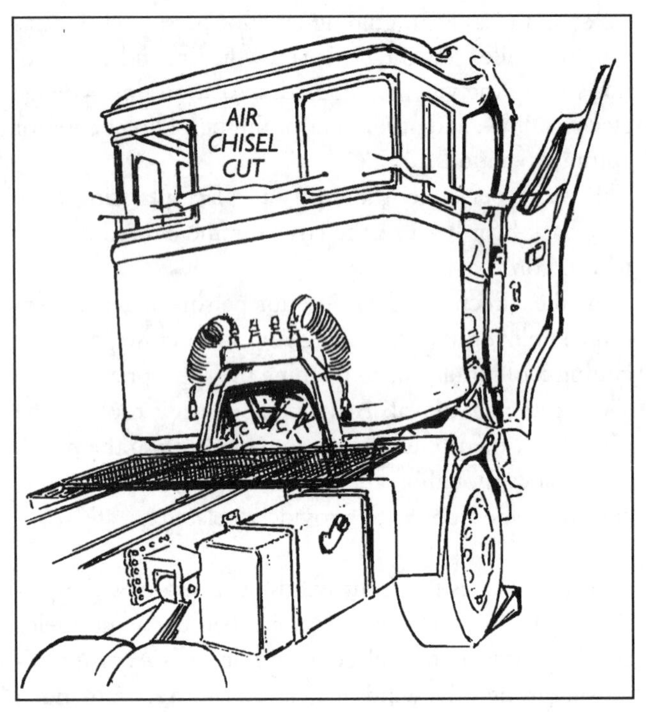

Figure 16–2 Roof removal offers rescuers a sizeable advantage.

If the vehicle is upright you must make a decision regarding how you will remove the roof:

1. Partial removal
   - Front
   - Rear
   - Side
2. Complete removal
   - Direction
   - Personnel
   - Technique

When selecting tools to be utilized, take into account the weight of the tool, number of rescuers to operate the tool, the power supply, and safety of personnel. Place personnel on the roof, at chassis level, or at ground level. Remember, a safety person always has his or her feet on the ground and is touching the rescuers who are off the ground.

When removing the roof consider the victim's location and position. Try not to move the roof portion over the victim. Consider terrain and ensure that adequate personnel are in place. Removal techniques include:

1. Strip interior
2. Position personnel to receive roof
3. Mechanism to support roof
4. Cut posts
5. Remove panels
6. Lower to the ground with control

Points to remember when attempting roof removal:

- With large areas of panelling, use an air chisel to cut between shearing points (Figure 16–3).
- Physically support the roof structure and cut the rear roof pillars.
- Remove the windshield and fixed glazing to the cab where appropriate, and remove or locate drop windows within the confines of the doors. Because of the height of the cab it will be necessary to work from ladders or from a rear platform as shown in Figure 16–1.
- The height and weight of the roof structure will make it necessary to remove the structure with extreme caution. Where the option exists, windshield pillars need only be partly out close to the bulkhead. This will enable the roof structure to be flapped forward.
- Once flapped forward, the cuts to the windshield pillars can be completed and the roof placed in a convenient position away from the immediate area (Figures 16–4 and 16–5).

The *fourth priority* consistent with a successful extrication outcome is the process of dash relocation or displacement in conjunction with enlargement of openings. This activity involves making an opening around the oc-

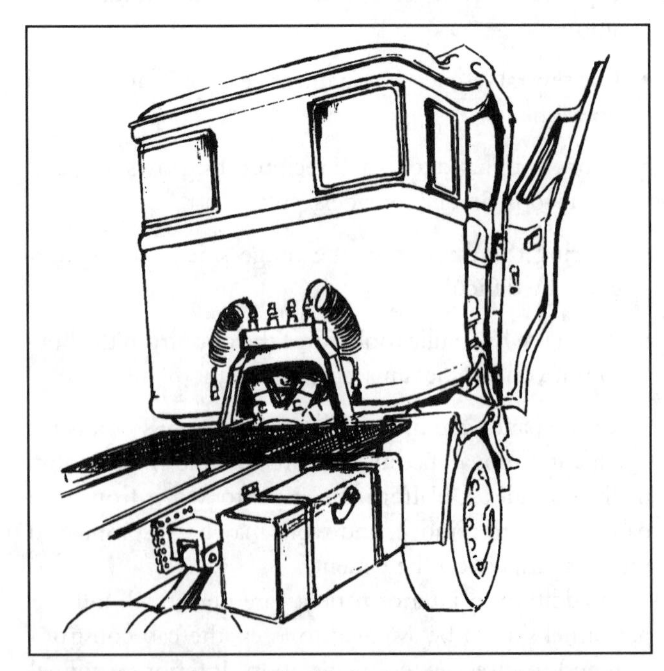

Figure 16–3 Use an air chisel to cut between shearing points.

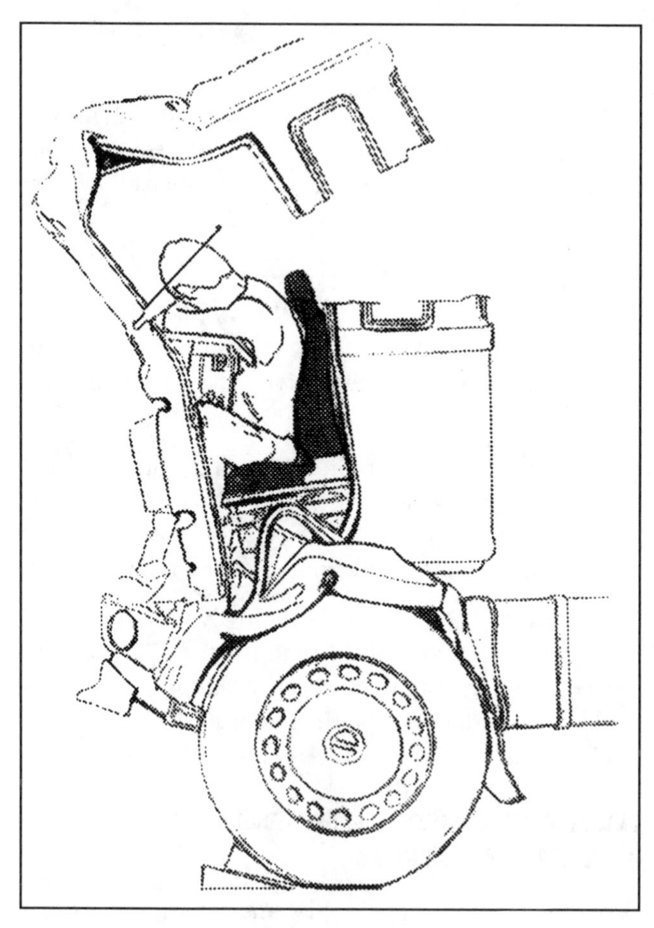

Figure 16–4 With roof flapped, cuts to windshield pillars can be completed.

cupant to make removal easier on the rescuers and safer for the occupant.

Cabover designs often lend themselves to complete frontal displacement of the bulkhead area away from the occupants. This can be accomplished with similar methods used in an automobile scenario. Unlike an automobile, normally only one side would need to be pushed. The door must be open on the side to be pushed. The roof must be separated, although not necessarily removed.

Late model trucks are equipped with crush-resistant cabs, necessitating the removal of the rear quarter section behind the occupants. Frontal displacement should be a rescuer's first choice, however, and is accomplished as follows:

- Position hydraulic power rams in the door openings and extend to the point of strain/firm contact. It may be necessary to use a spreader to obtain sufficient space to introduce the rams.
- Cut the windshield pillars at the top, nearest the roof structure (Figure 16–6).

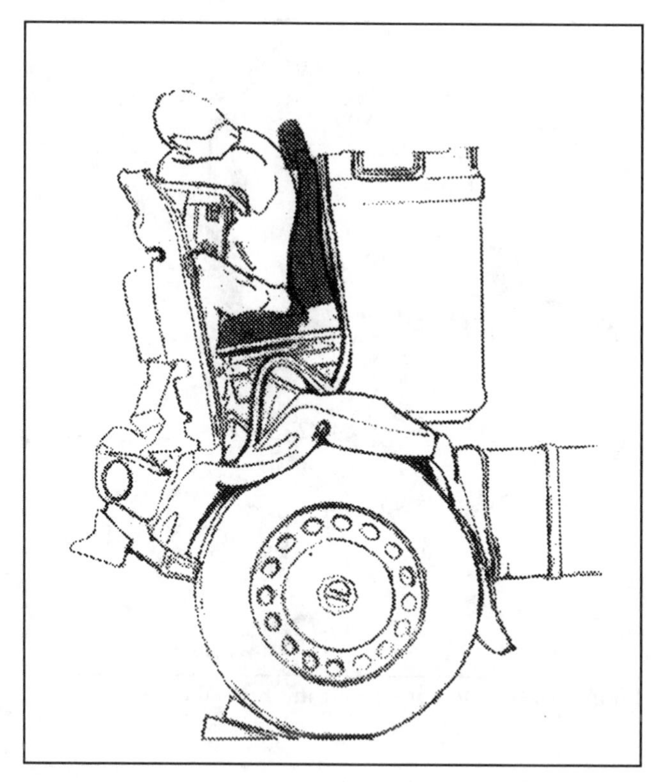

Figure 16–5 Roof is placed away from immediate area.

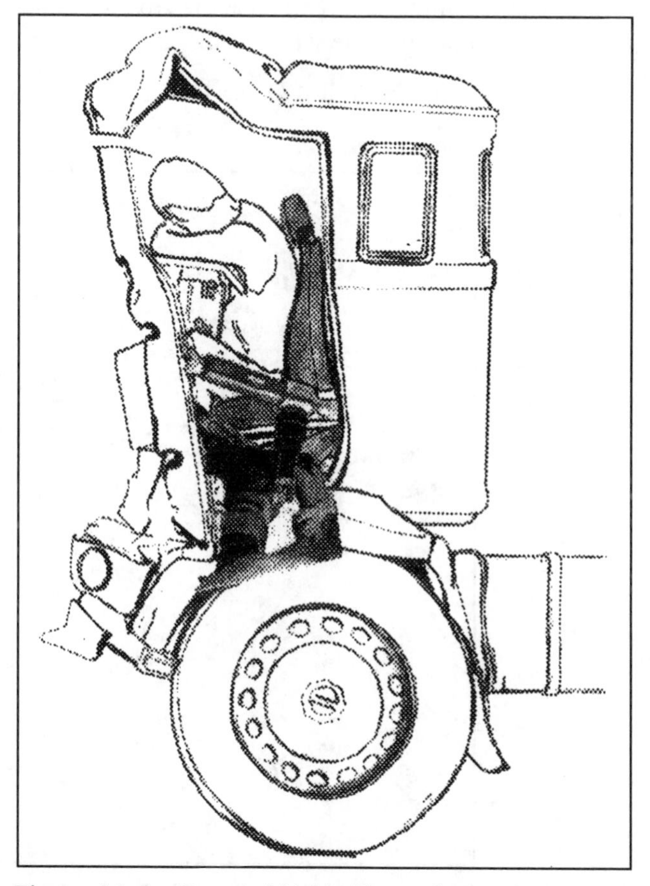

Figure 16–6 Cut windshield pillars at the top.

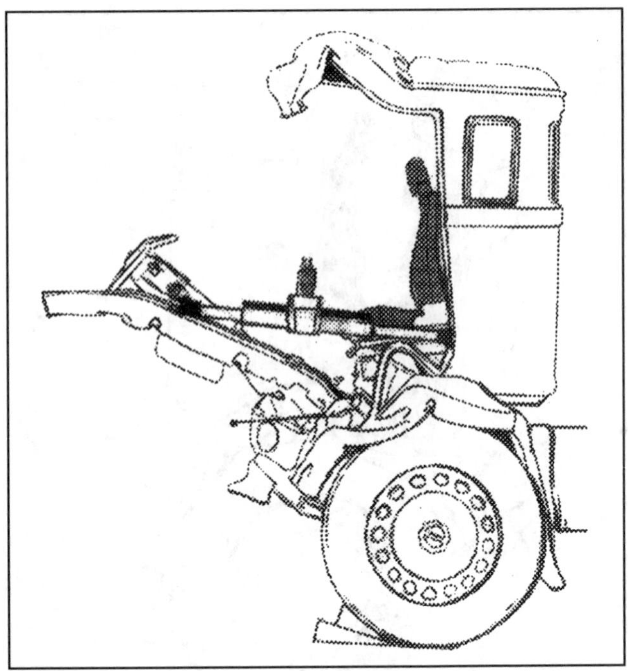

Figure 16–7 Do not extend rams beyond the relief cuts.

- To weaken the cabs superstructure, cut the door post level with the floorline or A post rocker panel. This will require a multicut operation as the cross-sectional areas of the door post are substantial.
- Extend the rams gradually. *Do not* extend any rams beyond the integrity of the purchase points/relief cuts (Figure 16–7).
- A winch can be used to take up the tension. This will give added security where a larger ram needs to replace a smaller one or in the event of ram slippage (Figure 16–8).

Caution Points to Remember

- When dealing with a tilt cab, the securing mechanism must be monitored at all times during winching operations.
- As ramming/extension progresses, it is imperative not to allow heavy-gauge moving metal to come into contact with the ram(s) as this may dislodge the purchase point(s) and put an undesirable strain on the plungers.
- Ramming must be carried out slowly, cautiously, and conducted in line with EMS instructions. The advantage of gaining optimum space in this way will be realized when lifting/lowering an occupant down from the truck's cab.

Cutting Away the Rear Quarter Section of the Crush-resistant Cab

When traditional frontal displacement measures are not feasible, removal of the rear quarter section of a crush-

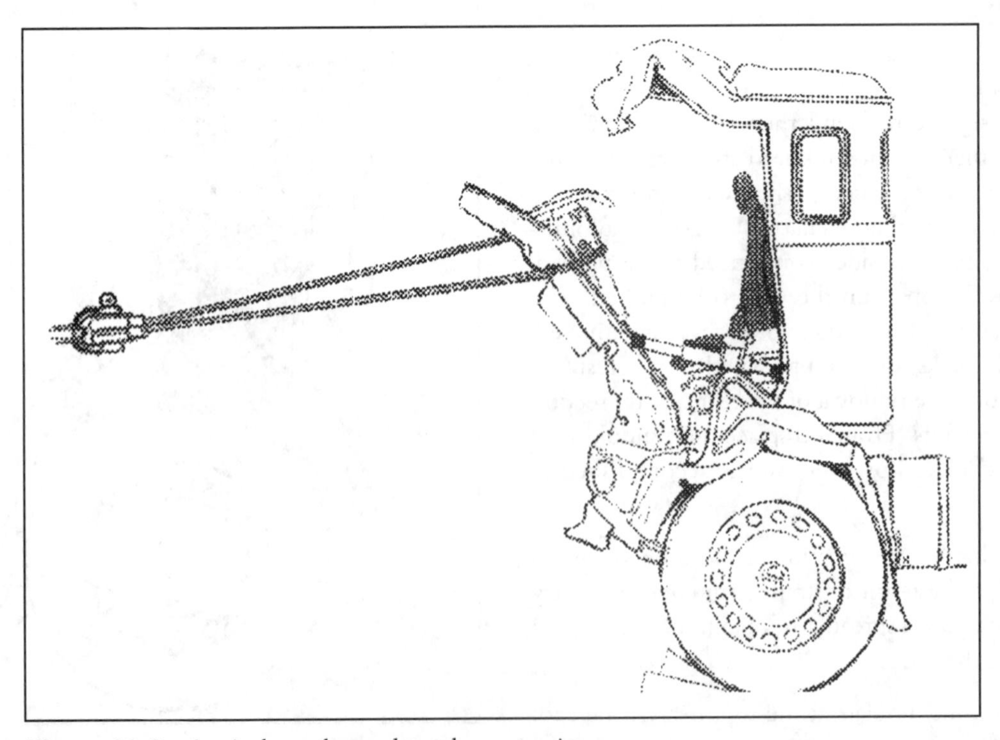

Figure 16–8 A winch can be used to take up tension.

resistant cab should be considered. The steps to accomplish this objective are:

1. Remove all necessary window glass.
2. Open all necessary doors.
3. Because of the metal panelling's composition, its removal using an air chisel will be prolonged. The panelling should be removed to the seam on the far side of the rear quarter window if present. All insulation, internal trim, and the furnishing of the sleeper cab should then be removed. With the outer skin removed, the structural ribbing to the rear of a crush-resistant cab will be exposed (Figure 16–9).
4. Cut the door posts at points A and B (Figure 16–9), at the rear of the door opening and the strengthening/reinforcement channel supporting the area that needs to be cut away, first at the top and then at the bottom C (Figure 16–10). The center strengthening bar should be cut at the far side of the rear quarter window D (Figure 16–10). The ribbed section, complete with the door post, can then be removed.

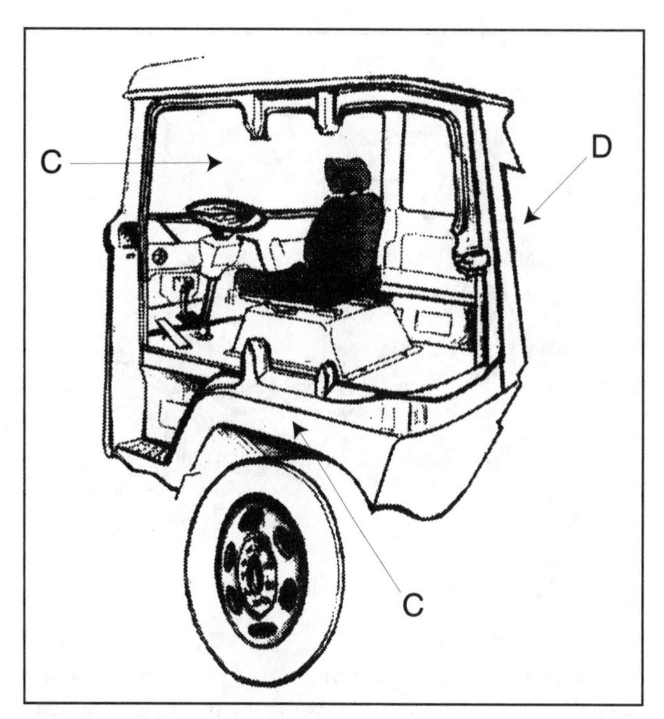

Figure 16–10 Cab's structural ribbing.

The American long-nosed tractor trailer unit, also referred to as the conventional cab, can be handled in much the same way as the European flat fronted, all steel tilt cab, that was just discussed. The fender may need to be removed to get a clearer look at the bulkhead area and door posts (Figures 16–11 and 16–12).

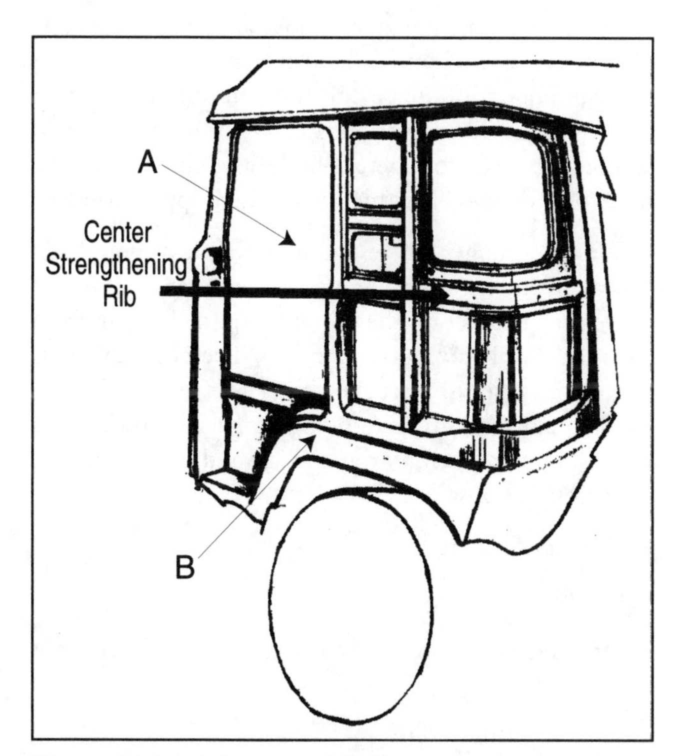

Figure 16–9 Cab's structural ribbing.

The super structure will need to be weakened by cutting the windshield pillars and the door posts, level with the floor line/rocker panels, otherwise the rear door posts will have insufficient strength and can give way as ramming begins (Figure 16–6). Likewise, the rear quarter section can also be cut away (Figure 16–10).

OCCUPANT HANDLING AND REMOVAL

Most cab seats are either mechanical or air controlled. The mechanically adjustable seat (Figure 16–13) features forward and reverse travel modes. It provides a reclining seat back and lumbar support. The height is also adjustable. Some manufacturers also provide a tilt/adjustment to the seats. The high back seat invariably has a built-in head rest and the passenger's seat may come fitted with arm rests. Where fitted, the seat suspension unit has a gas-filled strut.

The seat includes seat-track adjustment for forward/reverse directional movement. If you are going to remove the cab's roof in its entirety, then consider securing the occupant to traditional spinal immobilization devices suitable for lifting/hoisting, and removing the occupant and seat together as a unit. This will require apparatus suitable to the task (e.g., designated rescue vehicles with cranes or booms certified for this purpose).

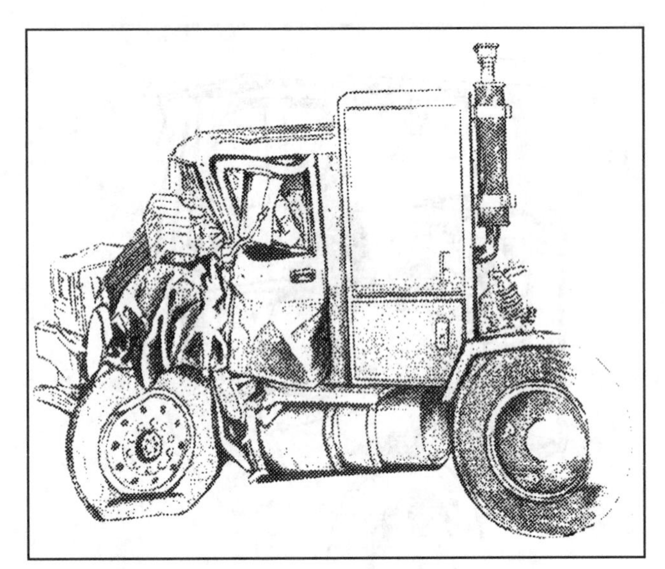

Figure 16–11 Fender into bulkhead area.

To remove an occupant in a seated position, it may be possible to unbolt the seat base from the height adjustment mechanism or the base pan from the floorboard. Alternatively, the seat can also be forcibly removed by other traditional methods.

Air-controlled, fully adjustable seats can be removed along with their air suspension unit by unbolting the seat-securing bolts. Alternatively, the rubber valance can be cut away with a knife and the seat base unbolted from the height adjustment frame.

The height adjustment configuration must not be cut until the air pressure is released from the system. The air suspension strut may be charged with up to eight bars of pressure. To purge the air suspension unit, press the air release button and hold in position until the system is empty of air (Figure 16–14).

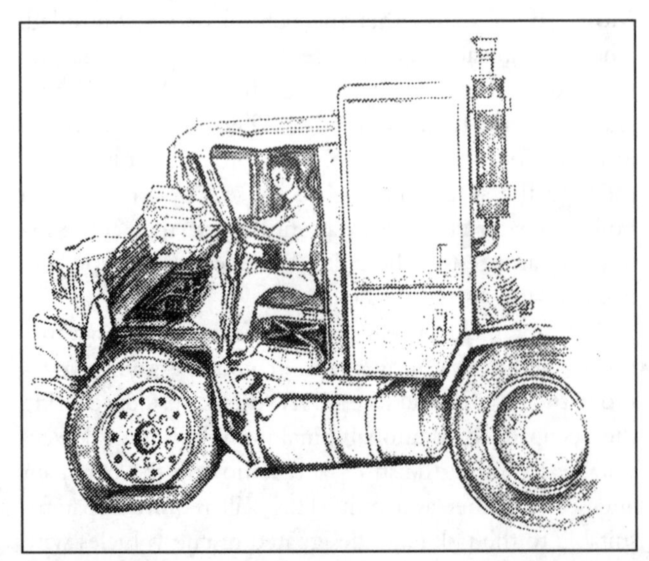

Figure 16–12 Removing fender.

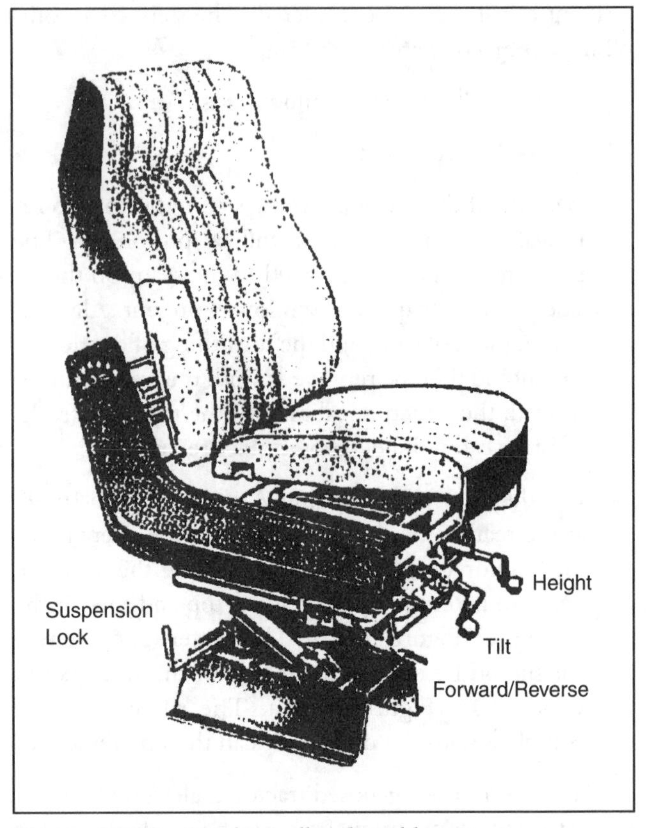

Figure 16–13 Mechanically adjustable seats.

Caution: If you are going to remove any type of seat configuration intact with the occupant, you must coordinate the immobilization phase and the removal process with EMS personnel on location. Life safety rope, approved webbing, and/or commercial bridle assemblies should be used for the lifting/hoisting effort where appropriate.

When dealing with rescue incidents involving large trucks, rescuers must remember that removing a patient from a cab ten feet off the ground is quite different from a conventional automobile scenario. The potential exists for back injuries to rescuers as well as fractures, dislocations, sprains, and strains resulting from falls, slippage, and off positioning when working in/around the occupants.

Factors to consider are:

- Height of the rig
- Confined working area
- Intensive personnel requirements to mitigate occupant removal
  - Interior personnel
  - Exterior elevated personnel

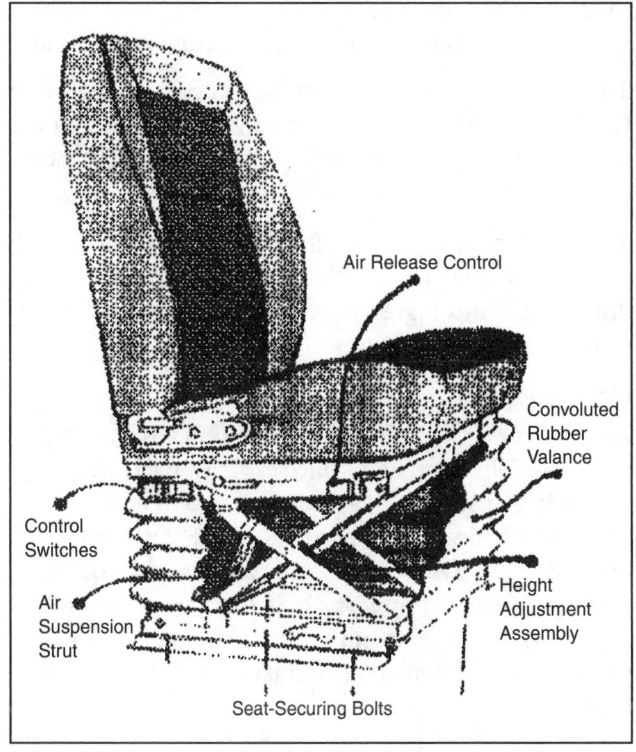

Figure 16–14 To purge the air suspension unit, press the air release control and hold in position until system is empty of air.

- Exterior ground level personnel
- Necessary equipment

- What removal techniques you intend to employ

Regardless of what your exposure has been, the bottom line is this: *When the big one happens you had better be prepared.* The challenges you face will prove worthy competitors to your skills proficiency level. How well you adopt the principles of extrication to large/elevated vehicles will determine the duration and success of the operation. The next time you are on duty at your station, gather a team of EMS/rescue providers together and conduct a company-level drill. Package and remove an occupant from the largest/highest piece of apparatus in your station and you'll begin to appreciate the tasks that lie ahead.

ISSUES IN BUS EXTRICATION

Three primary factors to consider when addressing the issue of extrication from buses are:

- Size
- Construction features
- Hazards

When addressing the issues associated with bus extrication, the problem of vehicle size directly impacts an operational plan along the same lines as big rigs. *Size* equates to numbers; *numbers* equate to injuries; *injuries* equate to patient packaging and removal. The bottom line? A nightmare for EMS/rescue personnel!

The mechanism of injury in bus accidents is wide and varying. The potential for serious trauma-related problems/deaths exists because of the lack of occupant restraints. Occupants usually impact with fixed objects within this conveyance and other passengers being hurled forward, sideways, etc.

How does bus construction influence extrication effort(s)? Buses can vary in construction and make-up. School buses have specific emergency exits, but transit/commercial conveyances generally do not. Instead, passenger windows will have to be used, so long as they are accessible to the rescuer(s). Seating on transit-type buses is far from uniform, in comparison to commercial coaches that feature front-facing seat arrangements. The aisles in transit-type buses are wider in comparison school buses and motor coaches. The width of the aisles in motor coaches range between 13 ins. to 18 ins. and pose some interesting challenges to rescuers attempting to remove occupants on backboards, scoop stretchers, and improvised devices.

Motor coaches also have higher seat backs and lower hanging luggage racks which severely hamper a rescuer's efforts to move occupants over the seat tops. It may be necessary to systematically remove rows of seats to provide a clear extrication path.

As with any bus construction, the framing members are markedly different between various types. They range from armored-car-like occupant protection as in the case of school buses, to rows of roof rivets in commercial coaches being more than 2 ft. apart. Rescuers attempting to access this area would probably find a rafter between two riveted members.

Hazards associated with buses in general stem from the fuel that propels them and the interior's finish. Also, buses, such as motor coaches, have a large storage area beneath the occupant areas. These storage areas are used for package delivery, personal property, and almost anything in small unregulated quantities. Remember also that commercial motor conveyances may be equipped with chemical toilets to the rear of the occupant/passenger area.

BUS CONSTRUCTION

School Buses

Introduction: On a national level approximately 400,000 school conveyances transport over 22 million children to and from public/private schools each day. During a school year cycle, these conveyances log approximately 4.1 billion miles. Despite their safety record overall, school conveyance accidents continue to occur.

Ronald E. Moore, an expert in the field of school bus rescue, notes that during one recent school year, 29,000 accidents occurred involving conveyances used for school-related activities. The majority (27,000) were classified as property damage only, while the remaining accidents caused 142 deaths and approximately 12,000 injuries. Interestingly enough, out of the 142 fatalities, 10 were children inside the bus, the rest were pedestrians and occupants of other vehicles involved in the accident. The biggest single cause of school conveyance accidents/injuries/deaths continues to be in the loading/unloading zones.

School conveyance construction features differ from automobiles. The extrication methodologies that the rescue service practices on automobiles may be impractical for a school conveyance. Knowing the construction, design, and regulations governing school conveyances will better prepare rescuers who are responding to these incidents.

School bus regulations are nationally mandated. The federal motor vehicle safety standards outline the minimum vehicle design and construction features required, along with the performance criteria for windows, exits, rollover protection, vehicle body joint strength, fuel system integrity, seat safety requirement, and the fire retardancy of interior materials. The National Highway Traffic Safety Administration has issued Highway Safety Program Standard #17 on pupil transportation safety to aid governments in regulating other aspects of school bus safety, such as vehicle color, lighting, markings, and procedures for onloading/offloading students.

Types of School Buses: There are basically four types of school conveyance vehicles:

Type A Smallest; gross vehicle weight (GVW) >10,000 lbs; suburban-type vehicle; seating capacity approximately 8 people; motor beneath or in front of the windshield

Type B Standard/chop van chassis; GVW >10,000 lbs.; body added by the manufacturer; seating capacity of 16 to 24 people; passenger door situated behind front wheels; motor beneath or behind the front windshield

Type C Engine compartment protrudes from the front; GVW >10,000 lbs.; seating capacity approximately 45 to 48 people; entrance door behind the front wheels; motor located in front of the windshield

Type D Referred to as a "flat nose" bus; super models carry up to 100 people; front/rear mounted engine; driver's seat and ingress/egress door located forward of front wheels

Construction

Body: Types B, C, and D school bus bodies consist of a roof, sidewall, floor, and front/rear area. Each area of the body is framed with a steel skeletal system hidden from view beneath the interior and exterior metal of the body. This system forms the basic structure of the entire school bus. It predicts how the conveyance will act during an accident and forms the basis of the protective envelope designed for occupant safety and survivability.

There are two basic construction methods used by school bus manufacturers:

- *Integral construction,* which essentially is custom built and is featured in the Type D bus design.
- *Body on chassis* method, where the body is installed onto a commercial chassis and is featured in the Type C bus design.

The strongest and most rigidly constructed area of a school conveyance body is the sidewall. This area is composed of a load-bearing vertical frame member of angle-iron steel that resembles the studding in the wall of a house. These vertical members also become the partitions between each of the passenger window units. Running horizontally inside each sidewall is an additional structural element, referred to as the "collision beam." This thick-gauge steel member, which resembles a highway guard rail, is strategically located to limit penetration of an object into the passenger compartment of the bus.

The interior and exterior walls of the bus consist of 20-gauge finish panels secured directly to the inner skeletal system of the sidewall. To meet requirements for interior noise levels and warmth, fiberglass or styrofoam insulation materials are sandwiched into the walls. To increase the impact resistance and the structural integrity of the sidewall, an additional item is installed on the exterior sidewall. As many as four 16-gauge steel W-shaped rub rails, each 4.75 ins. wide, are placed along the length of the sidewalls.

Forcible entry through the sidewall area of a school bus below window level is extremely difficult and time consuming due to the design and construction of the structural members.

The rear skeletal system is similar to the sidewall, with additional reinforcements installed to provide protection from rear-end collisions.

Roof: The skeletal system of the roof typically consists of heavy-duty 11-gauge curved steel frame members called "roof bows." These members are positioned in the roof structure running from side to side. Tied into each roof bow are 16-gauge one-piece steel angle-iron braces known as "stringers." There may be as many as three of these longitudinal members in the roof skeleton, running from the front header to the rear of the bus, strengthening the roof bows and the entire bus body structure.

Insulation material and wiring for sound and lighting equipment are located within the roof's skeletal framework. The outside and inside of the roof framing members are covered with 24-gauge sheet-metal panels. The seams of the metal panels can also indicate underlying roof bows or stringers.

Rescue personnel assigned to breach the roof structure can locate underlying roof bows and stringers by the pattern of rivets used to secure the outer and inner roof panels and by the seams of the metal panels.

Emergency escape hatches may be located in the roof structure. Molded of fiberglass or other lightweight materials, these hatches normally open by the activation of a release mechanism found inside the bus. At an emergency incident, simple forcible-entry techniques can open the roof hatch from outside. The hatches open 180° to provide a clear opening of at least 14 ins. × 18 ins. On some buses, particularly those used to carry physically disabled occupants, there may be larger hatches, opening 30 ins. × 30 ins.

Floor: The floor of a school bus consists of several important components. The heavy-duty vinyl or rubber floor covering that is visible inside the bus is commonly applied over half-inch or thicker plywood sheets. The plywood, if provided, covers the bottom floor layer, which is typically comprised of thick, 14-gauge metal panels. Type A suburban-style buses use only the original manufacturer's metal floor covered in vinyl, while Type B van-conversion buses generally use the same layered floor structure found in larger buses. Structural steel members that act as floor joists are spaced approximately every 17 ins. along the underside of the floor. These joists support the weight of the floor, seats, and occupant load, and are attached directly to the frame rails of the bus chassis.

Undercarriage: The undercarriage of the bus is a substantially reinforced area with an eight-gauge angle bar, 12-gauge channel stock, and 14-gauge sheet-metal construction. Forcible entry and access attempts to breach the floor should not be considered as a routine entry point due to the excessive time and effort necessary to accomplish such task.

Windows and Windshields: The rough openings for the side and rear passenger windows on buses are framed by the vertical wall members, the edge of the roof, and the top of the sidewall of the bus. The window posts are hollow, consisting of several layers of sheet metal shaped into a column. Any window post that is positioned between two side windows can be removed for extrication purposes with saws, chisels, or cutting tools.

The windows themselves are either laminated or tempered safety glass framed in extruded aluminum. The windows are of the split-sash design and are secured in the rough openings of the bus body with rivets or similar devices. School bus windows slide open from the top, providing an opening of approximately 9 ins. × 22 ins. or half the total window opening.

To provide a larger opening, selected side windows are designed to function as emergency exits and are so labeled inside the vehicle. (Exit windows may not be present in older buses or in states that do not require this feature.) From the exterior, the exit windows are readily identified by the appearance of hinges along the top side of the window frame. Once opened, they provide an approximate 22-in. × 22-in. opening.

Emergency exit windows do not have hold-open devices to secure the window and frame in the open (or "up") position. Rescue personnel operating at the scene of a bus incident must therefore either provide their own means of securing these windows in the open position or remove the entire swing-out window unit. Even in states that require emergency exit windows for buses that carry large numbers of students, emergency exit windows are not mandated on the smaller Types A and B school buses.

Windshields are set into the vehicle body by means of a multipiece rubber mounting gasket. On smaller school buses, the windshield is a single laminated safety-glass pane, while full-size buses have two or more sheets of glass in their windshield assemblies. Rescue personnel can readily remove windshield glass from the inside or outside of the bus either by chopping, pushing, or prying out the glass or by cutting and peeling off the windshield mounting gasket. Opening the windshield makes for a very efficient emergency-exit opening in the vehicle.

Rear window glass (found in the rear doors as well as to each side of the door in the rear wall of the bus) is either tempered or laminated safety glass. These relatively small window panes are also secured to the bus body by a readily removable rubber mounting gasket.

Doors can be two-part split or center hinged. They may be manual or air operated. Buses may also have a rear exit door.

Seats are of tubular steel, bolted to the floor. The seat bottom may be held on by removable clips.

Aisles range from 10 ins. to 15 ins. unless designed for wheelchairs, in which case the aisle is 30 ins.

Features for the Disabled in School Conveyances: Vehicles designed to transport the physically disabled have some unique design features and equipment that will challenge rescuers at an emergency scene. In addition, wheelchair-bound passengers add new complications to rescue and medical work inside the vehicle. The rescuer inside the bus needs to know how to handle special equipment such as the mechanism that secures the wheelchairs to the bus, the wheelchair hydraulic lift assembly, and the special restraint harnesses that secure passengers in their seats.

The vehicle's appearance may give yet another clue as to the special passengers who may be on board. If the vehicle can accommodate passengers in wheelchairs, an enlarged exterior door will be present, usually on the passenger side of the bus. In addition to the wheelchair door, rescue personnel may also see the wheelchair lift assembly inside the bus and realize that disabled people may be on board.

Transportation of Wheelchair Passengers: The wheelchair lift door is always larger than the conventional entrance door because it must have sufficient height and width not only for the disabled passenger but for a wheelchair as well. Due to the wheelchair size, the exterior door and wheelchair lift structure provide a minimum clear opening width of 30 ins. and a minimum head room height of 48 ins.

Wheelchair lift doors, similar to the conventional school bus entry and exit doors, typically have glass windows mounted on the doors with rubber gaskets. The doors have a mechanical latch assembly similar to that on the rear exit door of a conventional school bus, with both outside and inside door handles. It can be difficult for someone inside the bus to use the interior door release mechanism because the release handle is obstructed when the wheelchair ramp are in the stowed position.

Ramp Lift Assemblies: The wheelchair lift assembly can be found just inside the door. The lift assembly typically consists of an electric/hydraulic pump, several pairs of hydraulic cylinders, a heavy-duty metal framework and support structure, a movable floor structure and a hand-held electric trigger control device. The floor, or lifting platform, stores vertically inside the bus and typically has a minimum load carrying rating of 650 lbs.

The wheelchair lift assembly typically uses electricity and hydraulic fluid under pressure to operate. Under normal conditions, the system uses power from the vehicle's electrical system to energize the hydraulic pump. The pump pressurizes the cylinders that pivot the wheelchair lift floor in and out or lower and raise the floor for loading or unloading. The wheelchair door may be damaged enough during a crash to become jammed shut or otherwise inoperable, forcing rescue teams to employ various bus rescue techniques to open the door.

All hydraulic lift units contain a manual backup pump with a separate handle that functions similarly to a standard hydraulic jack. With the valves opened or closed manually, the backup pump can move the lift to any position desired, but this effort is extremely slow and tiresome. In addition, it will only work if the crash or fire has not disabled the lift assembly's hydraulic system or bent the lift's structure. This backup pump system is primarily intended for use by bus operators in case the lift malfunctions during routine loading or unloading.

For emergency situations, a special feature on the wheelchair lift allows the platform section to be lowered without using the electric/hydraulic system. The system uses either a strategically located emergency disconnect lever or a special pull-pin attached directly to the top of one of the hydraulic cylinders. The lever or pin is typically red for better visibility and ease of recognition and is accessible when the platform is stowed inside the bus.

Removing the release pin or operating the release lever disconnects the hydraulic mechanism from the floor section of the wheelchair lift. Then, rescue personnel can pull the floor out and down to its horizontal position. At this point, medical and rescue crews can move patients onto the deployed floor unit, where others outside the bus can receive them.

Emergency Windows and Roof Hatches. Side windows on disabled transport buses may be either the standard 22-in. × 22-in. school bus style units or specially sized, double-width windows. The window may be made of laminated safety glass, tempered safety glass, or plastic Lexan-type materials. All window frames are constructed of lightweight aluminum. As with conventional bus vehicles, side windows designed as emergency escape windows typically have swingout hinges along the top and decals or labels indicating the window's operation.

Additional emergency access openings may be available if the bus is provided with one or two roof hatches. These hatches are either the standard 14-in. × 18-in. size or the larger 30-in. × 30-in. size. All hatches are provided with inside release levers, although the latest generation of roof hatches is now equipped with both inside and outside release handles.

Interior Riding Positions: Bus passengers may be seated in a wide variety of arrangements. While passengers with normal mobility may sit in conventional school bus style seats (also referred to as utility or transit-style seats), occupants with impaired mobility may be in similar-looking seats that have incorporated additional body support equipment and some unique seatbelt body-restraint harnesses.

Wheelchair Attachments and Seat Equipment: When riding in buses, wheelchair-bound passengers remain seated in their wheelchairs. The bus operator must secure each wheelchair to the bus sidewall or floor at special attachment points. By using straps, buckles, and mechanical linkage pins, the most common wheelchair attachment system positions the wheelchair with the passenger's back to the sidewall of the bus, and feet extending well into the center aisle space. Newer systems, just now gaining acceptance, position the wheelchair-bound passenger in a forward-facing position.

The fastening device usually has a manually operated slide pin or lever and must be capable of holding the wheelchair in place during routine driving. Seatbelt systems provide additional security; these can be a simple lap belt unit or a shoulder harness/lap belt design similar to those found in automobiles.

Special note: Minimum standards require only that the wheelchair be secured to the vehicle. Regulations do not mandate that the wheelchair occupant be secured to the chair or otherwise restrained.

Due to the unique nature of bus transport for the disabled, there are a wide variety of individually designed seat arrangements. Standard child-safety seats may be used for small or young children, while a custom-fitted foam rubber seat, called a Carrie Seat, can be used for children with physical disabilities that require body support. A five-point restraint harness, similar to those used by race car drivers, may be used for passengers requiring upper-body restraint. Rescuers inside the bus may also find passengers secured in the lap-belt-only system provided on standard bench seats. The bus driver may be secured in either a lap-belt-only system or a shoulder harness/lap belt. If the vehicle transports people confined to wheelchairs, the standard aisle width is a minimum of 30 ins. in any area of the bus in which a wheelchair may be maneuvered.

Assessment and Extrication of a Disabled Passenger: When dealing with disabled patients, responders should remember that normal communication with these patients may be impossible. In fact, the injured person may not even be able to comprehend the events that are taking place around him/her, much less respond to them. Providers should also consider that traumatic injuries may be disguised by the disabled person's existing conditions. Internal injuries not immediately obvious during patient contact may remain undetected due to the patient's inability to perceive/experience pain.

Any bus that has disabled people on board may also be transporting people without disabilities. The bus driver and any adult chaperons are obvious examples of patients who should be cared for with routine medical assessment and treatment protocols.

Although several removal techniques are available, one successful method calls for cutting the patient free of the bus seat, leaving the restraint strapping or harness in place around him/her. With a pediatric patient transported in a child safety seat or a custom-fitted Carrie Seat, most EMS protocols require that the rescue team package and remove the patient and seat as a unit.

Dealing with a patient trapped by a damaged wheelchair presents yet another problem for rescuers. A typical electric wheelchair with battery can weigh as much as 400 lbs., not counting the occupant. During the dynamics of an accident, forces generated inside the bus can be severe, and a disabled person may be trapped not only by the bus structure but also by his/her own damaged wheelchair. This problem is best addressed through training and practice. The experience gained from extricating a training mannequin from entanglement in a wheelchair will prove very valuable during a real incident.

Transit/Commercial Buses

Transit buses are used for short distances, usually with no storage area or rest room. They generally seat 30 to 70 passengers. Commercial coaches travel longer distances, seat 50 to 60 passengers, and usually include storage areas and a rest room.

Overview of Bus Suspension System: The suspension system of a bus consists of air bags. These air bags replace the springs used in other suspensions systems.

There are four air bags in the front (two in front and two behind the front axle) and four air bags in the rear similarly positioned.

It is possible for an air bag to blow out. When this occurs the side of the bus with the blowout will drop down. It is still possible to drive the bus. Should someone be working under the bus, the bus may possibly drop low enough to cause injury.

The bus also has four shock absorbers, two front and two rear. There will be no hazard caused by excessive heat. There is oil in the absorbers but they are encased in steel and should pose no problem.

Door Operation: The front and rear doors of the bus operate off the air system. The door handle for operation is located to the left of the driver. This handle will operate the doors with or without the bus turned on.

Should this handle not function, an individual in the bus can turn the small door operation knob to manual and the air will be released from both the front and rear doors. This knob is located to the left of the driver in front of the door handle.

The door handle may be reached from the outside by reaching through the operator's window. The rear door may then be opened by slipping one's hand through the rubber guards on the door and grabbing the metal door bar. Doors may be broken if the above methods do not provide access to the inside.

Emergency Engine Shut-Off: To shut off the bus engine in an emergency from the outside: open the engine compartment door, locate the U-shaped valve, and pull down on this valve until the engine stops running. The valve is similar to that found on fire engines.

Engine: The bus is operated by a diesel engine. The fuel used is a mixture of #1 and #2 diesel fuel and will not ignite in most situations. There are different spark points, however, and caution should be used when operating around them.

If the engine is running, and the fan is not operating, *do not try to touch the fan to get it going*. The fan is operated by a thermostat and runs when necessary. Should the fan start while a hand is present, amputation could result.

If the engine is on fire and the compartment door cannot be opened, access can be gained by lifting the rear seats (which are on hinges) and removing a back panel.

There is also a switch on the dash that can be thrown to ensure no one will start the engine while the bus is not attended. This switch, called "emergency stop," can also be used to stop the engine if the engine fails to stop when the master control is turned to "off."

If this emergency stop switch is used, the engine can be restarted after manually resetting a cam on the air choke valve in the engine compartment at the rear of the bus.

Tires: Both tubed and tubeless tires are currently in use. All tires used will eventually be tubeless. Be careful if the tire area has been hit. There is no way to foretell a tire blowout. The force of a blowout could cause injury.

If the front tires or tire area have been hit, and the tires are tubed tires, extra caution must be used in working in this area. These tubed front tires have a lock ring that locks the tire into the rim. This ring can fly off from changes in pressure and cause serious harm. If you must do something to the front tubed tire, let the air out by the valve before doing anything else.

Air-conditioning: Freon is used in some air-conditioning systems. Freon itself is not poisonous. If you must get near a system that may have been damaged, wear goggles and protective clothing. Should a hose break or fluid be leaking, the freon will cause instant freezing to a temperature of −55°F. This will result in immediate and permanent damage to eyes, etc. When freon is leaking into a closed area, it absorbs all oxygen present and can cause asphyxiation. See that you have proper ventilation and that passengers are evacuated. Freon has been fazed out are non-CFC-type fluids are being utilized.

Windshield: The windshield is not held in place by mastic. To remove the windshield, remove the filler strip around the windshield and push it out around the rubber border.

Frame Style: There are four square pads, two on the front axle and two on the rear axle, where jacks can be placed if needed. A 12-tn. hydraulic jack is sufficient.

If the rear of the bus needs to be raised, place a hoist or cherry picker under the *inner bumper* and lifting the bus at that point. This is not the black rubber bumper that is visible.

Cutting into the body of the bus can be done anywhere along the sides between the beams, which are visible under the bus. The roof can be cut into at any point. The floor can also be cut through if necessary; it is plywood, not metal.

Ventilation: The only air intake is located in front in the driver's area. To ventilate the bus quickly of fumes, all the windows may be opened from the inside by either pushing out at the base or pulling the release handle and pushing at the base.

If the windows must be opened from the outside, merely pound out the pins or unscrew them and remove the windows. In an emergency, break the windows if time is of the essence.

Seats: The padded seats on the bus are made of a vinyl plastic. Both the exterior and filler in these seats will give off toxic fumes when burning. Protective masks should be worn if you must board a bus to evacuate and put out a fire.

BUS STABILIZATION

Every vehicle involved in an accident, including buses, must be stabilized before any other procedures are initiated. As emergency crews arrive at a bus accident scene, they may find the vehicle situated in any one of several configurations. Most frequently, the bus is found resting on its six wheels on the level surface of the roadway. It may, however, be on an incline or be partially or completely rolled over.

For a bus still on its wheels, initial stabilization efforts should focus on blocking or chocking the wheels to prevent the vehicle from rolling forward or backward. Then, teams must establish three or four contact points between the structural frame areas of the bus and the ground. This involves building box cribs (a crisscross pattern using blocks of wood) with hardwood blocking at the front and rear of the vehicle. Typically, a box crib at the bottom of the A or B posts at the front of the bus and a matching pair of box cribs at the rear bumpers are sufficient stabilization. Tighten with wedges or step chocks and check frequently.

Unlike automobile stabilization, bus bumpers may be used to assist in stabilization because they are bolted directly to the structural steel-frame channels of the bus chassis. One unique aspect of this procedure is that it may be necessary for rescuers to use more than 70 blocks of wood to construct the box cribs needed to stabilize a 40-ft. bus.

Buses that have rolled over may be stabilized with wood blocking, manual or power rescue tool rams, air bags or air cushions, winch lines or two-vehicle cables, or chain and come-along (hand-operated crank) tools.

Bus Conveyance Stabilization Reminders

- Always chock the wheels in both directions.
- Apply box cribbing to four sides and tighten with wedges or step chocks—monitor frequently!
- Never reach or crawl under a motor coach conveyance that is not fully cribbed. If the bus is equipped with an air suspension system, the bus may drop at anytime after the accident.
- Identify preestablished jack points on transit buses or motor coaches.
- Buses are more stable than automobiles in most positions because of their box-type design.
- Buses should be vertically stabilized which requires a large amount of cribbing. This is important because even though buses have heavy-duty suspension systems, it is still necessary to restrict excessive vertical bouncing.
- Air bags may be used, but only in conjunction with box cribbing.
- School buses and most motor coaches and transit buses are basically square in design and remain fairly stable when they come to rest on their sides. Cribbing and wedging will generally provide stabilizing support in these instances.
- Hi-lift jacks are ideally suited for the vertical stabilization of buses but should not be solely relied on to support the entire weight of the bus.

BUS ACCESS

- Front door
  1. Mechanical arm, try manual, or break glass
  2. Pneumatic, emergency release, or main control on driver side
  3. Latched emergency door, operate latch
- Windshield—remove rubber gasket and remove windshield.
- Side windows
  1. Operate emergency mechanism
  2. Side glass, break or pry open
- Side panels
  1. Identify structure
  2. Cut panels
  3. Cut structure
  4. Cover and protect exposed hazards
- Roof
  1. Emergency hatch
     a. Operate with normal mechanism
     b. Pry
  2. Breach
     a. Remove interior materials
     b. Identify structure
     c. Cut sheet steel

d. Cut structure
e. Cover and protect exposed surfaces

OCCUPANT HANDLING AND REMOVAL

Rescuers should remember that occupant handling and removal is difficult in buses. Narrow aisles make it difficult to move. It is also difficult to use the door for removal of packaged patients. The exception is the rear door. Plan on how you will handle these incidents before they occur.

SUMMARY

Remember, always try before you pry! Whenever possible, open doors by operating them in the normal manner. Windshields, side windows, side panels, and roofs provide a means of occupant access. IFSTA's *Principles of Extrication* provides a step-by-step methodology for these access points.

For those of you who have never responded to an accident involving a bus, and may have the responsibility of riding the "front seat" to an incident, this poem is for you. Some words of wisdom to *live by* for EMS and rescue providers, especially if the bus conveyance happens to be on fire.

When you're dealing with buses and the on-going fusses, occurring both inside and out

Take a moment of time to survey the line that separates chaos from clout

Don't charge in there blind, rather, protect your behind, from the obvious elements of strife

When that propane explodes as the story is told, it will be a significant emotional event in your life!

Robert J. Schappert III
MFRI

REFERENCES

Carr, T. 1994. *Big rigs/buses training program.* Montgomery County, MD: Montgomery County Department of Fire/Rescue Services.

Moore, R. E. 1991. *Vehicle rescue and extrication.* St. Louis: Mosby Yearbook, Inc.

Wilson, J. Jr. 1994. *School bus rescue.* Columbus, MO: University of Missouri Extension Division.

Watson, L. M. 1990. *RTA-persons trapped.* Essex, England: Greenwave LTD.

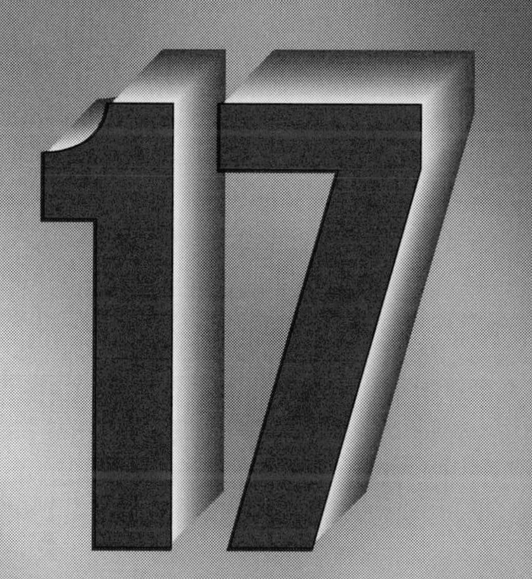

Skills Proficiency Evaluation: Passenger and Commercial Conveyance Rescue—Patient Packaging and Transfer

OBJECTIVE

The student will be able to demonstrate knowledge and understanding of the skills learned in sessions 1 through 6 and session 16, necessary to perform duties as a rescue technician, without assistance, to an accuracy of 70% and the satisfaction of the instructor. **This is a pass/fail point in the program.** Satisfactory completion permits the student to continue in the program.

OVERVIEW

Passenger and Commercial Conveyance Rescue—Patient Packaging and Transfer

- Commercial Conveyance Vehicles
- Passenger Conveyance Vehicles

ENABLING OBJECTIVES

17-1-1 Demonstrate patient removal from commercial conveyance vehicles.

17-1-2 Demonstrate patient removal from passenger conveyance vehicles.

Skill Station 1
Commercial Conveyance Vehicles (Team Evaluation)
Correctly demonstrate the following:

38. Establishing incident command
39. Circle check
40. Stabilizing on wheels
41. Constructing a safe platform to gain access
42. Stabilizing the patient
43. Packaging and removing the patient to the ground

(Evaluator will specify type of transfer device.)

Skill Station 2
Passenger Conveyance Vehicles (Team Evaluation)
Correctly demonstrate the following:

44. Establishing incident command
45. Circle check
46. Stabilizing on wheels
47. Constructing a safe platform to gain access
48. Stabilizing the patient
49. Packaging and removing the patient to the ground

(Evaluator will specify type of transfer device.)

REFERENCES

See Sessions 1-1 thru 6-1 and Session 16-1.

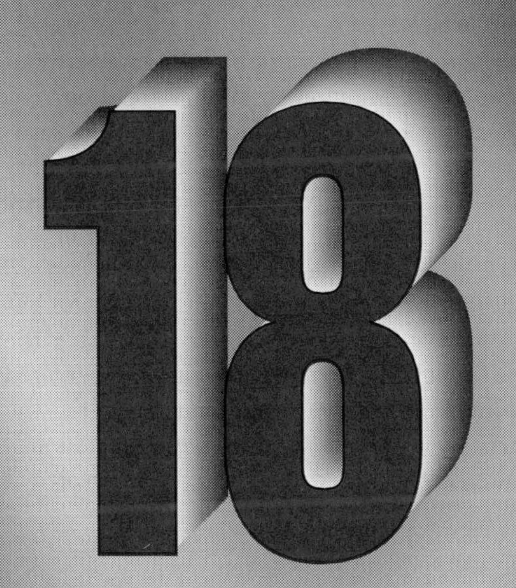

Compliance Issues of Confined-Space Rescue Operations: First Responder Awareness

OBJECTIVE

The student will be able to define and describe the hazards, equipment, and procedures for entering a confined space, from memory, without assistance, to an accuracy of 70% and the satisfaction of the instructor.

OVERVIEW

Compliance Issues of Confined-Space Rescue Operations: First Responder Awareness

- Confined Space Defined
- Hazards of Confined Space
- Accidents in Confined Space
- Monitoring Activities
- Entry Procedures
- Isolation Process
- Entry Permits
- Logistical Support Equipment

ENABLING OBJECTIVES

18-1-1 Define confined space.

18-1-2 Describe the hazards associated with confined-space rescue operations.

18-1-3 Identify the reasons why confined-space accidents occur.

18-1-4 Describe how to conduct monitoring activities in a confined-space rescue operation.

18-1-5 Describe the process associated with the entry phase of confined-space rescue operations.

18-1-6 Describe the isolation process of confined-space rescue.

18-1-7 Describe the information required for confined-space entry permits.

18-1-8 Describe the logistical support equipment required/necessary for conducting confined-space rescue operations.

INTRODUCTION

As a member of the first responding rescue unit to a confined-space incident, rescuers and officers alike must accept the fact that a potential killer awaits the unsuspecting or untrained good samaritan individual(s). This hidden killer can spell the end to your fire service career—and your life—if you don't heed the words of noted experts in this specialty field.

Under no circumstances, should any rescuer/officer responding to a confined-space incident enter a confined-space area to attempt victim rescue/extrication unless you have the proper equipment, supervision, and are trained in OSHA/MOSH laws.

There is absolutely no debate, discussion, or compromise when it comes to operational procedures/mandates relating to confined-space incidents. OSHA/MOSH inspectors will respond to your incident, observe your operations, and cite you for failing to be in compliance. The risk to human life and the likelihood of liability is too great to ignore. All rescuers/officers must be properly trained in entry/safety procedures to carry out these tasks. If you lack definitive operational training and certification, your role is strictly that of a first responder, which is:

- Conduct an initial size-up of the incident and report findings.
- Seal off the area and deny entry.
- Establish the hot zone and associated warm and cold zones.
- Stand by in a predetermined staging area until a specialty rescue unit or unit with expertise arrives to relieve you of responsibility.

Rationale

Any confined space is considered oxygen deficient until an appropriate assessment and monitoring process determines otherwise. This process must be conducted by a trained, competent person.

This student manual is written with one thing in mind: your safety and survival. If you choose to ignore its contents and freelance, you run the risk of losing your life and jeopardizing the lives of those you convince to follow you. Is this an acceptable consequence? If you allow emotions to overshadow sound judgement, reasoning, or objectivity, the end result will be catastrophic. Read on!

October 10, 1986: A utility company worker entered an underground vault to inspect a backflow prevention valve in a water line. The valve was located in an underground vault that was accessible through a 30-in. access hatch/cover. Upon entering the vault, the worker found the vault contained an excessive amount of water. Sometime later a pedestrian walking by the cover looked into the vault, and noticed the worker floating in the water.

Two other utility workers attempted a rescue without the use of protective equipment. Both were soon rendered unconscious. Two police officers, who were summoned to the scene, attempted a rescue of the utility workers without the use of protective equipment. They became disoriented and were assisted from the vault.

Paramedics, who were called to the scene, also entered the vault without protective equipment. They, too became disoriented and required assistance to leave the vault. When firefighters arrived at the site, they entered the vault using breathing apparatus and recovered the three workers. Two of the workers were pronounced dead at the site. The third recovered after being treated at a local hospital.

October 7, 1987: Boatyard workers opened the sealed hold of a leaky barge to locate the source of a leak. During the repairs, one of the workers climbed into the hold of the barge and became unconscious. Two co-workers, one of whom was the victim's uncle, attempted a rescue of the victim by entering the hold of the barge and also became unconscious. A fourth boatyard employee called the fire department for assistance. After calling for help, he was able to pull the second and third victims from the hold without entering the space himself.

A paramedic unit from the fire department arrived at the boatyard, and one of the paramedics attempted a rescue of the initial victim without breathing apparatus or evaluation of the conditions in the hold. The paramedic became unconscious. Additional units from the fire department arrived at the boatyard, and, while wearing breathing apparatus, fire department personnel removed the initial victim and the fallen paramedic from the hold of the barge.

The initial victim was pronounced dead at the boatyard by additional paramedics. The second and third boatyard workers who attempted the first rescue were transported by medevac helicopter to the trauma center and recovered fully. The paramedic was transported to the hospital for observation and released.

Both accidents described above stress the importance of identifying the presence of confined spaces and their associated hazards.

CONFINED SPACE DEFINED

According to OSHA's Standard for Permit—Required Confined Spaces for General Industry; Final Rule, 29 CFR 1910.146, a confined space:

1. Is large enough and so configured that an employee can bodily enter and perform assigned work.
2. Has limited or restricted means for entry or exit (e.g., tanks, vessels, silos, storage bins, hoppers, vaults, and pits).
3. Is not designed for continuous employee occupancy.

Permit-Required Confined Space (permit space)

A permit-required confined space has one or more of these characteristics:

1. Contains or has known potential to contain a hazardous atmosphere.
2. Contains material with potential for engulfing an entrant.
3. Has internal configuration such that an entrant could be trapped or asphyxiated by inwardly converging walls, or a floor that slopes downward and tapers to a smaller cross-section.
4. Contains any other recognized serious safety or health hazard.

Nonpermit Confined Space

A nonpermit confined space does not contain or, with respect to atmospheric hazards, have the potential to contain any hazard capable of causing death or serious physical harm.

In this space, it is unlikely that an Immediately Dangerous to Life or Health (IDLH) or engulfment hazard would be present, and all other serious hazards have been controlled.

HAZARDS OF CONFINED SPACES

Confined spaces can masquerade in many different shapes and sizes, and can be found in a multitude of configurations. Many are located below the ground, however, some are found above ground, inside buildings, on the roads, railways, and even on water.

There are many others that come to mind when using the definition. Confined spaces are found in all types of industries and occupations. Confined spaces have inherent hazards that can injure or take the lives of fire service personnel who are called to the scene of a confined space accident. It is important that all persons who enter confined spaces be able to recognize these hazards before entering the space. Not all the hazards are obvious but all are equally dangerous.

These hazards are divided into two groups: atmospheric and nonatmospheric hazards. OSHA has reviewed injury and fatality statistics and identified atmospheric hazards as the leading cause of deaths and injuries that occur in confined spaces. These hazards are explained in detail below.

Atmospheric Hazards

Atmospheric hazards result from:

- Oxygen deficient/oxygen enriched atmosphere
- Lack of ventilation
- Chemical reactions in confined spaces (rust)
- Oxygen is displaced by other gases. The most commonly encountered gases are carbon monoxide, carbon dioxide, hydrogen sulfide, and nitrogen sulfide.

The term "hazardous atmosphere" means an atmosphere that may expose employees to the risk of death, incapacitation, impairment of ability to self-rescue, serious injury, or acute illness from one or more of the following causes:

1. Flammable gas, vapor, or mist in excess of 10% of the lower explosive limit (LEL).
2. Airborne combustible dust at a concentration that exceeds its LEL (this concentration may be approximated as a condition in which the dust obscures vision at a distance of 5 ft. or 1.52 m or less).
3. Atmospheric oxygen concentration that is below 19.5% or above 23.5%.
4. Atmospheric concentration of any substance for

which a dose or a permissible exposure limit is published in Subpart G, Occupational Health and Environmental Control, or Subpart Z, Toxic and Hazardous Substances of Part 1910 and could result in employee exposure above the pertinent dose limit or permissible exposure limit (PEL). (An atmospheric concentration of any substance that is not capable of causing death, incapacitation, impairment of ability to self-rescue, injury, or acute illness due to its health effects is not covered by this provision.)

5. Any other atmospheric condition recognized as immediately dangerous to life or health (any condition that poses an immediate or delayed threat to life or that would interfere with an individual's ability to escape unaided from a permit space). For air contaminants for which OSHA has not determined a dose or PEL, other sources of information, such as Materials Safety Data Sheet (MSDS) that comply with the Hazard Communication Standard, 1910.1200 of this part, published information, and internal documents can provide guidance in establishing acceptable atmospheric conditions.

In order to account for their differing effects, atmospheric hazards are classified by OSHA into three categories: asphyxiation, flammable/explosive, and toxic. Rescuers must remember that some chemical substances present multiple atmospheric hazards.

Asphyxiation Atmospheres: Asphyxiation atmospheres are the leading cause of death in confined spaces. Asphyxia is a condition of severe impairment or suspension of respiratory function, resulting from interference with pulmonary respiration and cellular respiration. An asphyxiant is any substance which, by its action either on the body or in the breathing atmosphere, can cause asphyxia.

OSHA uses the term "asphyxiating atmosphere" when referring to an atmosphere that contains less than 19.5% oxygen. Oxygen levels under 19.5% are inadequate for an entrant's respiratory needs when performing physical work, even if the space contains no toxic materials. These are sometimes referred to as oxygen-deficient atmospheres.

Flammable/Explosive Atmospheres: Flammable or explosive atmospheres are defined as those presenting hazards to workers due to the presence of flammable vapors, dusts, or gases. Vapors or dusts can accumulate in confined spaces due to a lack of natural ventilation. Flammable or explosive vapors can originate from the flammable liquids stored in some types of confined spaces. Flammable vapors can be introduced into spaces as a result of underground storage tanks that develop leaks. Other sources of flammable vapors, such as methane or hydrogen sulfide, are the byproducts of biological processes. A confined space is considered to have flammable vapors when those vapors exceed 10% of their lower explosive limit (LEL) or if a combustible dust is present at a concentration greater than or equal to its LEL. A flammable atmosphere generally arises from enriched oxygen atmospheres (above 23.5%), vaporization of flammable liquids, byproducts of work, chemical reactions, concentrations of combustible dusts, and absorption of chemicals from inner surfaces of the confined space.

Toxic Atmospheres: This term refers to atmospheres containing gases, vapors, or fumes known to have poisonous physiological effects. The most common toxic gases are carbon monoxide and hydrogen sulfide.

Some toxic atmospheres may have severe harmful effects which may not manifest until years after the exposure, while others kill quickly. Some can produce both immediate and delayed health effects.

Toxic atmospheres may be caused by the manufacturing process, the product stored, or by the operation being performed in the confined space. This toxic effect is independent of the oxygen concentration, which may, in fact, be greater than 20%.

Atmospheric Hazards: Atmospheric hazards account for the majority of the injuries and fatalities that occur in confined spaces. Most could have been avoided if proper planning, training, and work procedures were in place and followed. Employers must develop written confined-space entry programs to allow compliance by workers. Fire departments need to establish standard operating procedures (SOPs) for operations involving confined space incidents. Such SOPs should include a provision for training firefighters in hazard recognition.

Nonatmospheric Hazards

1. Limited to ingress and egress because they are hard to get into and out of.

2. Excessive depths and heights encompass spaces below grade and elevated spaces above grade. This also takes into account horizontal traveling distances. If ladders are used, they require safety arrest lines for fall protection.

3. Poor visibility results from lack of lighting in a confined space area. Lights must be intrinsically safe, which means explosion-proof lights should be hand held/portable, not hard wired.

4. Lack of communications (radios must be intrinsically safe).
5. Wet and slippery surfaces.
6. Mechanical hazards, like failure to lock-out and tag-out compressors, pumps, etc., result in deaths and injuries from crushing, electrical shock, and other associated hazardous energy sources.
7. Harmful materials (aside from contents) include bacteria (especially in wastewater applications) and animal life (spiders, snakes, etc.).
8. Lack of specialized equipment
   - SCBA/SABA (Supplied Air Breathing Apparatus)
   - Body harnesses
   - Tripods/lifts
   - Atmospheric test equipment (meters)
   - Lock-out/tag-out devices

   Remember, firefighters' gear may be a hinderance if flammability is present, but you will still need hard hats, SCBA, gloves, hard sole safety shoes, and coveralls.
9. Lack of specialized training
   - Hazard awareness
   - Safe work procedures
   - Rescue techniques and procedures
10. Personal failures of workers results from medical conditions such as heart attacks, strokes, and injuries, and mental conditions involving claustrophobia and equilibrium.

    These conditions can be somewhat mitigated through medical surveillance of workers and proper training programs with practical evolutions.
11. Sharp and protruding objects and equipment
12. Environmental hazards
    - Dust
    - Heat, cold
    - Humidity
    - Noise, vibration
13. Unstable materials such as dry bulk materials that may engulf victims.
    - Death and injuries from asphyxiation
    - Death and injuries from crushing
    - Instability of crusted materials, silos, bins, etc.

ACCIDENTS IN CONFINED SPACE

In almost all accidents that involve confined spaces, victims fail to recognize and evaluate the hazards associated with working in such areas. In some cases, this is due to a lack of written entry procedures and training. In other cases, employees fail to follow safety procedures set forth by employers in confined-space entry programs. A high percentage of injuries and fatalities results from untrained, would-be rescuers attempting to rescue victims in confined spaces. Would-be rescuers account for more than 60% of all fatalities that occur in confined spaces. Statistics on confined-space accidents are not entirely accurate. Most accidents are only reported when they result in a fatality. The accidents that result in injuries (referred to as "close calls") are seldom reported.

Again, under no circumstances should firefighters or rescuers/officers, attempt or participate in any confined-space rescue operation unless they are trained operationally and functionally with a team wearing the appropriate personal protective equipment (PPE).

MONITORING ACTIVITIES

Prior to entering a confined space for a rescue, evaluate what hazards exist. Test the atmosphere for: adequate oxygen levels, presence and levels of flammable gases or vapors, and the presence and levels of toxic materials. Be sure to test the atmosphere at all levels of the space (top to bottom or end to end) due to differences in vapor pressures of gases. Test continuously during the entry phase due to the possibility of changing conditions within confined spaces.

Monitoring for Asphyxiation Hazards

Since the majority of all injuries and deaths in confined spaces are caused by atmospheric hazards, special attention must be given to monitoring the atmospheres in them. As discussed earlier, atmospheric hazards fall under three classifications: asphyxiating, flammable/explosive, and toxic. Because of a lack of natural air movement, dangerous gases can sometimes accumulate within confined spaces. Some atmospheric hazards can be classified into more than one class. Carbon monoxide, for example, is flammable but is also considered toxic, since it can contaminate air in a confined space leading to adverse health effects. The only way to ensure proper atmospheric conditions in confined spaces is by monitoring the atmosphere with a meter.

To properly use monitors and interpret the information they provide, one must have a basic understanding of matter and how matter can behave. There are three stages of matter: solids, liquids, and gases. As hazards, solids rarely pose any atmospheric hazards in confined spaces but can create serious engulfment hazards. Both liquids and gases can create atmospheric hazards in confined spaces. Some gases will sink to the low areas of confined spaces and others will rise to the high areas.

Evaluate Vapor Density: The value by which we can predict where a vapor will collect is called the *vapor density*. Vapor density is derived by comparing equal amounts of a vapor to an equal amount of air at the same temperature and pressure. The vapor density of air is given a value of one. If the vapor density of a vapor is greater than one, then the vapor is heavier than air and will collect in the low areas of a confined space. If the vapor density of a vapor is less than one, then the vapor is lighter than air and will collect in the high areas of a confined space. Liquids can also produce vapors that can collect in confined spaces.

Evaluate Boiling Point: The temperature at which a liquid will give off vapors is called its *boiling point*. Liquids boil when their vapor pressures are greater than the atmospheric pressure. Boiling point and vapor pressure are inversely proportional. That is, when a liquid has a low boiling point, it has a high vapor pressure.

Monitor for Oxygen Levels: When monitoring confined spaces, the first hazardous condition to check for is an adequate level of oxygen in the space. As you know, our bodies need oxygen to survive. Our bodies get that needed oxygen from the air we breathe. Normal air is a mixture of 79% nitrogen and 21% oxygen. Oxygen levels can change in confined spaces due to a variety of reasons. Some gases can force air from confined spaces. When this is done intentionally to lessen rusting inside reactor vessels, it is referred to as "padding a space." Some reactor vessels are purged with gases such as nitrogen to cleanse them of harmful byproducts after reactions occur. These purgings can remove air from the spaces also. Some work performed in confined spaces such as welding or brazing can alter the oxygen level in the air. It does not take a great change in the oxygen level in air to affect human performance.

Because slight changes in the oxygen level cause behavioral changes, a person can be overcome in an oxygen-deficient atmosphere and not be able to assist himself/herself. An atmosphere is considered to be oxygen deficient when the percentage of oxygen falls below 19.5%. The only safe and accurate method to measure oxygen content of a confined space is with a monitor. Most monitors that sense/measure oxygen levels will alarm at 19.5% oxygen in air. In addition to oxygen deficiency, a confined space can become oxygen enriched. In this condition, the oxygen level exceeds 23.5%. Most monitors will also alarm when atmospheric conditions become oxygen enriched.

Monitoring for Flammable/Explosive Hazards

The next hazard to monitor for is the presence of flammable vapors. Flammable vapors can accumulate in confined space for many reasons. Some flammable liquids stored in confined spaces will give off flammable vapors. Some types of work performed in confined spaces, like painting, can cause flammable vapors to accumulate. Some chemical reactions that occur in reactor vessels will release flammable vapors into those confined spaces. To understand the potential for injury from flammable vapors, you must have an understanding of some basic terms that explain how flammable liquids and gases behave. To begin with, most flammable liquids will only burn in their vapor state.

The temperature at which a flammable liquid will give off enough vapors to develop a mixture with air that will burn is called the *flash point*. There are limits to the concentrations of vapors that will burn. Each flammable vapor has its limits, both low and high. The low point is called the LEL and the vapors with concentrations below the LEL are said to be too lean to burn. The high point is called the upper explosive limit (UEL) and vapors with concentrations above the UEL are said to be too rich to burn. The concentrations between the LEL and UEL are in the flammable range and will burn. Monitors that measure flammable vapors register in the percent of the LEL (e.g., a percentage of a percentage). Some monitors used in the public utilities measure the actual concentration of gas in air. The only accurate method to measure the levels of flammable vapors is with a monitor. Most monitors used in confined-space entry are set to alarm at 10% of the LEL. When flammable vapor concentrations exceed this amount, no entry should be made into the confined space until the concentration has been lowered by ventilation or some other means.

Monitoring for Toxic Hazards

The last hazard class to monitor for in confined spaces is the presence of toxic substances. The term *toxic substances* refers to an extensive list of materials that have the potential to cause adverse health effects in individuals exposed to them. Exposure can be by inhalation, ingestion, injection, or absorption. Exposure to some materials can produce instantaneous health effects and other materials can cause delayed health effects. There are many factors that determine how toxic a material is. These include the concentration of the material, the route of exposure, the amount of time a person was exposed, and the health condition of the person exposed.

Exposure Limits: The National Institute for Occupational Safety and Health (NIOSH) has researched and formulated exposure limits for almost 400 different potentially dangerous substances. OSHA regulates these limits. Other agencies, such as the American Conference of Governmental Industrial Hygienists (ACGIH), publish exposure limits supported by their research. These values are product-specific and rely on proper identification and monitoring of the substance. There are three values used by these agencies to describe their recommended safe levels of exposure:

1. Threshold Limit Value (TLV)
2. Permissible Exposure Limit (PEL)
3. Immediately Dangerous to Life or Health (IDLH)

There are TLVs that pertain to 40-hour work weeks with 8-hour days (TLV—time-weighted average), 15-minute exposures (TLV—short-term exposure limits), and absolute limits for exposures (TLV—ceiling). PEL refers to values of exposure as determined by OSHA in federal law. IDLH levels are maximum levels that a person could escape from within 30 minutes, should their respiratory protection fail, without impairing the escape or causing irreversible health effects.

Use of Meters

There are a variety of meters available for monitoring the atmospheres in confined spaces. There are meters available for monitoring levels of all confined-space atmospheric hazards. Some meters can monitor more than one hazard class such as flammable vapors and oxygen concentrations, while some meters can only monitor one specific hazard class. Some meters use pumps to draw samples into the meter, while some use diffusion to sample the atmosphere. Meters can have a myriad of accessories and options as diverse as those found on the showroom of a car dealership. Because of the diversity of meters from manufacturer to manufacturer, it is not practical for this text to discuss operations of even a small portion. It is important for the firefighter to understand the principles of operation of the specific meter that his/her department uses.

Meters used to monitor confined spaces should be able to monitoring flammable vapors and oxygen concentrations simultaneously. They should be capable of calibration in the field by the user. They should be intrinsically safe and capable of operating for at least eight hours on a single battery charge. Meters should be able to sample a confined space from outside the space. They meters should be able to have the alarm setpoint set in the field by the user. Some meters have latching alarms. When a concentration of gas exceeds the alarm setpoint and the alarm sounds, the alarm will continue to sound, even if the concentration of gas reaches a safe level, until the alarm is reset manually.

Regardless of the manufacturer or style of meter, there are some basic instructions and precautions for using meters to monitor the atmospheres of confined spaces.

1. Gases can have different vapor densities and will be found at different levels in a confined space. This means it is important to slowly monitor all levels of a confined space prior to entry.
2. If a meter has a sample pump, care must be used to prevent liquids from being drawn into the meter if the probe is lowered into the liquid.
3. Meters are sensitive instruments that require care, attention, and periodic maintenance. Make sure that the batteries are charged.
4. Know how the instrument operates and how the reading is obtained. Use the proper type of instrument for the tests required, and understand that unit's particular limitations.

ENTRY PROCEDURES

When preparing to enter into confined spaces, certain procedures must be followed to ensure the safety of personnel. Most of these procedures are done to eliminate or detect the presence of hazards already discussed. Entry into confined spaces means the intentional passing into a confined space for purposes of conducting work. You are considered to have entered into a space as soon as any part of your body has broken the plane of an opening into a confined space. Procedures for safely entering confined spaces requires the use of a program outlining entry preparation and that employees be aware of hazards that exist in confined spaces.

Prior to entry, the confined space must be monitored. Since most injuries and fatalities associated with confined spaces are a result of atmospheric hazards, it is important to ensure the space has an atmosphere with a sufficient oxygen level, free of flammable vapors, and free of toxic

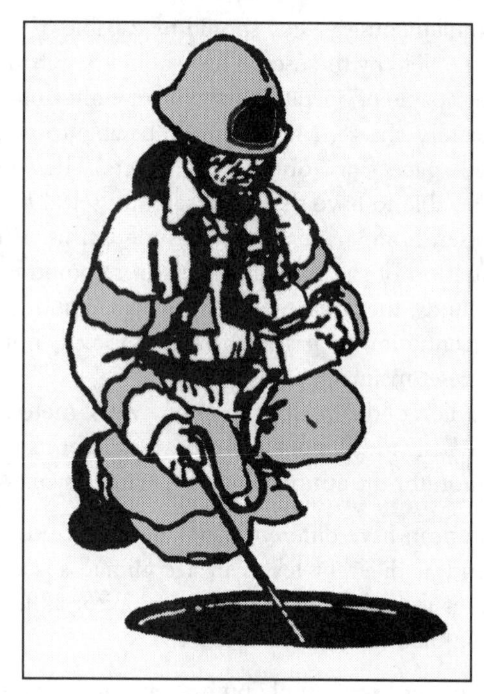

Figure 18–1 Sampling process.

vapors. The only positive method of ensuring a suitable atmosphere for entry is with the use of a monitor. Monitoring of the space must be done before entry, at all levels, and continuously during entry procedures. Proper attention must be given to the monitoring process. Too many times a monitor is placed in service only to be forgotten until conditions are severe enough to affect entry personnel. Figure 18–1 depicts the sampling process.

ISOLATION PROCESS

Whenever entering a confined space, efforts must be made to ensure that the space is and will remain free of any products that could be introduced while persons are in the space. Isolation means the separation of a permit space from unwanted forms of energy which could pose a serious hazard to permit space entrants. Isolation is usually accomplished by emptying the space, blanking or blinding, removal or misalignment of pipe sections or spool spaces, double block and bleed, or lock-out/tag-out.

Emptying the Space

The first and simplest means is to empty the space of its contents. Care must be exercised in emptying a space. Considerations should include where the contents will go where emptied and what effect moving the product will have on a victim in the space. Sometimes confined spaces can be off-loaded into other containers.

Blanking or Blinding

Blanking or blinding means the absolute closure of a pipeline or duct, by fastening across its bore a solid plate or cap which completely covers the bore; which extends at least to the outer edge of the flange at which it attaches; and which is capable of withstanding the maximum upstream pressure. Simply stated, for clarification purposes, blanking involves use of an impervious "blank" placed between a flange on the upstream line that feeds product to the space. If possible, the downstream side of the flange should be left unfastened to prevent any leakage through the blank from entering the space.

Line Breaking

Line breaking means the intentional opening of a pipe, line, or duct that is or has been carrying flammable, corrosive, or toxic material, an inert gas, or any fluid at a pressure or temperature capable of causing injury.

Double Block and Bleed

Double block and bleed means the closure of a line, duct, or pipe by locking and tagging a drain or vent which is open to the atmosphere in the line between two locked/closed valves. It involves the shutting down of two valves feeding product into the space and opening a valve between the two shut valves that would allow any leakage from the first valve from contacting the second valve. The open valve or "bleed" should be the same diameter as the feed line to allow for the maximum flow of product should a complete failure of the first valve occur. Figure 18–2 depicts the blanking process.

Electrical/Mechanical Lock-out and Tag-out

Some confined spaces exist solely to house mechanical/electrical devices such as agitators, pumps, fans, meters, and compressors.

Some of these devices activate automatically in response to changes in flows, levels, and pressures. They will activate independently of the presence of workers in confined spaces. It is important these devices be isolated. Always lock out their correct power sources with a lock-out device. The most ideal situation is when each worker has an individual lock, each keyed differently, and carries the key into the space with him/her. This will allow each person entering the confined space to apply a lock to the lock-out. This prevents unlocking of the power source while the worker is in the space. Once a lock-out is applied, it is important that the lock-out be tagged. The tag supplies information that worker's lives can be endan-

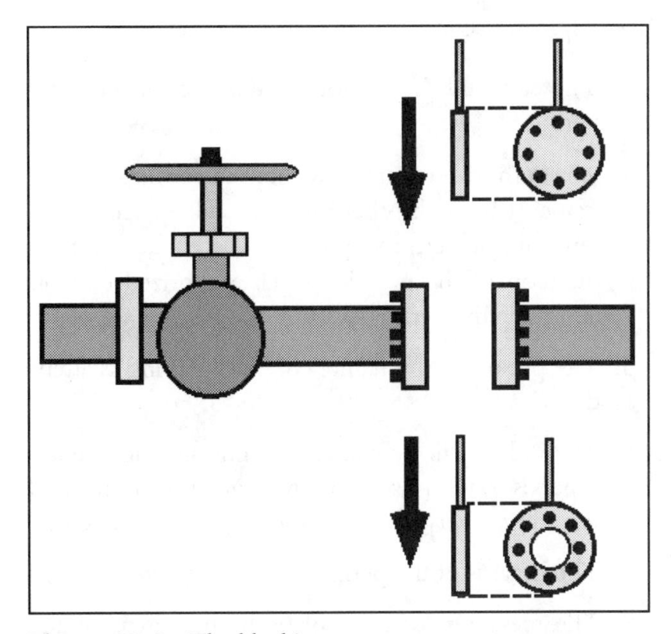

Figure 18–2 The blanking process.

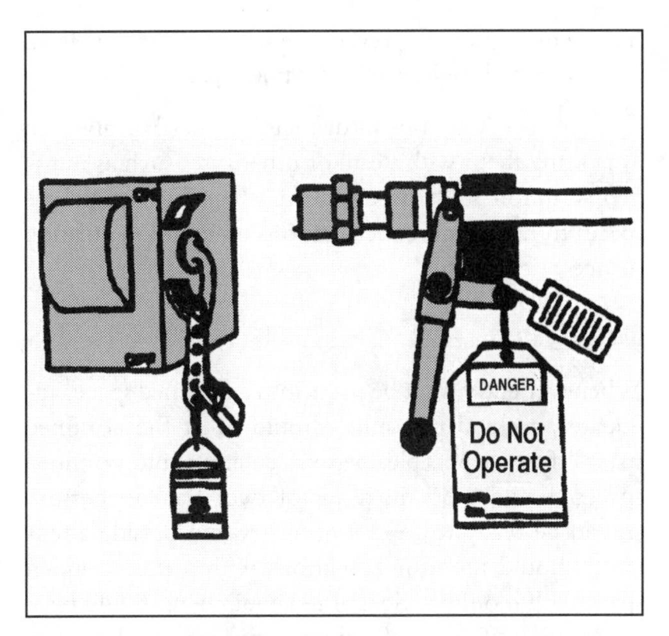

Figure 18–3 OSHA's regulation for lock-out/tag-out.

gered if the equipment is energized while workers are still in the space. Figure 18–3 depicts OSHA's 29CFR 1910.147 regulation required for the lock-out/tag-out process.

Secure Covers

During the isolation process it is important to remember to secure all covers. Some confined spaces have hinged covers or doors that could close, trapping workers in confined spaces. It is important to prevent these covers from closing.

Ventilation Process

When the atmospheric conditions in a confined space do not meet the limits for oxygen, flammability, and toxic vapors previously discussed, the confined space must be ventilated to bring the atmosphere into those limits. Since natural ventilation does not occur in confined spaces, ventilation exchanges the air in the space with fresh air within the limits of 19.5% oxygen, less than 10% of the LEL, and within or less than the permissible exposure limits of toxic materials. Figure 18–4 depicts this ventilation process. When using positive pressure ventilation (PPV) ventilation, always use electrically powered devices. Gasoline blowers introduce unacceptable levels of carbon monoxide into the confined space creating an unsafe atmosphere.

The air flow should be introduced into the space and the blower tube should be at the level at which persons will be working while in the space. When the fan is directed to exhaust air from the space, a slight vacuum is created that can draw other contaminants into the space. By directing the air flow into the space, a positive pressure is created and any contaminants are diluted by the addition of the fresh air. A ventilation fan should be allowed to operate long enough to exchange the air content of a space several times. If necessary, the fan should be left to operate during the entry into the confined space.

Note: the fan intake is positioned upwind of the man-

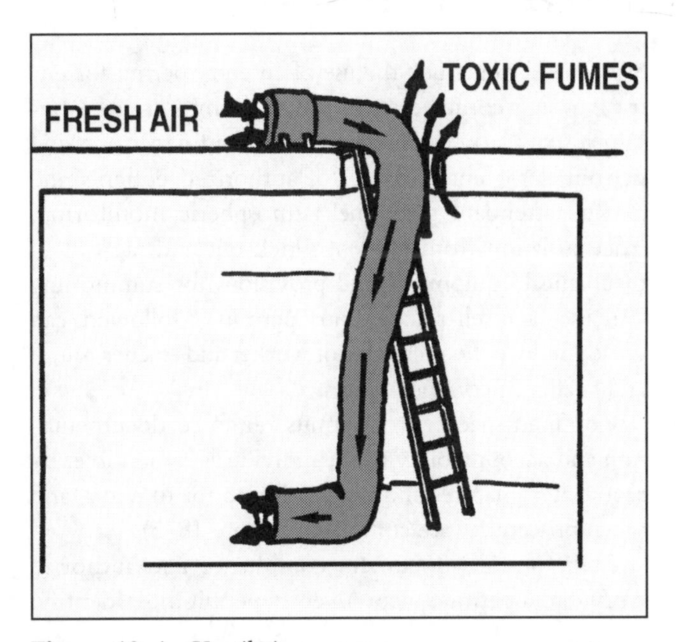

Figure 18–4 Ventilation process.

hole. This is done to prevent the exhausted vapors from being reintroduced into the confined space.

Some spaces must be made inert by special means such as purging them with steam or other gases such as nitrogen. Caution must be exercised when returning these spaces to natural air concentrations by use of ventilation devices.

Buddy System

Whenever entry must be made into a confined space, adequately trained personnel should be at the confined space. If at all possible, persons entering into confined spaces should work in teams of two. Backup persons should be ready to assist if necessary and outside attendants should monitor conditions within the confined space with monitors. Specialized equipment should be at the location of the confined space and persons should be trained in its use. Persons should be trained in cardiopulmonary resuscitation and have some means of summoning assistance if necessary.

Fire departments need to develop written SOPs to handle accidents involving confined spaces. Emergency services providers fail to recognize the hazards associated with confined spaces and rush into dangerous situations, often with disastrous results. Remember, 60% of all fatalities associated with confined spaces are the result of would-be rescuers (both co-workers and emergency services personnel).

ENTRY PERMITS

SOPs need to include the use of an entry permit for entry into any confined space. Entry permits are step-by-step instructions for preparing the confined space and personnel for entry, names of authorized entrants and backup attendant personnel, atmospheric monitoring, space isolation from contents, lock-out and tag-out of mechanical equipment, and provisions for summoning assistance and self-rescue. Entry permits, if followed, can greatly reduce the incidence of worker and rescuer injury and fatality in confined spaces.

Confined-space entry permits reinforce documentation and accountability to the individuals responsible, by requiring signatures and notifications prior to entry, and when procedures are completed (Figure 18–5).

Entry permits document compliance and authorize entry into a permit space. An entry permit must identify:

1. The permit space to be entered.
2. The purpose of entry.
3. The date and the authorized duration of the entry permit.
4. The authorized entrants within the permit space, by name or by such other means as will enable the attendant to determine quickly and accurately, for the duration of the permit, which authorized entrants are inside the permit space.
5. The personnel, by name, currently serving as attendants.
6. The individual, by name, currently serving as entry supervisor, with a space for the signature or initials of the entry supervisor who originally authorized entry.
7. The hazards of the permit space to be entered.
8. The measures used to isolate the permit space and to eliminate or control permit-space hazards before entry.
9. The acceptable entry condition.
10. The results of initial and periodic tests performed, accompanied by the names or initials of the testers, and an indication of when the tests were performed.
11. The rescue and emergency services that can be summoned and the means for summoning those services.
12. The communication procedure used by authorized entrants and attendants to maintain contact during the entry.
13. Equipment, such as PPE, testing equipment, communication equipment, alarm systems, and rescue equipment, to be provided for compliance with this section.
14. Any other information whose inclusion is necessary, given the circumstances of the particular confined space, in order to ensure employee safety.
15. Any additional permits, such as hot work, that have been issued to authorize work in the permit space.

LOGISTICAL SUPPORT EQUIPMENT

Respiratory Protection

A good and prudent rule of thumb is to never enter a confined space unless you are wearing positive pressure breathing apparatus (SCBA) or supplied air breathing apparatus (SABA). Keep in mind that some spaces may, in

CONFINED-SPACE ENTRY PERMIT

LOCATION OF SPACE ____________________

DESCRIPTION OF SPACE ____________________

PURPOSE OF ENTRY ____________________

PERSON IN CHARGE ____________________ PHONE ____________

AUTHORIZED ENTRANTS ____________________
____
____

WORK TO BE PERFORMED:
____
____

ATTENDANT(S) ____________________

TEST TO BE TAKEN	PEL	YES/NO	TIME	TIME	TIME	TIME	TIME	TIME
% OF OXYGEN	19.5%-23.5%							
% OF LEL	ANY % OVER 10							

PERSON PERFORMING TESTS ____________________

INSTRUMENTS USED	TYPE	IDS#	CALIBRATION BY AND DATE

SPECIAL REQUIREMENTS: CHECK IF REQUIRED TO BE USED/PERFORMED

LOCKOUT/DE-ENERGIZE______	HARNESSES________	LIGHTING________
LINES BROKEN, CAPPED, BLANKED______	LIFELINES________	PROTECTIVE CLOTHING______
PURGE, FLUSH AND VENT________	LIFTING DEVICE______	FIRE EXTINGUISHERS_______
VENTILATION__________	RESPIRATORS_______	OTHER, SEE REMARKS_______

REMARKS
____
____
____

ISSUED BY (PRINT)
____________________ SIGNATURE ____________________

IN CASE OF EMERGENCY CONTACT ____________________ PHONE ____________________ (DAY)
____________________ (EVE)

Figure 18–5 Confined-space entry permit.

fact, be safe, but some monitoring devices may not be functioning properly. Always opt for safety.

Harnesses

All persons entering confined spaces must wear a life safety harness and a retrieval line. Life safety harnesses are constructed in accordance with two different safety standards. These standards are the National Fire Protection Association (NFPA) 1983, *Standard on Fire Service Life Safety Rope, Harnesses, and Hardware,* and the American National Standards Institute (ANSI) A10.14, *Requirement for Safety Belts, Harnesses, Lanyards, Lifelines, and Drop Lines for Construction and Industrial Use.* Harnesses should be constructed from continuous filament nylon fibers and be adjustable over a variety of individual sizes.

The NFPA standard has three classifications and the ANSI standard has four classes. The NFPA classes are shown here.

Class I:

1. Seat-style harness for emergency escape or one-person loads
2. Not for rescue

Class II: Seat-style harness for rescue and other two-person loads

Class III:

1. Full-body harness for rescue and other two-person loads where inverting may occur
2. One or more parts
3. Only effective harness for victims/patients. Requires no skill/knowledge on patient's part once in harness

All harnesses should be inspected prior to use. They should be stored in a dry, cool area out of direct sunlight.

Mechanical Advantage Systems

When recovering a victim of a confined-space accident from a vertical space, the rescuers require some type of mechanical advantage (MA) system and an elevated anchor point from which to apply the MA to lift the victim. When selecting an MA system to rescue victims of confined-space accidents, remember that time is a critical element in the successful rescue. If your system can only be used to lift, not lower, then a separate system must be set up if the rescuers must be lowered into the confined space.

If the system can apply MA to both lift and lower, then precious time can be saved in the recovery of the victim. There are commercially available winches, hoists, and tripods that can be used to recover victims, and you have been taught several ways of applying MA to rope systems such as the Z-rig and the piggyback systems. Block-and-tackle systems can also be used to apply MA.

Vertical Lowering: An elevated anchor point must be selected to anchor whatever MA system is selected when recovering a victim in a vertical confined space. Anchor points in interior spaces such as tanks and pits can sometimes be found in the ceilings of buildings. Elevated anchor points can be constructed from ground ladders such as the ladder gin and the ladder sheerlegs.

Tripods are also commercially available for confined-space entry. There are several brands of tripods on the commercial market today. When selecting a tripod for rescue and recovery use, look for a tripod that is lightweight, adjustable over a variety of heights, has multiple points for anchoring MA systems, has nonslip footing on the legs, and whose legs will lock in the open position. When using a tripod, remember the strongest point of a triangle is where two of the sides meet. Likewise, the strongest points in a tripod are the legs. When using a tripod, for maximum stability, apply the MA in line with one of the legs of the tripod. Figure 18–6 depicts removing a victim using a hand winch attached to one of the legs of the tripod. Figure 18–7 depicts removing a victim using an MA attached to the center of the tripod.

Whenever lifting a victim where the potential for falls exists, a second lifeline should be attached to the victim. This belay line would hold the victim from falling should the MA system fail. This belay line should be attached to a suitable anchor and belay device and kept free of slack in case of a fall.

When recovering victims from confined spaces, it is sometimes necessary to reduce the dimensions of the victim by raising his/her arms above the head. If the victim is suspected to have suffered a spinal injury, care must be exercised not to worsen the condition by moving the victim's limbs. In a vertical confined space, wristlets can be used to raise the victim's arms. Attach a separate line, such as a tag line or utility line, to the wristlets to lift the victim. The wristlets can be used to maneuver the victim from a horizontal confined space using the SKED stretcher. The victim's arms can be raised over his/her head while being placed in the SKED to reduce the victim's dimensions.

DEFINITIONS

Acceptable environmental conditions: Confined-space workplace conditions in which uncontrolled haz-

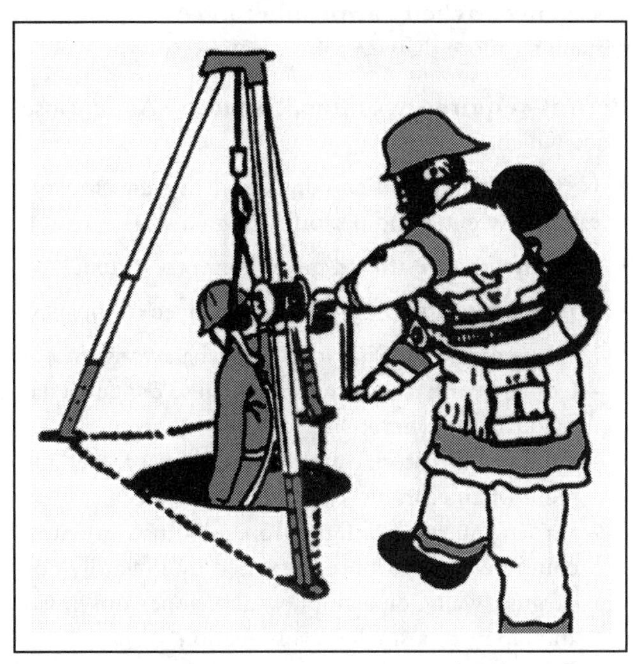

Figure 18–6 Removing a victim using a hand winch attached to one leg of the tripod

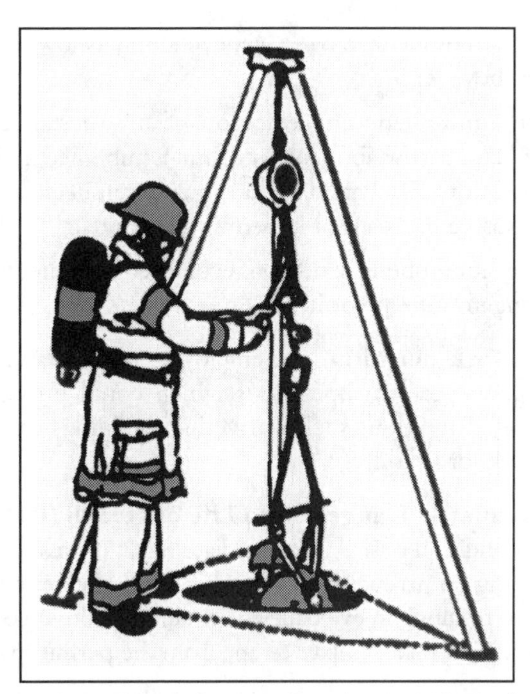

Figure 18–7 Removing a victim using an MA attached to tripod's center

ardous atmospheres are not present, and which include any additional environmental criteria the employer may require for employee entry into a permit-required confined space.

Attendant: An individual stationed outside the permit-required confined space who is trained as required by the OSHA standard and who monitors the authorized entrants inside the permit-required confined space. An attendant cannot monitor more entrants or permit spaces than the entry permit specifically authorizes.

Authorized entrant: An employee who is authorized by the employer to enter a permit-required confined space.

Blanking or blinding: The absolute closure of a pipe, line, or duct, by fastening across its bore a solid plate or "cap" which completely covers the bore; which extends at least to the outer edge of the flange at which it is attached; and which is capable of withstanding the maximum upstream pressure.

Double block and bleed: The closure of a line, duct, or pipe by locking and tagging a drain or vent which is open to the atmosphere in the line between two locked/closed valves.

Emergency: Any occurrence or event(s) internal or external to the confined space which could endanger entrants.

Engulfment: The surrounding and effective capture of a person by a liquid or finely divided solid substance.

Entry: The act by which a person intentionally passes through an opening into a permit-required confined space, and includes ensuing work activities in that space. The entrant is considered to have body entered as soon as any part of the entrant's body breaks the plane of an opening into the space.

Entry permit: The written or printed document established by the employer, the content of which is based on the employer's hazard identification and evaluation for that confined space, and is the instrument by which the employer authorizes employees to enter that permit-required confined space.

Entry permit system: The employer's written procedures for preparing and issuing permits for entry and returning the permit space to service following termination of entry, and designates by name or title the individuals who may authorize entry.

Hazardous atmosphere: An atmosphere exposing employees to a risk of death, incapacitation, injury, or acute illness from one or more of the following causes:

- A flammable gas, vapor, or mist in excess of 10% of its lower explosive limit.
- An airborne combustible dust at a concentration that obscures vision at a distance of 5 ft. or less.

- An atmospheric oxygen concentration below 19.5% or above 23.5%.
- An atmospheric concentration of any substance for which a permissible exposure limit is published in Subpart Z of CFR Part 1910 and could result in employee exposure in excess of its permissible limit(s).
- Any atmospheric condition recognized as immediately dangerous to life or health.

Hot work permit: The employer's written authorization to perform operations which could provide a source of ignition, such as riveting, welding, cutting, burning, or heating.

Immediately Dangerous to Life or Health (IDLH): Any condition posing an immediate threat or loss of life; resulting in irreversible or immediate severe health effects; resulting in eye damage, irritation or other conditions which could impair escape from the permit space.

Immediate-severe health effects: Any acute clinical sign(s) of a serious, exposure-related reaction manifested within 72 hours after exposure.

Inerting: Rendering the atmosphere of a permit space nonflammable, nonexplosive, or otherwise chemically nonreactive by such means as displacing or diluting the original atmosphere with steam or a gas that is nonreactive with respect to that space.

In-plant rescue team: A group of two or more employees designated and trained to perform rescues in permit spaces in their plant.

Isolation: The separation of a permit space from unwanted forms of energy which could be a serious hazard to permit space entrants.

Line breaking: The intentional opening of a pipe, line, or duct that is, or has been, carrying flammable, corrosive, or toxic material, an inert gas, or any fluid at a pressure or temperature capable of causing injury.

Low-hazard permit space: A permit space where there is an extremely low likelihood that an IDLH or engulfment hazard could be present, and where all other serious hazards have been controlled.

Not-permitted condition: Any condition or set of conditions whose hazard potential exceeds the limits stated in the entry permit.

Oxygen-deficient atmosphere: An atmosphere containing less than 19.5% oxygen by volume.

Oxygen-enriched atmosphere: An atmosphere containing more than 23.5% oxygen by volume.

Permit-required confined space: An enclosed space which:

- Is large enough and so configured that an employee can bodily enter and perform assigned work.
- Has limited or restricted means for entry or exit.
- Is not designed for continuous employee occupancy.
- Has one or more of the following characteristics:
  - Contains or has a known potential to contain a hazardous atmosphere.
  - Contains a material with the potential for engulfment of an entrant.
  - Has an internal configuration such that an entrant could be trapped or asphyxiated by inwardly converging walls, or a floor which slopes downward and tapers to a smaller cross-section.
  - Contains any other recognized serious safety or health hazard.

Permit-required confined space program: The employer's program for preventing unauthorized employee entry and for ensuring safe entry into and work within permit spaces by authorized employees.

Retrieval line: A line or rope secured at one end to the worker by a chest-waist or full-body harness, or wristlets, and with its other end secured to either a lifting device or to an anchor point located outside the entry portal.

REFERENCES

Maryland Fire and Rescue Institute. 1991. *Rescue specialist.* Berwyn Heights, MD: MFRI.

Maryland Fire and Rescue Institute, Special Programs Section. 1996. *Confined space program.* Berwyn Heights, MD: MFRI.

NFPA 1983: *Standard on Fire Service Life Safety Rope and System Components,* 1995 ed., American National Standards Institute, National Fire Codes, Vol. 9, Rev. 11/96.

OSHA 29–Labor, Code of Federal Regulation: Permit-Required Confined Spaces, 1910.146; The Control of Hazardous Energy (Lock-out/Tag-out), 1910.147. Published by The Office of the Federal Register, National Archives and Records Administration, as a special edition of the Federal Register. 1997. Washington, DC: US Government Printing Office.

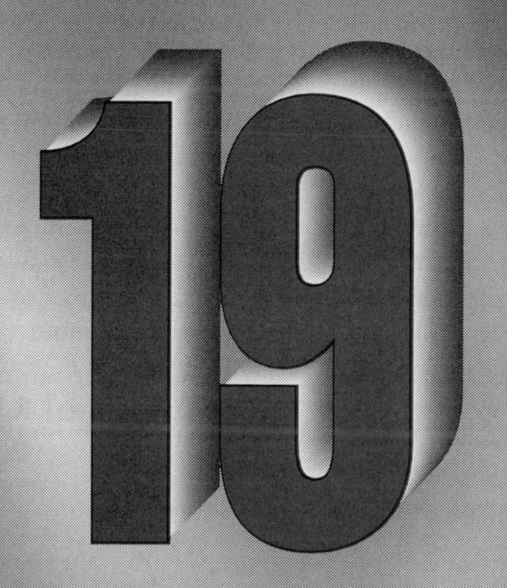

Compliance Issues of Trench/Excavation Rescue Operations: First Responder Awareness

OBJECTIVE

The student will be able to identify and describe the awareness issues and related safety risks inherent to trench-/excavation-type rescue incidents, from memory, without assistance, to an accuracy of 70% and the satisfaction of the instructor.

OVERVIEW

Compliance Issues of Trench/Excavation Rescue Operations: First Responder Awareness

- Trench/Excavation Defined
- Specialized Training Requirements
- Trench/Excavation Accidents
- Soil Facts to Consider
- Causative Factors
- Trench/Excavation Components
- Trench/Excavation Collapses
- First Responder Policies
- Specialized Rescue Equipment
- Code of Maryland Regulations (COMAR)/OSHA Review

ENABLING OBJECTIVES

19-1-1 Define the differences between trench- and excavation-type incidents.

19-1-2 Identify and describe the need for specialized training relating to trench/excavation incidents.

19-1-3 Identify and describe the operational perspectives relating to trench/excavation accidents.

19-1-4 Identify and describe the factors relating to soil characteristics.

19-1-5 Identify and describe the causative factors associated with trench/excavation accidents.

19-1-6 Identify and describe the trench/excavation components and the shoring that would be used to stabilize the trench.

19-1-7 Identify and describe the types of trench/excavation collapses.

19-1-8 Identify and describe the policies of a first responder when confronting a trench/excavation accident.

19-1-9 Identify and describe the specialized rescue equipment and procedures necessary to address a trench/excavation accident.

19-1-10 Define the current COMAR/OSHA laws that are applicable to trench/excavation accidents.

INTRODUCTION

This session is designed to illustrate and depict the awareness issues confronting a trench rescue incident. It incorporates descriptions of trench rescue equipment with a "chalk talk" approach to entering a trench/excavation scenario. Samples of jurisdictional standard operating procedures (SOPs) for first responders are provided for your review and consideration. This session is *not* intended or designed to train operational-level providers. The training you receive in additional modular training will provide the means to accomplish this objective.

This session is provided as a "wake-up" call for basic rescue providers and officers because the rules of engagement have drastically changed as they relate to trench/excavation accidents. Sand and dirt—our friends during adolescent years—is now the enemy. The depth and width of holes and the potent force of mother nature have sharply altered the way in which we do business. Excavation sites pose serious dangers to would-be rescues because of the unknown variables that lie in waiting. Rescuers must now use a systematic and approved methodology in dealing with trench/excavation scenarios.

For a first responder awareness session, the enabling objectives are very aggressive. In fact, they exceed what may be considered a standard overview. This is deliberate in order to make a case for seeking additional training in this specialized area. You will see that it contains a wealth of reference information, yet at the same time sends the message that trench rescue incidents can quickly overwhelm you if allowed to go unsupervised in strict compliance with current OSHA standards.

The bottom line is that when operating on a trench/excavation accident, you must have your act together. These accidents do not allow, nor make provisions for, shortcutting and freelancing. As with confined-space rescue, trench accidents are ready-made and freshly dug grave sites for untrained and unqualified rescue personnel. The end result of noncompliance is serious injury, death, liability for incident participants, and criminal prosecution/penalties. Our approach to these incidents is changing because of state and federal mandates. Traditionally, the fire service has been reluctant at times to accept this regulatory process. The alternative, unfortunately, may well be your demise. The philosophy associated with trench/excavation rescue is very simple. When in doubt, stay out!

TRENCH/EXCAVATION DEFINED

A *trench* is defined as: an excavation that is deeper than it is wide.

An *excavation* is defined as: an opening in the ground from a digging effort.

SPECIALIZED TRAINING REQUIREMENTS

The collapse forces of a trench are tremendous. Because of these forces, specialized training is necessary.

- Shear wall collapse speed = 45 mph.
- 1 cubic foot of soil = 100 lbs.
- Clay can weigh 140 lbs., dry sand as little as 65 lbs.
- 24 in. soil on chest = 750 lbs. to 1,000 lbs.
- 18 in. soil covering body = 1,000 lbs. to 3,000 lbs.

Respiratory distress, crush injury, and total body impact relate to victim injuries and severity. In the past, an untrained rescuer's first inclination is to jump in the trench on arrival. This untrained rescuer then becomes part of the incident management problem. Inadequate shoring also poses serious life safety hazards to victims and rescuers.

Increased Potential for Trench/Excavation Rescuers

Underground utilities
Thousands of open trenches throughout the state
Lack of contractor training
Lack of enforcement
More complex underground engineering
Amount of construction on-going
Home improvement projects
Toxic atmospheres in trench

TRENCH/EXCAVATION ACCIDENTS

Question: What depth/width do most incidents occur?

Response: Between six ft. to eight ft. deep, less than six ft. wide.

Question: Most incidents occur in bad weather.

Response: **False.** Most incidents occur in good weather. Crews are more careful during bad weather.

Question: Clay is the least dangerous soil type.

Response: **False.** Most fatal trench accidents occur in clay soil. Clay looks strong but is very deceptive.

Question: Once a collapse occurs the trench is safe.

Response: **False.** Don't just jump in and get the victim out. When a collapse occurs, the same trench has a 50–50 chance of collapsing again.

Question: He's just buried to his legs, let's just yank him out.

Response: **Don't.** As described earlier, the forces of moving earth are tremendous. You will only hurt the victim if you pull on him. Completely uncover the victim before trying to remove him. Energy imparted to the victim by moving soil pulverizes the body.

SOIL FACTS TO CONSIDER

If one cubic foot of dirt weighs about 100 lbs., then:

- One cu. yd. of dirt weighs about 2,700 lbs.
- One gal. of dirt weighs approximately 13 lbs.
- One cu. ft. of dirt would fill about 8 1-gal. buckets.
- One cu. yd. of dirt would fill nearly 203 1-gal. buckets.

CAUSATIVE FACTORS

Causative factors associated with trench/excavation accidents include:

1. Narrow spoil clearance
2. Excess weight close to walls
   a. Vehicle parked
   b. Roadway
   c. Other equipment/supplies
3. Vibrations
   a. Vehicle (road)
   b. Train
   c. Working equipment (outside)
   d. Working equipment (inside)
   e. Factory close by
4. Disturbed soil
   a. Previous excavations
   b. Underground lines
   c. Dump sites
5. Layered soil
   a. Natural soil layers
   b. Disturbed soil conditions
6. Too much water
   a. Seepage
   b. Eroding (rain/broken line) top, center, bottom
7. Not enough moisture/drying
   a. Soil-binding concept
   b. Stress cracks
8. Freezing/thawing

TRENCH/EXCAVATION COMPONENTS

As shown in Figure 19–1 trench/excavation components include:

Trench lip—2 ft. each direction from the top (down and out)

Belly—Center portion of a trench wall

Toe—2 ft. from the bottom

Floor—Base of trench

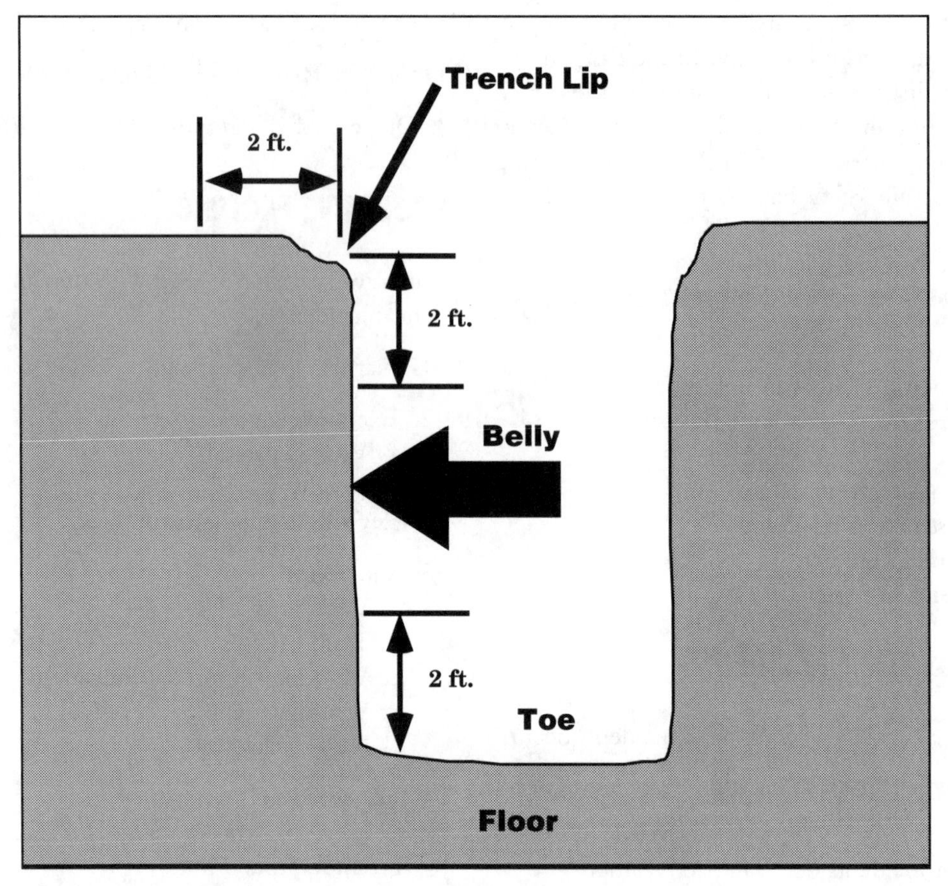

Figure 19–1 Trench/excavation components.

TRENCH/EXCAVATION COLLAPSES

Types of trench/excavation collapses include:

- Slough-in
- Spoil pile
- Shear

Slough-in Collapse

The loss of the trench belly occurs in a slough-in collapse (Figure 19–2). This type of collapse is dangerous because an improper approach can easily cause a secondary collapse. A slough-in collapse is difficult to shore. The patient is found on the floor or impaled on the far wall.

Spoil Pile Collapse

In a spoil pile collapse, the most common type of collapse, additional pressure is exerted from the pile downward and towards trench opening (Figure 19–3). The patient is found on the floor or impaled on the far wall. The law requires the spoil pile to be a minimum of 2 ft. from the lip of the trench.

Shear Collapse

A shear collapse involves the loss of the entire side wall (Figure 19–4). This type of collapse frequently occurs in area of previous excavation. The patient is found on floor of the trench or against opposite wall from where shear occurred.

FIRST RESPONDER POLICIES

First responder policies do not permit any form of entry level operations on the part of first responders. Rescuers must receive advanced training in operations/entry level operations before they would be permitted to function in a trench/excavation.

- Provides an awareness to untrained rescuers as to procedural guidelines in the event of a response to trench/excavation accidents
- Sets forth the specific functions that a first responder can perform prior to the arrival of "operations level" personnel
- Focuses on securing the incident and preparing the way for the arrival of "operations level" personnel

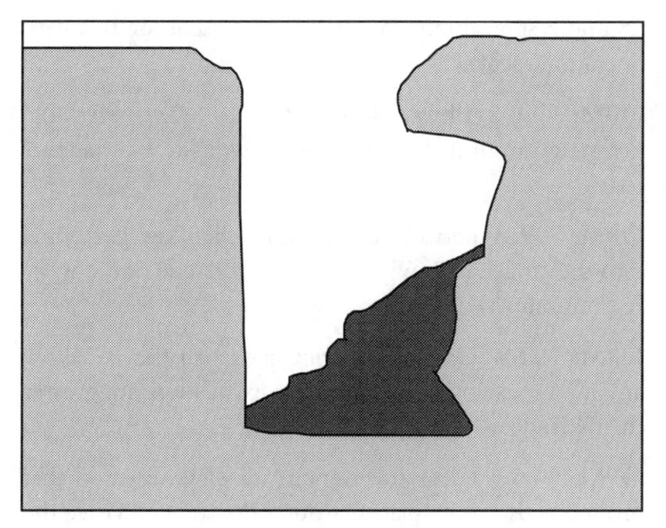

Figure 19–2 Slough-in collapse.

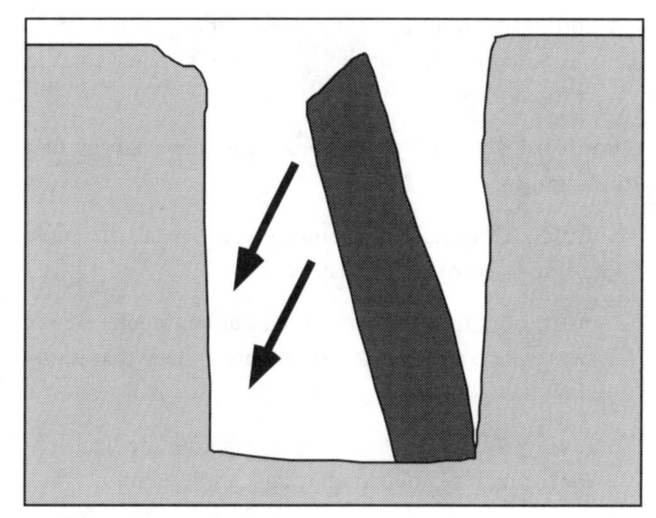

Figure 19–4 Shear collapse.

- Stresses the "pre-entry" aspects for initial responders
- Authorities having jurisdiction (AHJs) should have SOPs in place to comply with OSHA/COMAR regulations

Anne Arundel County Fire Department

First Responder Trench Safety and Cave-in Entrapment Procedure OPM #70

OPM: 70.1 This operating procedure is intended to provide guidelines for all first responding units at trenching and excavation site collapse and cave-in incidents.

OPM: 70.2 The primary purpose of the first arriving units and incident commander (IC) is to secure the incident area and ensure the safety of both victims and rescue personnel. Under *no circumstances* will the incident commander allow anyone in an unshored trench or excavation site which is greater than 4 ft. deep.

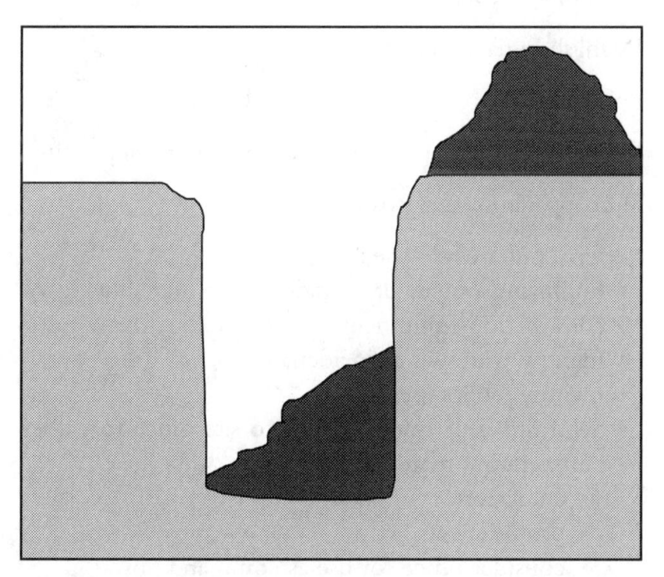

Figure 19–3 Spoil pile collapse.

OPM: 70.3 The majority of collapse and cave-in incidents involving trenches are body recovery operations due to the physical forces involved: 1 cu. ft. of dirt weighs about 100 lbs., therefore any victim who is completely buried or has only their head visible can not expand their chest to breathe and succumbs to suffocation. Victims buried only to the waist have the greatest chance of survival. The IC should establish an operational plan using the "risk-benefit" analysis approach.

OPM: 70.4 *The first arriving unit shall:*

OPM: 70.4.1 Establish initial command and position the unit at least 250 ft. from the incident scene. All personnel are to walk to the incident scene.

OPM: 70.4.2 Establish an off-site staging area at least 500 ft. from the incident scene for all other responding apparatus. Apparatus should be shut off if possible.

OPM: 70.4.3 Conduct an outer circle scene survey of a 500 ft. radius. Utilize first responder personnel to:

1. Eliminate sources of vibration, stop and shut off all construction equipment, and stop road traffic within 500 ft. of the incident scene.
2. Identify witnesses to incident and establish time when incident occurred.
3. Identify the job foreperson and request pertinent information such as site plans, cut sheets, profile sheets,

and exact number of workers working the trench. Consider the use of the foreperson's trailer for the command post.

OPM: 70.4.4 Conduct an inner circle scene survey of a 100 ft. radius:

1. Approach trench from end only. Sidewalls are most prone to secondary collapse.
2. Assist nonentrapped personnel out of trench. *Do not enter* trench which is greater than 4 ft. deep that is unshored.
3. If you have multiple victims, establish a medical sector for patient collection, triage, and treatment.
4. Establish number of trapped victims and their exact location. Once contact has been made with a conscious victim, maintain the contact.
5. Establish trapped victim(s) condition if possible. Is the victim(s):
   a. Totally buried, if so how deep
   b. Buried to neck
   c. Buried to waist
   d. Trapped by utilities
6. Utilize on-scene construction personnel to assist with ground-level activities (gather lumber, move equipment, etc.).

OPM: 70.5 *Report incident status to fire alarm:*

OPM: 70.5.1 Identify command.

OPM: 70.5.2 Confirm entrapment and number trapped.

OPM: 70.5.3 Confirm apparatus staging.

OPM: 70.5.4 Request needed resources:

1. Request MOSH compliance officer for technical assistance.
2. Request police assistance for crowd, traffic control, and incident investigation.
3. Request utility company of involved utilities.
4. Request any additional resources you feel necessary at this time.

OPM: 70.6 *Trench Rescue or Recovery Operations:*

OPM: 70.6.1 Establish command structure and assign sectors. The first arriving "Trench Safety and Rescue" trained officer or firefighter to arrive on location will assume responsibility for the trench rescue or recovery operation sector.

OPM: 70.6.2 Physically secure a 100 ft. operational perimeter around the inner circle with fire line tape or rope.

OPM: 70.6.3 Permit no one other than key personnel into the circle circle who have trench rescue or recovery responsibilities.

OPM: 70.6.4 Under *no circumstances* will the IC allow anyone in an unshored trench or excavation site greater than 4 ft. deep.

OPM: 70.6.5 Clear the trench site of spoilage so that ground pads can be placed around the trench. Move the spoilage away from the trench a minimum of 2 ft. Sheets of plywood can be used as ground pads. *No* personnel will walk around the trench site without ground pads being in place.

OPM: 70.6.6 Be *extremely* cautious of a secondary cave-in or collapse. Prior to the arrival of the cave-in unit, any temporary structure, shoring, and sheeting put in place to protect the victim must be in compliance with the MOSH *Trenching and Excavation* operations handbook.

OPM: 70.7 For technical support see, *Trenching and Excavation* by MOSH.

Montgomery County Fire Department

First Responder Policy for Trench Collapse and Cave-in Incidents Trench Collapse Incidents Procedure

First Arriving Unit Must:

Establish initial command.

Position unit no closer than 250 ft. to the scene.

Establish off-site staging for other responding apparatus.

Shut apparatus off, if possible.

Perform outer circle check:

- Eliminate sources of vibration, stop and shut down construction equipment, stop traffic.
- Identify witnesses to incident.
- Identify job foreperson.
- Send fire department person to site office to gather pertinent information, such as:
  - cut sheets
  - profile sheets
  - consider office for use as command post

- Begin to establish incident perimeter, 100 ft. minimum

Perform inner circle check:

- Approach site from end of trench.
- Identify victim location using signs and witnesses.
- Identify number of victims.
- Establish victim condition if possible. *Do not enter trench over 4 ft. without adequate shoring.*
- How is victim trapped?
  - Totally buried, if so how deep
  - Trapped by utilities
- Assist nonentrapped personnel out of the trench.
- Encourage construction workers to assist at ground level, gathering lumber, etc.
- Establish full command structure.

Complete physical perimeter 100 ft. (barrier tape).

Establish and maintain contact with victim.

Verify that all necessary utilities have been contacted by the Emergency Communications Center (ECC).

Utilize personnel from the staging area (leave apparatus in staging area) to begin clearing site for ground pads.

Personnel will not walk around trench site without ground pads in place.

Notes to the First Responder of a Trench Collapse

1. Under *no* circumstances will any personnel enter a trench that is deeper than 4 ft. that has not been safely shored.
2. The initial actions taken by the first responding unit have a direct impact on the outcome of the overall incident. An organized approach is critical!
3. This policy is intended to provide guidelines for the first responder to follow prior to the arrival of the Cave-in Unit and the Collapse Rescue Team.
4. Many other areas need to be addressed but this list will allow fire and rescue personnel to operate in a relatively safe manner for both the victim and rescuer.

Cave-in Unit Incident Procedures

Incident Procedures

First response procedures should be followed by first responding units.

When the first cave-in personnel arrive on the scene, they will report to the IC.

Cave-in personnel will assist on-scene units in the implementation of first response procedures as well as identify a possible approach for the cave-in team.

The cave-in unit will be placed as close to the incident as possible without jeopardizing trench security.

Upon arrival of the unit, the cave-in officer in charge (OIC) will report to the IC.

With approval from the OIC, the cave-in officer will assign positions to cave-in personnel.

Ground pads must be placed before personnel walk around the trench.

Ground pads should be placed from the end of the trench, always placing *pads* ahead of the work area.

Ground to be covered by *ground pads* must be leveled prior to *pad* placement.

While placing *pads* note any abnormality in the surface covered (i.e., stress cracks, makeup of soil, moisture content etc.).

The cave-in OIC will assist the OIC with the establishment of a "hot zone" (the area immediately surrounding the incident site); limited personnel are allowed in this area. These personnel include: the cave-in rescue sector officer, cave-in rescue safety officer, rescue EMS officer (patient care person preferably a paramedic), and approximately three additional workers who are cave-in trained.

This area will have a physical barrier, such as barrier tape, around it.

A ladder must be maintained in the trench any time personnel are in the trench as a quick means of egress.

The atmosphere in the trench must be monitored before entry and the trench must be ventilated prior to entry.

Generally two or three officers are on duty in the hot zone (Figure 19–5) at any given time: the cave-in rescue sector officer responsible for the actual trench site and rescue strategy; the cave-in rescue safety officer who has numerous responsibilities; and the rescue EMS officer who is responsible for the patient.

The rescue safety officer is responsible for:

- Acting as a second set of eyes for the rescue sector officer.
- Establishing a personnel control sheet, which serves to track personnel in the "hot zone."
- Maintaining an overall safety watch to include personnel actions and soil conditions, etc.

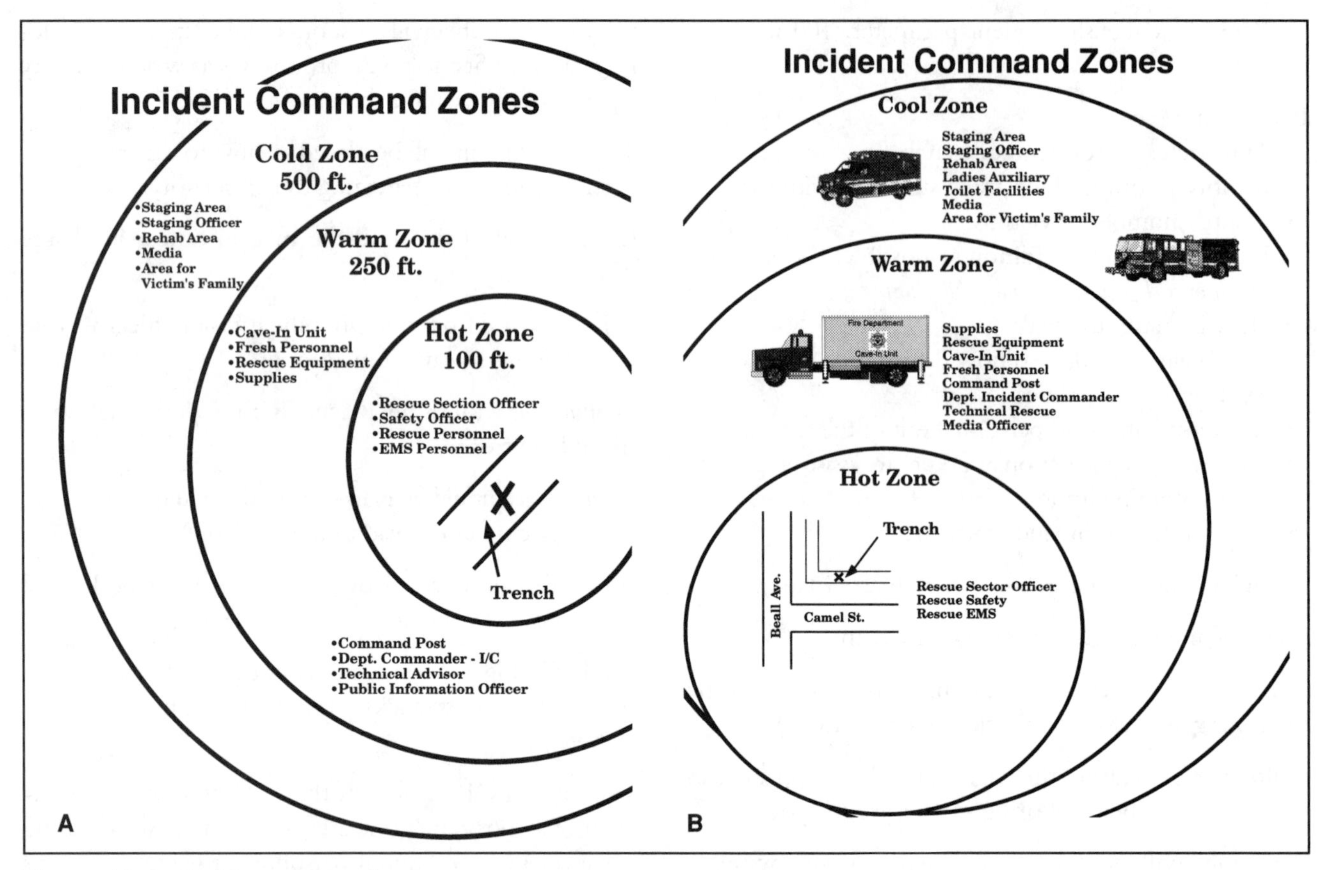

Figure 19–5 Incident command zones.

- Watching for a secondary collapse.
- Monitoring trench atmosphere for contamination.
- Acting as the rescue EMS officer, if appropriate.

The rescue EMS officer is responsible for patient care, handling, and monitoring. Concerns include: hypothermia, respiratory distress, and spinal immobilization. Monitoring specifically by the rescue EMS officer does not have to be continual.

Tools and equipment which must be in the hot zone will be carefully placed so as not to present a hazard to personnel. Tools and equipment should be placed a minimum of 15 ft. from the trench lip. *The rule, 2 ft. back for every 1 ft. of trench depth, should be utilized.*

A "warm zone" will also be established surrounding the hot zone (see Figure 19–5). The warm zone is established immediately outside the hot zone. It, too, should have limited access. This is a work area. Equipment is gathered by the rescue equipment officer and readied for utilization in the hot zone.

This area also houses the command post. Included in the command post are personnel such as: the departments ICs, the technical rescue officer who serves as an advisor to the IC, the public information officer, police representatives, and other personnel whom the OIC determines are needed.

Personnel are also gathered in this area and briefed and readied for assignments in the hot zone. Concerns include: how the problem is being handled, progress made, hazards, and what is expected of the fresh crew. Crews relieved from the hot zone pass on information to fresh crews in this area.

The third established area, the "cool zone" (Figure 19–5) is for personnel who are not going to be immediately utilized and for the rehab of personnel who have been previously used. Also included in this area are such concerns as: apparatus staging, media, victims' family gathering area (separate from public), ladies auxiliary, and toilet facilities.

SPECIALIZED RESCUE EQUIPMENT

Many departments have specialty/jurisdictional response units designated for trench, excavation, cave-in incidents only. These units carry OSHA recommended/approved equipment to deal specifically with trench, excavation, cave-in incidents in compliance with 29 CFR 1926.650 and 651.

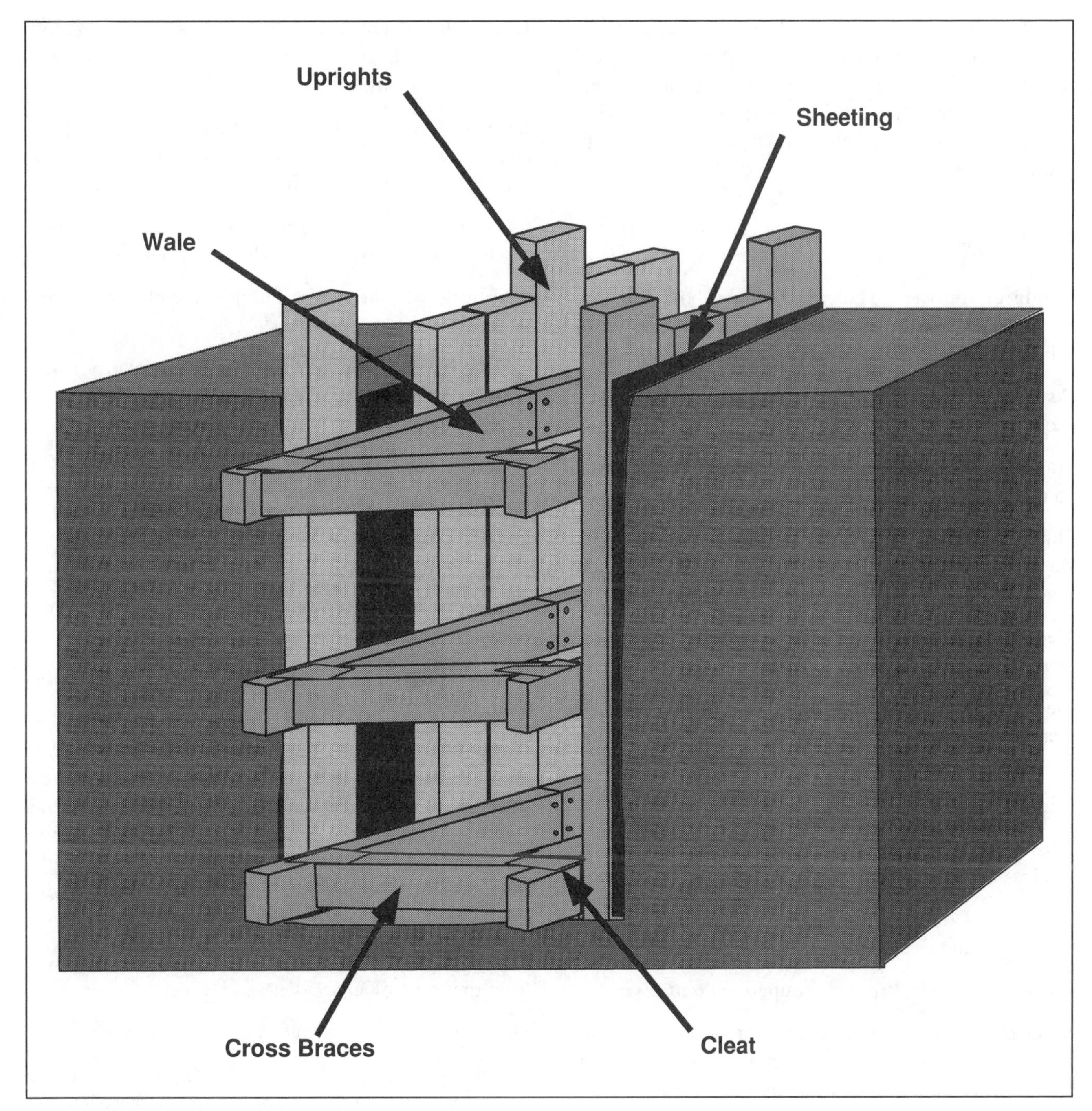

Figure 19–6 Timber shoring components.

Following is a list of some specialized rescue equipment:

- Shoring
- Panels
- Assorted hand tools
- Lifting/hoisting devices
- Air knives
- Extrication/removal devices
- Timber (Figure 19–6)

CODE OF MARYLAND REGULATIONS AND OSHA REVIEW (COMAR)

MOSH (COMAR standard for Maryland) establishes inspection procedures and provides clarification to ensure uniform enforcement of the excavation standards contained in Subpart P, 29 CFR 1926.650, 651, and 652, and Maryland amendments. OSHA (29 CFR 1926.650 through 652) excavation standard applies to all open excavations made in the earth's surface, including trenches, all surface encumbrances that would create a hazard, and protective systems.

DEFINITIONS

Angle of repose: The greatest angle above the horizontal plane at which loose material (such as soil) will lie without sliding.

Asphyxiant: A gas capable of causing death due to oxygen deficiency.

Backfill: The refilling of a trench or the material used to refill a trench.

Bater boards: A series of horizontal boards spanning the trench, used by the contractor to set the line and grade of the pipe.

Bedding: Sand or fine stone placed in the bottom of a trench as a foundation for the pipe.

Bedding stone: Small rocks spread over the floor of a trench as a foundation for sewer pipes and other utility lines.

Bisect: Cross or intersect.

Blockade: A barrier placed to halt the flow of vehicle traffic.

Boxed end of the shore: The end of a timber shore that is held in place against the sheeting with scabs.

Cave-in: The collapse of unsupported trench walls.

Check: A lengthwise separation of wood fibers, usually extending across the annular rings. Checks commonly result from stresses set up in wood during the seasoning process.

Choker: Another term for wire rope sling.

Clampstick: A nonconducting lineworker's tool essential to safe movement of energized electric wires.

Cohesive: Holding together firmly.

Command post kit: A briefcase, trunk, or other container filled with maps, standard operating procedures, directories, community resource lists, inventories, and other items that will help an officer to best utilize emergency service forces at the scene of a large-scale incident.

Community resource: A firm or other organizations that can provide personnel, equipment, and machines at the time of an emergency.

Compact soil: Soil that is hard and stable in appearance. Compact soil can be readily indented by the thumb, but penetrated only with great difficulty.

Confined area: Any space that lacks ventilation; usually the space is larger in area than the point of entry.

Cribbing: Short pieces of lumber used to support and stabilize an object.

Cul-de-sac: A dead-end street, but usually provided with a turnaround at the end.

Cut sheet: A job foreperson's daily plan. Shows depth and grades for pipe.

Damage: With regard to lumber: injuries such as gouges, splits, and punctures.

Danger zone: The area surrounding an accident site. The site of a danger zone is proportional to the severity of on-the-scene hazards.

Decay: The decomposition of wood substances caused by fungi.

Deep-well systems: A means for dewatering the ground around a trench. In a line parallel to the trench, pipe casings with screens are driven into the ground to a level below that of the trench floor. Electric submersible pumps lowered into the casings continually dewater the work area. The water is collected in a header and discharged at a point distant from the site.

Detour: A plan or procedure for routing traffic away from the scene of an accident.

Dewatering: Removing water from the work area.

Diaphragm pump: A positive displacement pump that has a diaphragm instead of a piston; an excellent device for moving water in which foreign matter is suspended.

Disrupted utilities: Broken water mains, gas mains, service lines, electrical conduits, etc.

Disturbed soil: Ground that has been previously excavated.

Double-head nail: A nail with a flange close to the head. The flange prevents the nail from being driven all the way into lumber. Removal is easy because the head remains exposed.

Driving home pipe: Connecting together pieces of slip-joint pipe.

Engineer's hubs: Stakes placed on a utility construction job site by a layout crew. Symbols on the stakes tell the contractor where and how deep to dig.

Excavation: An opening in the ground that results from a digging effort.

Extrication collar: A cervical collar with high sides; it provides additional protection for the cervical spine.

Eye of the sling: A loop fashioned into the end of a wire rope.

Fissure: A narrow opening in the ground; a crack of some length and considerable depth.

Flag stake: A piece of lath with a colored ribbon attached to mark the location of an engineer's hub. On the stake will appear information about the centerline and depth of the trench.

Floatation: The distribution of weights and forces over a larger area.

Free-standing time: The period of time during which trench walls remain standing unsupported after excavation.

Frost line: The depth to which frost penetrates the soil.

Grade crossing: A railroad crossing at highway level.

Grade pole: A wood or fiberglass pole that is either cut to a certain length or provided with markings. It is used by workers when they are setting pipes on grade.

Ground cover: A tarpaulin placed on the ground for an equipment layout.

Ground pads: Full sheets of ⅝ in. or ¾ in. plywood placed adjacent to the trench lip. Ground pads distribute weight and forces over their surface area and thus minimize the possibility of rescuers creating a secondary cave-in.

Header: A large, diameter pipe with inlets for suction hoses and a connection for the suction side of a pump.

Hydraulic shoring: Trench shores or jacks with movable parts that are operated by the action of hydraulic fluid.

Hydrostatic pressure: The force generated by a liquid.

Kiln dried (lumber): Lumber that is artificially dried in an oven-like structure.

Laser blower: A motor-driven fan (usually 12 V) used by contractors to purge a pipe of stale air when a laser instrument is being used.

Laser target: A square or triangular plastic device used in conjunction with a laser instrument to set the line and grade of pipe.

Loam: A combination of sand and clay.

Lower explosive limit (LEL): In a range of percentages, the point below which a mixture of flammable gas and air will not ignite because there is an insufficient concentration of the gas.

Manifold: A pipe fitting with several inlets and/or outlets.

Mechanical strut: An adjustable support. When it is made up into a solid support, it resists forces exerted in the direction of its length.

Mechanism of entrapment: Any object that confines (or traps) an accident victim.

Methane gas: The chief component of natural gas; colorless, odorless, and flammable.

Mine drift: A nearly horizontal mine passageway.

Offset: The distance (in feet) measured perpendicular from an engineer's hub to the pipeline.

One-call system: A service from which contractors, emergency service personnel, and others can obtain information on the location of underground utilities in any area.

Operating radius (of a crane): The horizontal distance from the centerline of rotation (the center pin of the cab) to a vertical line through the load's center of gravity.

OSHA: The Occupational Safety and Health Administration, a division of the U.S. Department of Labor.

Panels: Multilayered sheets of wood, usually 4 ft. × 8 ft. by various thicknesses, used to support the walls of a trench.

Parallel trench: A previously excavated and backfilled trench close to and paralleling the trench being dug.

Perimeter: A real or imaginary line established to control the movement of spectators.

Pipe: A conduit for fluids, gases, and finely divided solid materials.

Pipe string: Lengths of pipe laid parallel to the trench lip in preparation for being joined and buried.

Pneumatic shoring: Trench shoring or jacks with movable parts operated by the action of a compressed gas.

Primary assessment: The initial determination of what has happened in an accident situation; the "size-up."

Profile: A job blueprint that shows sectional elevations.

PVC pipe: A lightweight pipe made of polyvinylchloride.

Release tool: A hand-held device used to depressurize hydraulic shoring.

Replacement sewer line: A new pipeline installed adjacent to an existing line for the purpose of taking over the original line's function.

Rescue area: Generally the area 50 ft. in all directions from the accident site.

Right-of-way: A strip of land temporarily granted to the contractor to perform work.

Running soil: Loose, freely flowing soil such as sugar sand.

Safing: Making a portion of a trench safe by the installation of sheeting and shoring.

Sanitary sewer: A buried pipeline that carries sewage.

Saturated soil: Soil that contains an unusually high quantity of water. Easily identified because of seeping.

Scab: A short piece of lumber, generally cut from 2 in. × 4 in. stock, that is nailed to an upright to prevent the shifting of a shore.

Screw jack: A trench shore or jack with interchangeable threaded parts. The threading allows the jack to be lengthened or shortened.

Secondary cave-in: A collapse of another portion of a trench wall after the initial accident.

Select fill: Soil that is specially chosen to replace that which has been excavated.

Self-dumping valve: A spring-loaded valve that is part of a pneumatic shoring system. When the valve handle is depressed, the system is pressurized; when the valve handle is released, pressure is released.

Shackle: A U-shaped, round piece of steel that is provided with a pin or a threaded bolt. Used to join rigging devices.

Shake: A separation along the grain of lumber.

Shear: In trench/excavation rescue, force-caused stress that results in a section of trench wall sliding from the main body of earth.

Sheeting: Generally speaking, wood planks and wood panels that support trench walls when held in place with shoring.

Shoring: The general term used for lengths of timber, screw jacks, hydraulic and pneumatic jacks, and other devices that can be used to hold sheeting against trench walls. Individual supports are called shores, crossbraces, and struts.

Shotgun: Another term for a clampstick, so named because of the slide action of the wire grip.

Skip shoring: The procedure for supporting trench walls with uprights and shores at spaced intervals.

Sliding choker: A steel hook provided on a wire rope sling. The hook enables the sling to adjust for loads of various sizes and shapes.

Slough-in: The collapse of a portion of trench wall in such a fashion that an overhang remains.

Snatch block: A wood or steel-shell, single-pulley block that can be opened on one slide to accept a rope or cable.

Soil typing: Determining properties of soil such as strength, in-place unit weight, compressibility, and permeability.

Solid sheeting: The procedure for supporting trench walls with sections of sheeting butted together.

Spoil pile: The heap of material excavated from a trench.

Spot bracing: Another term for "skip shoring."

Spot dewatering: The technique of drawing water from localized portions of the ground around a trench.

Spray deflector: The plate on the end of the release tool that deflects hydraulic fluid lost during the depressurizing operation.

Staging area: A gathering point; in rescue cases, for emergency service and support apparatus, equipment, and personnel.

Storm sewer: A buried pipeline that carries surface water (such as rain water).

Story pole: See "Grade pole."

String lines: Strings placed on one side of and parallel to the trench. Used to determine grade.

Strongback: See "Uprights."

Sump: A pit dug at a low point in the trench floor; it serves to keep the screened end of a suction hose below the water level.

Supplemental sheeting and shoring: Additional sheeting and shoring installed as the level of the trench floor is lowered during digging operations.

Tension cracks: Cracks in the ground adjacent to the trench. Tension cracks indicate that the ground has shifted and should be considered as warning signs.

Tight sheeting: Another term for "solid sheeting."

Trash pump: A centrifugal or diaphragm pump designed to move water that contains mud, stones, and other debris.

Trench: A temporary excavation in which the length of the bottom exceeds the width of the bottom. The term "trench" is generally limited to excavations that are less than 15 ft. wide at the bottom and less than 20 ft. deep.

Trench box: A steel, fiberglass, or aluminum structure placed in a trench to protect workers from the collapse of the trench walls, and which can be moved along as work progresses.

Trench lip: The edge of a trench.

Unbroken utilities: Water mains, gas mains, electrical conduits, and pipelines that remain intact (although they may be exposed) during a trenching operation.

Underground utilities: Conduits carrying water, gas, electric, transmission lines, sewage, etc.

Upper explosive limit: In a range of percentages, the point above which a mixture of flammable gas and air will not ignite because there is not sufficient oxygen.

Uprights: Generally speaking, planks that are held in place against sections of sheeting with shores. Uprights add strength to the shoring system. They distribute forces exerted by trench walls and counterforces exerted by shores over wider areas of the sheeting.

Utility hole: An access way to sewer pipes; an opening used for maintenance and inspection.

Ventilating the trench: Using a powered fan to replace stale or contaminated air in a trench with fresh air.

Virgin soil: Ground that has never been excavated.

Wales: Braces placed horizontally against sheeting. Wales transmit loading from the sheeting to shores. Also called "walers" and "stringers."

Wall: The side of a trench from the lip to the floor. Also called the "face."

Wane: An edge or corner defect in lumber characterized by the presence of bark or the lack of wood.

Warp: A twist or curve in lumber that was originally straight.

Water table: The upper limit of a portion of the ground that is wholly saturated with water from underground sources. May be very near the surface or deep in the ground.

Wedged end of the shore: The end of a timber shore opposite the boxed end. It is between this end and the uprights that wedges are driven to make the structure rigid.

Well casing: A large, diameter pipe (12 ins.) that is used in deep-well systems.

Well-point system: A series of pipes driven into the ground around a trench for the purpose of dewatering the work area. Water is drawn through the pipes, into a header, and finally into the suction side of a pump.

Whip hose: In a pneumatic shoring system, the length of hose that carries air from the self-dumping valve to the quick-disconnect coupling.

Wire rope sling: A lifting device made of wire rope. An eye is provided at both ends.

REFERENCES

Anne Arundel County EMS/Fire/Rescue Department . 1995. *Operational Procedures Manual: 70-Trench Rescue-First Responder.* Anne Arundel County, MD: Anne Arundel County EMS/Fire/Rescue Department.

Montgomery County Department of Fire/Rescue Services. 1994. *First responder policy for trench collapse incidents.* Montgomery County, MD: MCoDFRS.

OSHA 29–Labor, Code of Federal Regulation: Excavation Requirements, 1926.650; Specific Excavation Requirements, 1926.651; Requirements for Protective Systems, 1926.652. Published by The Office of the Federal Register, National Archives and Records Administration, as a special edition of the Federal Register. 1997. Washington, DC: US Government Printing Office.

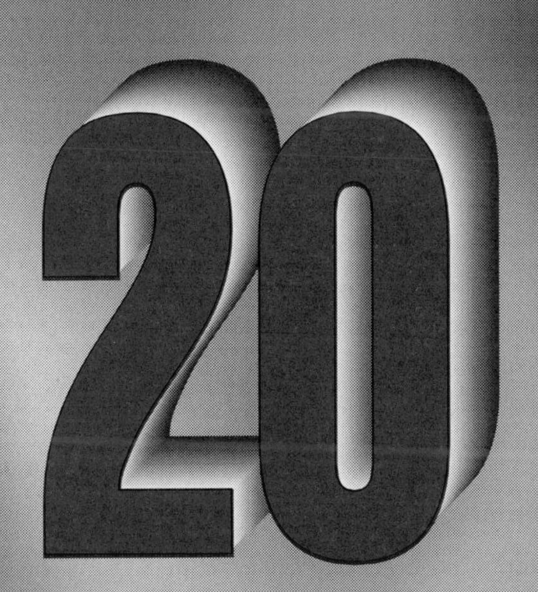

Aquatic Emergency First Responder: Awareness and Exam #3

OBJECTIVE

The student will be able to define the role of the aquatic emergency first responder and identify the features that make aquatic emergencies unique, and be able to demonstrate knowledge and understanding of the skills learned in sessions 16 through 20 on a written exam, from memory, without assistance, to an accuracy of 70% and the satisfaction of the instructor. **This a pass/fail point in the program**.

OVERVIEW

Aquatic Emergency First Responder: Awareness

- First Responder's Role
- Characteristics and Hazards
- Immersion-related Injuries
- Aquatic Emergency Scenarios
- Specialized Patient Care
- Safety Practices and Safety Equipment

ENABLING OBJECTIVES

20-1-1 Define the first responder's role on an aquatic emergency scene.

20-1-2 Identify the characteristics and hazards of the aquatic emergency environment.

20-1-3 Describe immersion-related injuries.

20-1-4 Describe factors associated with aquatic emergency scenarios.

20-1-5 Describe the specialized patient care requirements associated with aquatic emergency scenarios.

20-1-6 Describe the safety practices and equipment requirements for aquatic emergencies.

INTRODUCTION

It has been said among the ranks of emergency service providers/rescuers that "the difference between a hero and a fool is training." Across the United States, the fire service decorates both its heros and its fools. One wears a ribbon proudly on their chest, the other holds it posthumously in folded hands lying in a flag-draped casket. Given the choice, one would opt for his/her moment of glory rather than the lead column in the obituary section of the hometown newspaper.

In spite of this reality, well-meaning rescuers continue to lose their lives during the initial contact phase of water and ice emergencies. Why? Because sound judgement, good reasoning, and a disciplined plan of action was not used. The temptation to enter an uncertain environment to rescue an animal, child, or adult was too great—resulting in the ultimate catastrophe: a senseless loss of a rescuer's life because they lacked the training and expertise to effectively bring an aquatic emergency to a successful conclusion.

As a result, there are an average of seven public safety drowning deaths annually across the United States. OSHA regulation 29 CFR 1926.21 mandates that employees (first responders) be trained in "the recognition and avoidance of unsafe conditions and the regulations applicable to his/her work environment to control or eliminate any hazards." Furthermore, since fire/rescue-based first responders are charged with the task of saving lives, they must also be trained to treat patients who have been injured in aquatic emergencies.

The bottom line to addressing aquatic-related emergencies from a first responder perspective is very simple: Never trade lives for any reason. Never jeopardize your personal safety or that of your co-workers/rescuers. Never attempt a rescue from water or ice scenarios unless you are trained and proficient in the use of required resources, and have the means to conduct any such effort safely and prudently.

FIRST RESPONDER'S ROLE

A firefighter would never advance attack lines for an interior extinguishment activity without first conducting an incident size-up which would include hazard identification and analysis. Why then would a rescuer enter or attempt to enter water and/or ice conditions without conducting an initial size-up operation? When you provide an answer to this question, you will also identify the issues that result in fire service personnel losing their lives. These issues are:

- Allowing emotions to override good sense, and objectivity.
- Failing to weigh the potential risks v. benefits associated with a course of action.
- Failure to adhere to established standard operating procedures (SOPs) governing incident scene management or water and ice scenarios.
- Rescuer complacency.
- Rescuer freelancing with a wanton disregard for supervision and accountability.
- Allowing the dynamics of an incident to run *you*—not *you* controlling the dynamics.

With these issues in mind, let's examine, in closer detail, the role of the first responding rescuer during an aquatic-related emergency.

Size-up Activities

First and foremost, never approach within 10 ft. of the water's edge. This negates potential slippage/fall potential to the rescuer. Conduct an assessment of upstream and downstream hazards to the patient. Survey the shorelines, routes of safe access to the patient, and the surf, current, and icy conditions. Remember, current is the most frequently underestimated hazard. Determine if you have a rescue situation or a body recovery operation. Establishing safety at the incident also involves securing routes of access to prevent bystander mishaps. Remember the example of the Air Florida Flight 90 in Washington, D.C. where a bystander dove into the icy waters of the Potomac River to save a member of the flight crew? He did this because he was frustrated by the perceived ineffectiveness of rescuer efforts.

During size-up activities, attempt to establish eye contact and voice communication with a viable patient(s) to calm and reassure them. A patient's "will to live" can dramatically influence their immersion survivability. Encourage the patient to attempt self-rescue, if doing so does not put the patient at greater risk, and if there are sufficient personnel on hand to assist with throw ropes.

CHARACTERISTICS AND HAZARDS

To better understand hazards/risk assessment, a rescuer/first responder must be familiar with the terms and definitions of:

- Oceans, large lakes, and surf zones
- Swiftwater/rivers and streams
- Flash flooding
- Ice formation

Oceans, Large Lakes, and Surf Zones

Waves Swells of energy transferred through deep water caused by wind. Can cause serious injury as surf at shorelines.

Undertow Return flow of water to point of origin before a wave, but no further.

Longshore/littoral currents Pile-up of water at beach caused by incoming waves that flow along the beach at approximately ankle-knee depth.

Rip current "Escaping" littoral current that develops sufficient force to overpower incoming waves. "Rips" usually do not extend much past the breaking waves but can occasionally achieve speeds of 5 mph. or 6 mph. and carry swimmers hundreds of yards out to sea.

Tidal wave Cyclic rising and falling water level in seas and oceans caused by the gravitational pull of the moon. Generally benign unless coupled with a gale-force wind.

Rip tides Extremely dangerous, fast, choppy, seaward current created by escaping water from tidal basins that overcomes incoming tides. Also a clash created where two tidal flows meet such as Oregon Inlet, the Outer Banks of North Carolina, or the inlet at Ocean City.

Runout Similar to a rip current, the runout is an "escaping" current of offshore water released by a break in a sand bar.

Sunami Japanese term meaning *harbor wave.* Giant destructive waves that radiate from the epicenter of some seismic activity at up to 500 mph. and as much as 50 miles between wave crests. As they approach shore, they are thrust upward to heights that can reach 200 ft. Rare; usually occur in Alaska, Hawaii, and on Pacific coast.

Swiftwater/Rivers and Streams

Laminar flow Water flowing down the center of a smooth flowing, straight stream in successively faster "layers" from bottom to surface. The fastest flow is just below the surface where there is no friction with the air.

Helical flow Water flowing in a downstream coil. As laminar flow approaches the shoreline, it wells up from the stream bottom toward the surface, out toward the center of the stream, and then back toward the bottom.

Hydraulic (hole) A swiftwater hazard which traps floating objects and forces them through recirculating cycles, pushing them underwater, forcing them downstream, pushing them to the surface, and then pushing them back upstream to repeat the cycle. Caused by water pouring vertically over an obstacle, displacing the water on the downstream side, and surface water flowing back upstream to fill the void. Whitewater in a hole may contain from 40% to 60% entrained air.

Backwash Water moving backward; caused by water pouring over an obstruction which creates a "hole" in the downstream surface, causing downstream water to flow backward to fill the hole.

Boil (line) The interface of downstream water below a hydraulic where the backwash and outwash separate. The characteristic "boiling" appearance is caused by the release of entrained air.

Outwash The downstream component of the hydraulic below the "boil" that continues downstream.

Chute or downstream "V" The fastest, clearest channel through rapids in swiftwater, recognized by a characteristic V shape which points downstream, as well as the darker shiny appearance of the water in the chute.

Standing wave Aerated water found at the bottom of chutes as a result of high-velocity water being poured into the same spot in a continuous manner.

Eddy Water moving opposite the river vector, caused by water flowing around an obstruction. Found on the downstream side of the obstruction.

Eddy line Line of whitewater between an eddy and the downstream current.

Upstream "V" A characteristic V pattern in swiftwater which points upstream, caused by water parting as it flows downstream around an obstacle.

Ferry angle A 45° angle to the river vector that a boat or swimmer would assume, with the bow of the boat or the swimmer's head inclined upstream, toward the desired shoreline.

River vector The angle of the current relative to the shoreline. The current does not necessarily flow parallel to the shoreline.

River right/left A means of identifying the two shorelines of a stream or river by looking downstream during orientation.

Upstream/downstream A means of identifying a stream's or river's direction of flow as being either "up," toward the source, or "down," away from the stream source.

International scale of river difficulty A classification of river navigability from "easy" to "extreme risk of life" using a scale of I to VI.

Class I Moving water with few riffles and small waves.
Class II Easy rapids with waves up to 3 ft. high.
Class III Rapids with high waves capable of swamping an open canoe.
Class IV Long, difficult rapids, requiring precise maneuvering in turbulent water.
Class V Extremely difficult, violent rapids that require scouting.
Class VI Class V hazards to the extreme. Nearly impassible.

Pillow An apparent "mound" of water formed by moving water flowing over a submerged object that is just below the surface.

Strainer A buildup of debris in swiftwater that allows water to pass through, but traps and holds solid objects such as swimmers.

Funnel effect Acceleration of swiftwater caused by a narrowing or constriction of the stream bed.

Swiftwater dynamics To better understand the effect of reducing or increasing the size of the stream bed on the velocity of the water, it is important to be able to calculate the volume of water that physically occupies the stream bed at any given time.

1. Multiply river width by river depth = area (ft. squared).
2. Pace off 40 paces on the shoreline to approximate 100 ft.
3. Drop a float in the current even with the start of the 100 ft. measured area.
4. Measure the time required for the float to travel 100 ft.
5. Divide 100 by the number of seconds required for the float to travel the 100 ft. course to determine the rate of water movement in ft./sec. (fps.).
6. Multiply fps. by ft. squared (as determined in No. 1) to determine cubic feet of flow per second (cfs.).

As the speed of the water changes, the force that the water exerts on any resisting object also changes. Water has mass and weight. Each gallon of water weighs approximately 8.35 lbs. and there are approximately 7.5 gals/cu. ft. Water in motion, therefore, exerts force. The information above shows that as the speed of travel increases, the force of the water increases exponentially (at a much greater rate). To convert the speed from fps. to mph. multiply by 3,600 and divide by 5,280.

Flash Flooding

No communities are totally free of swift water. Flash floods occur in every state in the United States. They account for more loss of life and more property loss than any other natural disaster. Flash floods usually occur as a result of extremely heavy rainfall during a short period of time. The flash flooding condition in California during January 1995, for example, resulted, in part, from lack of vegetation to prevent erosion. Terminology associated with flash flooding and water movement and dynamics includes:

Catch-basin effect Collection of water through the convergence of water from a variety of confluences including ground runoff, storm drains, etc.

Confluence A flowing together of two or more streams; the point where they flow together.

Buoyancy A force exerted by liquids equal to the weight of the liquid that is displaced by an immersed body. Buoyancy means a body which is immersed in a liquid contained in a vessel will displace a volume of liquid which is equal in mass to the immersed body. The surface of the liquid contained in the vessel will exert a lifting force equal to the weight of the displaced liquid. The weight of the immersed body is effectively reduced by the weight of the displaced liquid. If the weight of the immersed body is less than the weight of the displaced liquid, then the body will be held afloat at the surface.

- Any passenger vehicle which is driven into water will be swept away by approximately 2 ft. water. The weight of the average passenger vehicle is less than 3,000 lbs. Since the volume of water that is displaced by such a vehicle is approximately 3,000 lbs. at 2 ft. in depth, most vehicles would become neutrally buoyant at the surface and would float.
- Heavier vehicles such as fire apparatus should also avoid driving over flooded roadways. The effect of churning/flash flood water on bridges, bridge supports, and roadways would be an erosion or undermining of the earth and gravel base, resulting in the loss of structural integrity on the road surface. Debris carried by the flood water would cloud the water and conceal any structural damage.

Surface loads Floating debris carried on the surface of swiftwater which is particularly prevalent in floodwater. Surface loads pose a hazard to navigation and pose a major threat to rescuers and patients who may be in the water.

Suspended loads Floating debris carried in a partially submerged state that poses the same threat to rescuers and patients but is more insidious due to the fact that it may be concealed from rescuers posted as lockouts.

Bottom loads Debris that has lost all buoyancy but is being swept along on the bottom of the stream bed by the force of the current.

Ice Formation and Characteristics

A variety of actions influence ice formation and strength. There is no foolproof way of determining ice integrity. The only absolute certain way of guaranteeing personal safety is to stay off of the ice!

Frazil ice The first ice crystals form at 39°F. They appear on the surface of puddles on cold mornings as a shiny film. These first crystals of frazil ice do not fully consolidate into solid sheets of ice until water temperatures drop to approximately 32°F.

Turnover As still water in ponds and lakes is cooled or warmed by the weather, cold water, being denser than warm water, sinks to the bottom while warm water remains at the surface. At 39°F, water begins ice formation in the form of crystals. These crystals are larger and less dense than the water from which they were formed. As a result, these crystals follow the rules of buoyancy and rise to the surface.

Clear ice Ice formed after one continuous, long hard freeze. This is usually the strongest type of ice.

Snow ice Opaque or milky-looking, weak ice formed by freezing water-soaked snow.

Layered ice Ice formed by multiple layers of frozen and refrozen snow, giving it a characteristic layered or striped appearance.

Frazil slush Slushy covering formed over moving water where current prevents a solid freeze.

Anchor ice Ice formed on obstructions, such as rocks or bridge pilings, which are cooled at night forming ice at the water's surface but are warmed during the day by passive solar heat. Once warmed, the ice bond is melted and the ice which was attached is then freed to become drift ice.

Pack ice Ice chunks driven together by wind, waves, or current. Pack ice can pile up in chunks with thicknesses varying from less than 1 in. to several feet.

Drift ice Floating ice that is not attached to the shore; free-floating ice.

Ice cracks May be either wet or dry, caused by excess weight on the ice or by expansion and contraction caused by temperature fluctuations. Should be anticipated to be weak spots.

Thaw hole A vertical hole in the ice formed when warmer surface puddles melt through to the underlying water.

Ice Strength: Thick ice is generally stronger than thin ice:

1 in. = keep off

2 ins. = one person

3 ins. = three cross country skiers

4 ins. = one ice fisherman

5 ins. = one snowmobile

6 ins. = ice boating

7 ins. = group activities

8 ins. = one automobile

9 ins. = several snowmobiles

10 ins.–12 ins. = light truck

New ice is stronger than old ice. Ice grows stronger and thicker during formation. As ice deteriorates, the bond between ice crystals breaks down, sometimes causing old ice to take on a black appearance. Old, deteriorating ice may be thick but still lack structural integrity. Warm weather causes ice to deteriorate. The inverse of those factors that form ice cause ice to weaken. Light wind enhances ice formation by accelerating cooling of lakes and ponds. Heavy winds retard ice formation and keep holes open through wave action. Heavy winds can also force water under ice edges, accelerating ice deterioration from underneath.

How Does Snow Affect Ice Conditions and Formation? Snow can insulate ice by reflecting sunlight off the surface which helps to retain the strength of the ice. It can also insulate the underlying ice and protect it from sudden cold temperatures to slow ice formation. Snow can reduce the weight-bearing capacity of ice by weighing it down with the weight of the snow. It often conceals thaw holes and areas of open water, endangering ice travellers.

Water Dynamics and Other Factors That Affect Ice Formation: Water on top of ice erodes it. Fractures are sometimes caused by water "percolating" through ice. Ice closer to shore is weakest. Movement of the ice sheet due to expansion and shifting, coupled with the absorption of passive solar heat by shallow bottoms and heat generation from rotting vegetation, tends to weaken ice at the shore.

Currents also weaken ice. River ice tends to be 15% weaker than lake ice. Water chemistry is a major factor in ice formation. Pure water freezes faster and deeper than water containing chemicals or pollutants. Underground springs also weaken ice. Rising warmer water tends to erode ice from underneath. Fish and water fowl weaken ice. Schools of fish churn up warmer bottom water causing ice erosion from underneath. Flocks of swimming waterfowl keep water from freezing by keeping it in a constant state of motion.

IMMERSION-RELATED INJURIES

Drowning literally is suffocation in water. In the truest sense of the word, the patient's mouth and nose must be submerged long enough to interfere with normal breathing. Exact figures on the number of true drowning deaths are difficult to obtain. Most deaths secondary to an immersion are listed as drownings regardless of the cause of death.

The fatalities from the sinking of the *Titanic* are a prime example of this erroneous thinking. Of 1,489 fatalities, over 300 were found afloat on the surface with their faces out of the water, one hour and fifty minutes after they entered the 32°F water, yet their cause of death was listed as drowning. Post-immersion resuscitation due to advances in prehospital care are lowering the numbers of waterside DOA pronouncements. Patients are transported to hospitals and tertiary care centers where they may die days, weeks, or even months later. In these cases the cause of death is usually listed by the pathophysiology that ultimately won, rather than the precipitating event (drowning) that put them in that condition.

About 85% of all drownings are *wet drownings*. Wet drownings result in relaxation of the epiglottis and larynx, allowing water and vomitus to enter the airway and lungs causing asphyxiation. About 15% of all drownings are *dry drownings*. In dry drownings the epiglottis and larynx do not relax, which prevents the aspiration of more than minute amounts, if any, of water, causing in-water suffocation.

The complications that may result from wet drownings are directly related to the type of water from which a patient is retrieved (e.g., salt water or fresh water). In salt water, fluid is drawn into lungs from vascular space resulting in Acute Respiratory Distress Syndrome (ARDS). ARDS may be caused by the aspiration of salt water, vomitus, or other contaminants and results in shortness of breath, rapid breathing, damaged lung tissue, hemorrhage, and fluid accumulation in the lungs. On the other hand, fresh water draws water from the lungs into vascular space. It may cause kidney failure, heart failure, breakdown of red blood cells, and clotting disorders. A variety of infections can result from aspiration of fungi, bacteria, and other pollutants and contaminants.

Secondary drowning, also known as *parking lot drowning,* results in death from one of the complications mentioned above. Near drowning implies recovery from immersion-induced suffocation. Successful resuscitation is generally predicated on the type and clarity of water, age of the patient, temperature of the water, duration of immersion, and aggressiveness (techniques) used in the prehospital and hospital treatment protocols. Typically, the signs and symptoms of cold water near drownings that may be displayed are:

C—Cold to the touch

C—Cyanosis or bluish skin color

P—Pulseless (either very slow or barely detectable)

P—Pupils equal, dilated, and unresponsive

R—Rigid muscles

R—Respirations absent or so slow and/or shallow as to be nondetectable

Each year approximately 700 persons suffer permanent, partial, or complete loss of use of their limbs or body functions as a result of trauma to their spinal cord. This is usually caused by impact against the bottom of a body of water or impact with some in-water obstruction (including other swimmers) after head-first diving or jumping. Some patients recall being able to swim to the surface unaided, but are impaired after being yanked from the water by well-intentioned bystanders. The number of fatalities from this cause is nearly impossible to ascertain due to a failure to conduct post-mortem autopsies. This results in erroneous cause of death determinations involving drowning incidents.

Cardiac arrest usually occurs in older, fearful, out-of-shape nonswimmers who are suddenly and unexpectedly plunged into very cold water that is over their heads.

Hypothermia, a lowering of the core temperature of the body, is also a complication of cold water immersion and the profound affects on the body's ability to function. Mild hypothermia occurs when the body core temperature is between 99°F and approximately 96°F. Patients exhibit vigorous shivering, but remain conscious and oriented.

In moderate hypothermia, body core temperature is between 95°F to 86°F. Patients cease shivering, muscular coordination diminishes to muscular rigidity, and level of consciousness deteriorates from being stuporous to being unconscious.

In cases of severe or profound hypothermia, the patient's core temperature is less than 85°F. Patients are unconscious with diminishing to nondetectable vital signs. Patients in severe hypothermia have lost all ability to compensate for lost body heat and frequently display a dramatic "afterdrop" or sudden drop in body temperature. This is a true medical emergency. At core temperatures of approximately 70°F, patients will go into cardiac dysrhythmia leading to arrest.

Terrestrial or chronic hypothermia results from prolonged exposure to cold weather as experienced by winter outdoor sports participants, such as hunters, where they may spend extended periods of time motionless and in one spot. This should also be considered in any elderly person, child, or homeless/street person who displays stuporous or confused behavior after outdoor exposure in cold weather.

Immersion or acute hypothermia results from immersion in any water that is less than 98.6°F but is particularly rapid in onset in cold water. Water rescue specialists, such as the U.S. Coast Guard, define cold water as 70°F or less. The following factors decrease the ability of a cold water immersion patient(s) to assist in their own rescue or maintain consciousness:

- Water is denser than air.
- Still water draws heat out of the body 25 times faster than air of the same temperature.
- If the water is in motion, or if the patient attempts to swim or struggle in the water, estimates suggest that body heat may be lost at a rate of 35 to over 100 times faster depending on the velocity of the water and the physical makeup of the patient.

AQUATIC EMERGENCY SCENARIOS

An understanding of the events that precipitate an aquatic emergency can provide the first responder with clues to the patient's injuries and ability to self-rescue. The role of alcohol and drugs in aquatic emergencies is significant because:

1. Advertising for alcoholic beverages targets recreation, in general, and water sports, in particular.
2. Traditional customs and practices have included some amount of imbibing during boating, swimming, and fishing outings.
3. Estimates of aquatic fatalities that have *some* blood alcohol content (BAC) run as high as two-thirds.
4. Estimates of aquatic fatalities that are legally intoxicated run as high as 50%.
5. Alcohol is a central nervous system (CNS) depressant and it:
   - Slows reaction time.
   - Reduces muscular coordination.
   - Impairs gag reflex.
   - Elevates BAC and impairs balance.
   - Impairs judgement.
   - Dilates peripheral blood vessels, accelerating the onset of hypothermia.

Immediate Disappearance Syndrome

Immediate Disappearance Syndrome (IDS) accounts for approximately 20% of all fatal submersions. The IDS patient enters the water and never returns to the surface. The rescue "window of opportunity" for IDS patients is zero seconds for surface rescue. Interviewing witnesses to determine a "point last seen" for rescue divers is critical if the patient is to have any chance for resuscitation. The steps to problems in IDS interviewing are:

1. Isolate each witness and interview at observation point.
2. Use rescue swimmers or boats as reference points for witnesses.
3. Have law enforcement personnel conduct interviews. (They are trained in interviewing techniques.)
4. Determine a probable time of submersion. The longest known time of submersion with full recovery after resuscitation is 66 minutes. The standard accepted philosophy of dive teams across the United States is to shift modes of operation from rescue to recovery after approximately one hour of known submersion, or one hour of on-scene time, whichever comes first.

Causes of IDS: The primary cause of IDS is cervical spine trauma or head injury as a result of jumping or diving into shallow water, or striking an underwater obstruction including other swimmers.

A second cause of IDS is hyperventilation prior to extended underwater swims. This results in loss of consciousness or "shallow water blackout."

The third cause of IDS, caloric labyrinthitis, is a condition whereby an individual is suddenly plunged into cold water, either as a swimmer who dives through a *thermocline* or someone who falls into cold water that is over his/her head. In either case, the patient becomes disoriented due to the physiological effect of cold water on nerve centers, and cannot determine which way to swim to the surface. Breath-holding time is also diminished resulting in a patient who is out of air and does not know which way to swim to safety. Thermocline is a phenomenon where water settles into layers, divided by temperatures and density. Cold water, which may be as much as 20°F colder than warmer water above it, presents as a mirrored surface as it is approached from above.

Physiological overload describes a variety of causes of IDS that are physical responses to sudden, unanticipated immersion in cold water that is over the patient's head. Persons with a previous history of cardiac disorders may experience cardiac dysrhythmia such as fibrillation and/or cardiac arrest. An undiagnosed enlarged heart may result in tachycardia, hyperventilation, and seizures.

Sudden, unexpected immersion in cold water often triggers an involuntary gasp, known as the *torso reflex*. If the patient's face and air passages are covered with cold water at the moment of inhalation, the surprised patient inhales cold water instead of air, which either fills the patient's lungs or stomach with cold water. In either case, the patient has exhaled whatever air that was in his/her lungs and lost their buoyancy, and either the stomach or the lungs now contain a volume of cold water which accelerates the onset of hypothermia.

Distressed Nonswimmers

Distressed Nonswimmers (DNS) unintentionally slip, step, or fall into water that is over their heads. DNS patients account for approximately 60% of all fatal submersions. The rescue "window of opportunity" for DNS patients is 20 to 60 seconds. Researcher and career lifeguard Frank Pia has determined that small children may only struggle at the surface for 20 seconds and adults usually last no more than 60 seconds.

DNS patients do not wave their arms and cry out for help. The primary function of the airway is the exchange of air. Patients that do not have enough air to breathe have no air to use for cries for help. The arms are involuntarily extended laterally and are pushed down on the surface of the water in futile efforts to raise the airway above the surface. Witnesses often report mistaking this "instinctive drowning response" for playing. The head is tilted back in a position similar to the characteristic "sniffing position" that croup patients demonstrate to straighten and elevate the airway above the water level. The patient's mouth is opened wide to facilitate maximum air exchange. Patients bob vertically above and below the water as they struggle to stay afloat.

Potential rescuers can neither communicate or reason with DNS patients. Anyone who approaches within arm's length will be grabbed violently and be pushed under as the DNS patient struggles to climb up and out of the water over their would-be rescuers.

Sudden Disappearance Syndrome

Sudden Disappearance Syndrome (SDS) accounts for approximately 20% of all fatal submersions and is frequently boat related. SDS patients clad in heavy winter clothing (e.g., layered hunting clothes or snowmobile suits) fall overboard from small craft (e.g., canoes, rowboats, or small motorboats), or fall in from some above water location and make the fatal mistake of attempting to swim to shore. As the patient swims, air trapped in the bulky clothing is displaced and buoyancy is lost. The swimmer suddenly shifts to DNS behavior and disappears.

The rescue "window of opportunity" for the SDS patient is usually 5 minutes to 10 minutes. Since there is no way of determining when clothing will surrender its buoyancy, persons struggling in the water under these circumstances should be treated with highest priority before they shift to DNS.

All watercraft that are 20 ft. or less in length, and are manufactured in the United States, are required to have adequate intrinsic floatation to float upright and level when filled with water. They are designed to carry all the occupants in this condition. Since the majority of drownings occur within 10 ft. of safety, patients of boating mishaps who are still within easy reach of their craft should be instructed to crawl back into the swamped craft to await rescue.

Hypothermia Induced Debility

Hypothermia Induced Debility (HID) embraces a variety of physiological responses to immersion in cold water. Hypothermia kills less than 1% of fatal submersions. However, water rescue experts agree that hypothermia plays a role in most aquatic deaths. Alcohol consumption, anti-hypertension drugs, and some other medications amplify the cooling effect of cold water. The rescue "window of opportunity" for HID patients can be as short as 15 minutes for patients that are immersed in 32°F water. Just as HID patients are unable to participate in their own rescue, so are they unable to grab a potential rescuer due to rigid muscles and diminished levels of consciousness.

SPECIALIZED PATIENT CARE

It is not the intent of this section to address the "how to's" of prehospital patient care for patients of aquatic emergencies. However, certain specialized patient care skills are reiterated here to reinforce them in the setting (environment) where they may be required.

IDS When available information from bystanders describes an IDS scenario, first responders should alert all rescue personnel to the potential for c-spine injury and head trauma. Procedures for in-water turning and c-spine stabilization should be practiced by rescuers during patient removal from the water.

Hypothermia Whether in the aquatic emergency environment or in the terrestrial setting:

1. Remove the patient from the source of cooling to a warmed environment. Emphasize the importance of handling the hypothermia patient gently. Rough handling during rescue, transportation, or treatment may trigger a lethal dysrhythmia in the profoundly hypothermic patient.
2. Remove clothing, especially when it is cold and/or wet as it will serve as a continued source of heat loss through conduction.
3. Apply blankets in a "hypothermia wrap" (refer to session 6).
   a. If patients must be managed for extended periods of time in a cold and/or wet environment, the addition of an insulating pad (e.g., Thinsulite) under the patient and a weather-resistant wrap (e.g., tarpaulin or salvage cover) wrapped around the patient and sealed at the edges with duct tape improves the efficiency of the hypothermia wrap. Supplemental warmed towels placed at any exposed area such as the head or neck further enhance the effectiveness of the wrap.
   b. The application of passive rewarming aids such as heat packs should be used judiciously and then only on patients exhibiting signs and symptoms of mild or moderate hypothermia. Heat packs that have been insulated with towels to prevent thermal burns of cold, heat-sensitized skin may be placed at the armpits, axilla, neck, and groin if medical consultation directs. Care must be exercised in the selection of heat packs as some reach temperatures as high as 140°F and should not be used.
4. Check ABCs. Respirations and pulses should be checked for one full minute. Faint pulses and respirations at subnormal rates may be overlooked in 15 seconds.
5. Supply supplemental oxygen in 100% concentrations. Oxygen should be warmed and humidified if possible. Nonrebreather masks are appropriate for patients with spontaneous respirations. Ventilation via bag-valve mask may be required if there are no respirations.
6. Begin aggressive CPR on pulseless patients. Remember that rough handling (including performing CPR) on a profoundly hypothermic patient with a slow, faint pulse may trigger a lethal dysrhythmia.

Near-drowning patients Without exception, all near-drowning patients must be seen by a physician in a hospital. Patients who are allowed to leave the scene of the near-drowning experience risk becoming a parking lot drowning hours later without medical resources to combat the injury to his/her system.

SAFETY PRACTICES AND SAFETY EQUIPMENT

OSHA regulation 29 CFR, part 1926.106 establishes safety practices for employees working over *or near* water where the danger of drowning exists. In Maryland, MOSH is responsible for the promulgation of safe practices in the workplace. Its regulations can be no less strict than OSHA regulations but they can be stricter. Public safety organizations such as fire departments and rescue squads are exempt from compliance with OSHA regulations. However, public safety workers are included in the regulations in Maryland and some other states. Since MOSH has adopted all of the OSHA regulations instead of rewriting their own, Maryland fire and rescue personnel are bound to comply with OSHA regulations.

1. "Employees . . . shall be provided with Coast Guard approved life jackets or buoyant work vests." Water rescue specialists across the United States generally agree that anyone within 10 ft. of the shoreline or embankment where a fall would put that person in the water, is required to wear a Personal Floatation Device (PFD). An acceptable alternative to wearing a PFD would be an attached lifeline and harness to prevent the wearer from falling into the water.
2. "Prior to and after each use, the buoyant work vests or life jackets shall be inspected for defects which would alter their strength or buoyancy. Defective units shall not be used." General guidelines for "defects" are:
   a. Free of any major rips or tears in the fabric which would allow the floatation to escape when jumping into water or when worn in rough water.
   b. All fabric in the PFD must be free of mildew or dry-rot.
   c. All zippers must slide freely and be free of missing teeth.
   d. All buckles and fasteners must be attached and work freely.
   e. All straps must be attached and must be free of rot, mildew, or other signs of deterioration.
   f. As a practice, PFDs with Kapok-filled bladders should be avoided in favor of PFDs with closed-cell foam floatation. However, if Kapok bladders are used, they should be tested for leaks before and after each use by squeezing each bladder and listening for any escaping air. If air does escape, the PFD should be replaced.
   g. All stitching should be intact.

PFD Classifications

PFDs must be properly sized to be effective. A loose-fitting PFD will ride up and even slip off the wearer in moving or swiftwater. Proper fit check requires the wearer to don the PFD and fasten all fasteners. While exhaling, a partner should lift the device at the shoulders. Wherever the wearer ends up inside the PFD in this exercise is where they will be in the PFD in the water. "*Too tight is just right.*"

The U.S. Coast Guard has established five classifications of PFDs.

Type I—Offshore Life Jacket: Characteristics of the Type I PFD are:

1. 22 lbs. of buoyancy.
2. Comes in two sizes: wearers who weigh less than 90 lbs., and those who weigh greater then 90 lbs.
3. Designed to turn an unconscious wearer and maintain them in a vertical and slightly backward position.
4. Easiest to don in an emergency because it is reversible.
5. Most effective in all types of rough water and should be worn where there is a probability of delayed rescue.

Type II—Nearshore Life Jacket: Characteristics of the Type II PFD are:

1. 15 lbs. of buoyancy.
2. Available in a variety of sizes including:
   - Adult (>90 lbs.)
   - Medium-framed child (50 lbs. to 90 lbs.)
   - Small-framed child (<50 lbs.)
3. Designed to turn and maintain an unconscious wearer in a vertical and slightly backward position.
4. More comfortable to wear than Type I, but due to its lower amount of flotation, does not have as pronounced turning and righting action as Type I, and does not perform as well in rough, open water.

Type III—Floatation Aid: Characteristics of the Type III PFD are:

1. The preferred PFDs for water rescuers due to the ease of movement and limited bulk, in addition to ease of sizing, comfort, and hypothermia protection.
2. 15 lbs. of buoyancy.

3. Available in a variety of sizes and styles.
4. Designed so the wearer can place himself/herself in a vertical and slightly backward position and the PFD will maintain them in that position.
5. Styles are designed to complement specific water sports such as hunting, fishing, paddling, and skiing. Should only be worn where the probability for quick rescue exists.
6. While not part of the Coast Guard specification, Type IIIs are usually designed to provide some degree of hypothermia protection that neither Types I nor II offer.

Type IV—Throwable Device: Characteristics of the Type IV PFD are:

1. Designed to be thrown to patients who can then clutch the device.
2. Only suitable where the probability of immediate rescue exists and even then are not suitable for non-swimmers and children.

Type V—Special Purpose Device: Characteristics of the Type V PFD are:

The label specifies *exactly* what activities this type can be used for. A distinction should be noted between immersion suits and exposure suits. Immersion suits provide floatation and hypothermia protection for the wearer who expects to be in cold water. Exposure suits are insulated coveralls for wear out of the water, but offer some floatation where the danger of drowning exists. Neither of these suits is appropriate for swiftwater use; however, of the two, immersion suits provide the most floatation. Case studies of white-water emergencies have demonstrated that the floatation provided by exposure suits is inadequate for personal protection in swift moving, aerated water.

Type V—Hybrid: Characteristics of the Type V PFD are:

1. Special-use device that incorporates an inflatable bladder to achieve its maximum buoyancy.
2. These are the least bulky type and are the most comfortable for continuous wear. However, they do not achieve full floatation unless inflated, which further requires the wearer to be conscious and oriented to perform this task.

First Responder Clothing

First responders are to wear helmets along with PFDs to provide slip, trip, and fall protection whenever they are working at waterside. Injury reports show that the majority of rescuer injuries occur at the shoreline, and that the most serious are head injuries.

Helmets should be:

1. Of a brimless design to provide maximum visibility while also providing temple protection.
2. Equipped with a quick-release type buckle or fastener such as a Fastex-type buckle that can be released under tension.
3. Equipped with impact protection of a closed-cell foam lining rather than a web-type suspension. The majority of the impact protection would be from the sides, back, and front, rather than from the top as a firefighter helmet is designed to withstand.
4. Designed with holes to drain water away from the wearer.
5. Of a design that would not further compromise the rescuer if he/she fell into the water hazard. (Firefighter helmets are not designed for this type of application or hazard.) The same justification applies to turnout or bunker gear. Firefighter turnouts become negatively buoyant in moving water and are inappropriate protective equipment to be worn where rescuers are at risk of falling in.

First responders should prepare for weather conditions they expect to encounter during a rescue that may require them to stand by for an hour or more.

During extreme hot weather first responders should make certain that all emergency workers on the scene are well hydrated and monitored for signs of heat-related illness. During cool and/or inclement weather, first responders must be alert to the potential for emergency workers to develop terrestrial hypothermia.

Precautions for temperature-related illness and/or injury include dressing emergency workers in layers:

1. The layer of clothing that is next to the skin is referred to as the *wicking layer*. Fabrics of choice for this layer include polypropylene, wool, and silk. These fabrics "wick" moisture away from the skin to prevent heat loss through conduction.
2. The next layer consists of as many layers as necessary dependent on the insulating properties of the garment, the level of activity of the wearer, and the temperatures at the emergency scene. Fabrics of choice for this "insulating" layer are chosen for their inherent ability to trap air. They include wool, synthetic pile material, and down.

3. The outermost layer, the weather-resistant layer, is designed to exclude wind and water only. It may have a semi-permeable membrane material such as Gortex to enhance the wicking action of any underlying layers of garments. The weather-resistant layer may or may not have any insulating properties which will impact on whether it is an all-season garment or a garment to be worn only during cold months.

SUMMARY

This session has attempted to place in proper perspective, the process associated with aquatic emergencies and the role *you* play as a first responder to such incidents. The bottom line, of course, is rescuer safety and survival. You are now armed with a wealth of information that will hopefully motivate you to pursue additional levels of water/ice rescue training as your commitment to emergency services work flourishes.

You are now in the limelight with the eyes of the public and your peers upon you. You will be judged by what you say, how you look and perform, and what you write. A successful career in rescue is predicated on good judgement, level of expertise, confidence, and competence.

You should function as a role model for your organization and the other members of your crew. Complacency often results in serious injuries and/or death to rescuers. Water and ice environments are no place to drop your guard. Drowning is the second leading cause of accidental death in Americans between the ages of 1 and 44, and the fourth leading cause of accidental death for all age groups. Statistics suggest that firefighters/rescue personnel are more likely to respond to aquatic emergency than a fatal fire. This period of instruction has been the first step in preparing you to meet this challenge. When in doubt, just secure the scene and wait for the calvary to arrive.

REFERENCES

National Safety Council. *Accident facts*. Chicago, IL: National Safety Council.

Ohio Department of National Rescue Division of Watercraft. 1980. *Ice rescue–training manual for rescue personnel.* Edited by Instructional Materials Laboratory. Columbus, OH: Ohio State University.

Ohio Department of National Rescue Division of Watercraft. 1980. *River rescue–training manual for rescue personnel.* Edited by Instructional Materials Laboratory. Columbus, OH: Ohio State University.

OSHA 29–Labor, Code of Federal Regulation: Working on or Near Water, 1926.106. Published by The Office of the Federal Register, National Archives and Records Administration, as a special edition of the Federal Register. 1997. Washington, DC: US Government Printing Office.

Segerstrom, J., B. Edwards, and M. Croslin. 1995. *Swiftwater rescue technician I.* 2nd ed. Elk Grove, CA: Rescue 3 Inc.

Smith, D. S. and S. J. Smith. 1994. *Water rescue: Basic skills for emergency responders*. St. Louis: Mosby Lifeline.

Index